EMPATHY AND READING

This pioneering collection brings together Suzanne Keen's extensive body of work on empathy and reading, charting the development of narrative empathy as an area of inquiry in its own right and extending cross-disciplinary conversations about empathy evoked by reading.

The volume offers a brief overview of the trajectory of research following the 2007 publication of *Empathy and the Novel*, with empathy understood as a suite of related phenomena as stimulated by representations in narratives. The book is organized around three thematic sections—theories; empathetic readers; and interdisciplinary applications—each preceded by a short framing essay. The volume features excerpts from the author's seminal works on narrative empathy and makes available her harder-to-access contributions. The book brings different strands of the author's research into conversation with existing debates, with the aim of inspiring future interdisciplinary research on narrative empathy.

This book will be of interest to students and scholars in such fields as literary studies, cognitive science, emotion studies, affect studies, and applied contexts where empathetic practitioners work.

Suzanne Keen serves as President of Scripps College, USA, where she is a member of the English Department. Her interdisciplinary work on narrative empathy draws on the novel, narrative theory, neuroscience, developmental and social psychology, and affective science.

EMPATHY AND READING

Affect, Impact, and the Co-Creating Reader

Suzanne Keen

Routledge
Taylor & Francis Group
NEW YORK AND LONDON

Cover image: © Getty Images

First published 2022
by Routledge
605 Third Avenue, New York, NY 10158

and by Routledge
4 Park Square, Milton Park, Abingdon, Oxon, OX14 4RN

Routledge is an imprint of the Taylor & Francis Group, an informa business

Library of Congress Cataloging-in-Publication Data
Names: Keen, Suzanne, author.
Title: Empathy and reading : affect, impact, and the co-creating reader / Suzanne Keen.
Description: New York, NY : Routledge, 2022. |
Includes bibliographical references and index. |
Summary: "This pioneering collection brings together Suzanne Keen's extensive body of work on empathy and reading, charting the development of narrative empathy as an area of inquiry in its own right and extending cross-disciplinary conversations about empathy evoked by reading"– Provided by publisher.
Identifiers: LCCN 2022001165 (print) | LCCN 2022001166 (ebook) |
ISBN 9781032205366 (hardback) | ISBN 9781032205335 (paperback) |
ISBN 9781003264071 (ebook)
Subjects: LCSH: Reading, Psychology of. | Empathy. | LCGFT: Essays.
Classification: LCC BF456.R2 K44 2022 (print) |
LCC BF456.R2 (ebook) | DDC 418/.4019–dc23/eng/20220323
LC record available at https://lccn.loc.gov/2022001165
LC ebook record available at https://lccn.loc.gov/2022001166

ISBN: 978-1-032-20536-6 (hbk)
ISBN: 978-1-032-20533-5 (pbk)
ISBN: 978-1-003-26407-1 (ebk)

DOI: 10.4324/9781003264071

Typeset in Bembo
by Newgen Publishing UK

for Fran,
who heard and read every word of these essays,
and whose attention improved them,
just as his loving regard
burnishes me

CONTENTS

ACKNOWLEDGMENTS

The essays and chapters reprinted in complete or excerpted form in this volume appear with the permission, gratefully acknowledged, of the publishers of the journals and books in which they originally appeared.

"Affect and Empathy Studies." *Oxford Companion to Law and the Humanities*. Ed. Simon Stern, Maksymilian Del Mar, and Bernadette Meyler. Oxford and New York: Oxford University Press, 2019. 181–97.

"Affective Trollope." *Routledge Research Companion to Trollope*. Ed. Deborah Denenholz Morse, Margaret Marwick, and Mark Turner. Routledge, 2017. 166–76.

"Empathic Inaccuracy in Narrative Fiction." *Topoi* 39.4 (Sept. 2020): 819–25. Published online 31 Jan. 2019.

"Empathy in Reading: Considerations of Gender and Ethnicity." Focus on Reception and Reader Response. *Anglistik: International Journal of English Studies* 24. 2 (2013): 49–65.

"Empathy Studies." *A Companion to Literary Theory*. Ed. David Richter. John Wiley & Sons, 2018. 126–38.

"Human Rights Discourse and Universals of Cognition and Emotion." *The Oxford Handbook of Cognitive Literary Studies*. Ed. Lisa Zunshine. Oxford and NY: Oxford University Press, 2014. 347–65.

"Intersectional Narratology: Queer, Feminist, Cognitive, and Affective Crossings." *Narrative Theory Unbound: Queer and Feminist Interventions*. Ed. Robyn Warhol and Susan S. Lanser. Columbus: Ohio State University Press, 2015. 123–46.

"Introduction: Narrative and the Emotions." *Poetics Today* 32.1 (2011): 1–53.

"Lifewriting and the Empathetic Circle." *Concentric: Literary and Cultural Studies* 42.2 (Sept. 2016): 9–26.

"Narrative and the Embodied Reader." *The Edinburgh Companion to Narrative Theories*. Ed. Zara Dinnen and Robyn Warhol. Edinburgh University, 2018. 43–55.

"Novel Reading and the Empathetic Angel of our Nature." *Rethinking Empathy through Literature.* Ed. Meghan Marie Hammond and Sue J. Kim. London and NY: Routledge, 2014. 21–33.

"Readers' Temperaments and Fictional Character." *New Literary History* 42.2 (Spring 2011): 295–314.

"Strategic Empathizing: Techniques of Bounded, Ambassadorial, and Broadcast Narrative Empathy." *Deutsche Vierteljahrs Schrift* 82.3 (Sept. 2008): 477–93. Rpt. *Empathie und Erzählung*. Previously reprinted in *Empathy and Narrative*, ed. Claudia Breger and Fritz Breithaupt. Freiburg/Breisgau: Rombach, 2010.

"A Theory of Narrative Empathy." *Narrative* 14.3 (October 2006): 207–36.

"Twenty-First-Century Fictional Experiments in Emotion and Cognition." *New Approaches to the Twenty-First Century Anglophone Novel*. Ed. Sibylle Baumbach and Birgitt Neumann. Palgrave Macmillan, 2019. 59–77.

INTRODUCTION

Sometime in the year 2000 I went to the library seeking the standard scholarly source on empathy and the novel, to support with a footnote some passages I had written in my book *Romances of the Archive in Contemporary British Fiction* (2001). About these works, I observed, "The emphasis on achieving empathy with human subjects denies sharp differences of the past from the present, suggesting instead that present-day researchers with the right identities and emotional qualifications can better comprehend those who were misunderstood in the past than anyone who coexisted with them. … [i]n an uncanny unhinging of agency, the researcher seems to be singled out by the quest, to be fated to be the one individual from the present who can reach into the dormant past to reanimate the interests of the silenced historical subject" (183). The novelists I was studying articulated a strong belief about the way shared identity boosted the powers of the empathetic imagination, or even uniquely qualified a researcher to discover the truth about the past. I had written, "Recognition of an earlier self marooned in the past verifies the imaginative insights of the archival romancer. The right pairing of subject and quester… makes a fetish of heritage. Paradoxically in fictions that emphasize their subjects' marginal positions and exceptional circumstances, continuities of nationality, location, religion, genealogy, gender, and sexual preference constitute privileged authorities that not only know, but also embody, the past" (206).

These sentiments ran counter to the general literary-critical attitude of the time, still under the strong influence of deconstruction, and I wondered whether it was feminist or queer theory that had reanimated what seemed to me like a quite old-fashioned faith in fiction's ability to forge connections over barriers of time and space. The empathy thematized in these works hinted that novel reading could make something happen in the real world, by changing readers' attitudes, or even moving them to action. I knew the canonical critiques of the *failings* of literary

DOI: 10.4324/9781003264071-1

works to move readers, as for example in Raymond Williams' *The Country and the City*, which documents apathy and inaction following on from novel reading, but where was the book that explained how empathy for imaginary worlds and fictional characters was thought to work in and on real readers?

I was aware of the philosopher Martha Nussbaum's claims about the positive impact of literary reading and her discussions of traditional realist fiction, but I couldn't accept her conflation of real-life empathy (which does sometimes lead to altruism) and narrative empathy for nonexistent beings. Where was the evidence that novel-reading really created "good world citizens," as Nussbaum contended (*Cultivating* 90)? The human rights track record of the twentieth century, arguably the peak novel-reading period since the rise of the genre in the West, did not inspire confidence in that claim. But even if it did, why did Nussbaum insist that only a few celebrated works of high literary realism would effect this important formation of good citizens? My writers wouldn't make the cut: they were the authors of time-slip fantasies, shlocky adventure stories, and as my title suggested, all sorts of romances. Yet in their popular genre fiction they proposed an impact of empathetic reading that at least bore a family resemblance to Nussbaum's ambitious brief for fiction. Was the promise of empathy, recognition, compassion, and altruism just a way of dignifying the habit of escapist fiction reading with the appearance of an improving regimen? I also had to entertain the possibility that fiction-reading did damage, as critics of the novel had been arguing since the eighteenth century. (The debate about the perils and powers of imaginative writing was older even than that, with Plato and Augustine cautioning, Sidney and Shelley cheering.) Could a habit of encountering other minds, even imaginary ones, change contemporary readers' attitudes and spur them into action on behalf of others? I was reminded of a deeper source in George Eliot's thinking about the novel, defending her creative practice against comparison with silly novels by lady novelists, elevating her ambition to use fiction to cultivate the sympathetic imagination of the reader, and bringing moral sentimentalism to bear on the literary arts.

But who had updated that claim recently, specifically for literary studies? It would have been quite an unfashionable stance at the time; indeed, when I was first talking about my research with university audiences in the early 2000s, I was often met with a quizzical response. "No one thinks that novels make readers into better people," I was frequently admonished. (Of course, lots of people did and do think exactly that: just not usually in English Departments, where the practice of critique tends more in the direction, then and now, of what Rita Felski has described as suspicious reading.) With a background in narratology, I had a reason for imagining that somebody might be working on empathy as an aspect of narrative impact or narrative communication. As a rhetorical narrative theorist with an interest in reader response, I was searching for a discussion finer grained than the broad and often defensive claims made for the impact of novel reading by defenders of the humanities. I hoped to find work closely examining the roles of authors and texts, specifically their narrative techniques, in evoking empathy in readers. I sought sources that would systematically reveal what had been theorized, what had been empirically tested, and what had been learned through interdisciplinary collaboration. Hard as it is now to believe, in 2000 I couldn't find what I was looking for: at least not in one place. Those sentences never got the footnotes I intended to write, in a book that meditated repeatedly on narrative empathy in response to a diverse group of contemporary British novelists' representations. After several days of searching, first in my decent small college library, then in the MLA bibliography, in Widener's online catalog, and finally in WorldCat, I had to concede that the source I was seeking didn't exist.

That was not to say that literary empathy was a neglected subject: far from it. Patrick Colm Hogan and Susan Feagin had written literary criticism centered on empathy. Wayne Booth's work on character identification, and scholars working on narrative ethics sometimes touched on empathy in relation to narrative impact on readers. Philosophers such as Noel Carroll, Gregory Currie, Jenefer Robinson, and Nancy Sherman engaged with empathic phenomena in relation to novels and films; Carroll, Currie, Peter Lamarque, Colin Radford, Murray Smith, Kendall Walton, and Robert Yanal debated the paradox of fictional emotions; in addition to Nussbaum, philosophers Eva Dadlez, Feagin, Peter Goldie, Derek Maltravers and others illuminated the nature of aesthetic emotion more broadly. Some of this philosophical work (mostly in the field of ethics) debated the influential cognitivists whose work dominated the philosophical study of emotions at the time. An affective turn underway in philosophy, but also in sociology, women's and gender studies, sexuality studies, and cultural studies, would make it more difficult to discuss cognition without at least acknowledging emotion and affect, as Antonio Damasio was energetically arguing at the time.

Empathy itself was sometimes studied as a matter of cognition, sometimes as a matter of emotion, and sometimes as involving both. When it came to narrative empathy, introspection told me that the emotions were certainly involved, and logic insisted that emotions evoked through *reading* must also involve cognition. So from the outset I treated empathy as both affective and cognitive, in its real-life and imaginative forms. Not every thinker on the subject acknowledged a difference between real-world empathy and the empathy for imaginary beings and worlds that I was interested in. Psychologist Mark Davis treated what he termed fantasy empathy as a sub-set of empathy, devoting one of the subscales of his Interpersonal Reactivity Index (IRI) to aspects of imaginary empathy: "Fantasy—taps respondents' tendencies to transpose themselves imaginatively into the feelings and actions of fictitious characters in books, movies, and plays" ("Multidimensional" 85). Others conflated fantasy empathy with the kind of empathy that involved reactions of an individual to the experiences, feelings, and reactions of another real person—or animal. This matters when theorists go on to attribute real-world impacts to empathy felt for fictitious beings. Cognitive science and the science of the emotions still to this day investigate radically different phenomena that share the common label of "empathy." The 1990s and 2000s had witnessed a renewed interest in empathy, as social neuroscientists developed a new understanding of the biological substrate for empathy. The mirror mimicry explained by Vittorio Gallese and others is a far cry from the altruistic concern spurred by an empathic response to another person in distress, perceiving their situation by means of matching emotion. In my view, empathy can best be understood as a *suite* of related phenomena, ranging from its historical roots in the *Einfühlung* of psychological aesthetics, to mind-reading (the empathic accuracy of role-taking and perspective taking), to motor-mimicry and emotional contagion, to shared feeling, to a prompt for sympathetic concern that leads to altruistic action, to aversive personal distress. Rich research traditions examining each of these phenomena exist in a variety of disciplines, though *Einfühlung* or "feeling into" inanimate objects has been largely eclipsed by interpersonal or inter-being versions of empathy.

But despite the burgeoning interest in empathy, aesthetic emotions, narrative impact, narrative ethics, immersion and virtual reality, and the exciting new neuroscience describing a shared manifold for intersubjectivity (after the discovery of mirror neurons), few authorities in any of those fields read one another or drew upon one another's research. At that time, the relatively new field of affect studies proceeded separately from the psychological science of emotion, a divide that still persists today in the manner of the Two Cultures. Many humanists and scientists worked on aspects of empathy and sympathy, but they rarely shared vocabulary or approaches. The theoretical allegiances of each discipline often blocked conversations, and well-known defections, such as Paul Ekman's conversion from social constructivism to the Darwinian view of universal human (and animal) emotions, resulted in the entrenchment of those who regard the expression of emotions as culturally determined. Even within psychological science, Antonio Damasio paddled against the current in his arguments, in scientific papers and popular books, that cognition could not be understood without considering emotion. Indeed, my reading of the influential cognitivists George Lakoff, Mark Johnson, and Mark Turner left me dissatisfied with the place of affect in their account of metaphor in embodied cognition. Emotions were there, to be sure, in metaphorical schemas, but in subordination to cognitive structures. Since I was interested in what kinds of fictional representations had actually been demonstrated to evoke empathic responses—affective and cognitive—in real readers, I found my way to the science of discourse processing, to empirical approaches to literary study, and to cognitive science, psychology, and neuroscience.

While I had been fairly confident in my preparation to read philosophy papers, I realized almost immediately that I would need to study hard in order to make sense of the psychology and neuroscience of empathy. With the gracious assistance of my Washington and Lee University colleagues in Psychology and Neuroscience, especially the late Dave Elmes, Tyler Lorig, Wythe Whiting, Julie Woodzicka, Len Jarrard, Jeanine Stewart, and Bob Stewart, I began studying the basics: brain and behavior, cognition, evolutionary psychology, and history and systems of psychology for starters. This preparation turned out to be essential as I began working on *Empathy and the Novel.* For it transpired, as interdisciplinary scholars know from experience, that experts in the other discipline(s) with whose work one attempts to engage would become the peer reviewers and gatekeepers who determined whether that work would see the light of day. Literary scholars might wonder what on earth I was doing reading the science of narrative impact or the social neuroscience of bias and dehumanization, but the researchers in those fields held me to their own high standards, exhibiting great patience as they welcomed me into their interdisciplinary conversations. I was especially fortunate to receive the encouragement, criticism, and pre-publication off-prints of psychologist Nancy Eisenberg, who had served as a peer reviewer of my book proposal in 2005. I have tried to pay that generosity forward.

Published by Oxford in 2007 and reprinted in paperback in 2010, my book *Empathy and the Novel* caught a wave of interest in empathy, affect, the emotions, and the potential impact of literary reading on the formation of readers' relations to other people in the real world. In it, I drew on interdisciplinary sources in psychology, neuroscience, philosophy, and narrative theory, and I revealed to my readers how little we really knew about how narrative empathy actually works. An aspect of author's creative imagining, of readers' immersion in fiction and co-creation of fictional worlds, and a matter of narrative techniques intended to evoke empathy, narrative empathy was at the time understudied, especially in empirical research about narrative impact. At the same time that cultural watchdogs were wringing their hands about dramatic declines in literary reading, robust beliefs in the power of novels to make readers into better people through empathy were often repeated. Along with Martha Nussbaum, Stephen Pinker is one of the most prominent advocates of this view, which links literary reading with the development of improved human rights, lower levels of violence, decreased prejudice against outgroups, and the development of good world citizens. In the book, I expressed skepticism about the reliability of the link between narrative empathy and altruism in the real world, and I examined all the studies that purported to demonstrate a causal relation between them.

The evidence at the time was scanty and unconvincing, though since then there have been solid demonstrations of at least short-term gains in prosocial behavior and more enduring impacts on readers' improved attitudes from empathic reading experiences. But the intention of *Empathy and the Novel* was not to take sides so much as it was to gather what was known into one place, consider its relevance to readers, authors, and fictional texts, and to expose the gaping holes in our knowledge. Not all literary scholars were open to the phenomenological, rhetorical, and reader-response approaches that made my bridge-building with the psychology of empathy possible. Though diminishing in influence at the time, psychoanalytic thought (Lacanian, Kleinian, Winnicottian) possessed an aura of legitimacy that psychological science lacked. Theory was one thing, empirical study quite another. I vividly recall one of my students, an English and Philosophy double major, declaring with a disdain bordering on disgust, "I understand now, Professor Keen. You are an *empiricist*." I am actually a theorist, but I do like to see corroborating evidence for our ideas about how narrative techniques and aspects of our reading experiences work. However, even assuming that the empirical disciplines had something to share with literary studies (and I was very interested in what we might learn from that conversation), so much more was *unknown* than I could have anticipated. Among the existing studies, many were bedeviled with what I had learned to recognize as confounding variables in the correlations or causes they examined.

As I documented these lacunae, I collected ideas from other researchers and augmented with my own queries a series of hypotheses that would require further study to validate or disprove:

Proposals about Narrative Empathy

- empathy for fictional characters may require only minimal elements of identity, situation, and feeling, not necessarily complex or realistic characterization;
- character identification often invites empathy, even when the character and reader differ from one another in all sorts of practical and obvious ways;
- spontaneous empathy for a fictional character's feelings opens the way for character identification;
- empathetic responses to fictional characters and situations occur more readily for negative feeling states, whether or not a match in details of experience exists;
- empathy with characters doesn't always occur as a result of reading an emotional evocative fiction;
- the capacity of novels to invoke readers' empathy may change over time (and some novels may only activate the empathy of their first, immediate audience);
- empathy for a fictional character need not correspond with what the author appears to set up or invite;
- situational empathy, which responds primarily to aspects of plot and circumstance, involves less self-extension in imaginative role-taking and more recognition of prior (or current) experience;
- readers' empathy for situations depicted in fiction may be enhanced by chance relevance to particular historical, economic, cultural, or social circumstances;
- generic differences are likely to play a role in inviting (or retarding) readers' empathic responses;
- (Miall and Kuiken) unusual or striking representations in the literary text promote foregrounding and open the way to empathetic reading;
- (Bourg) empathizers are better readers, because their role-taking abilities allow them to comprehend causal relations in stories;

- readers' perception of a text's fictionality plays a role in subsequent empathetic response, by releasing readers from the obligations of self-protection through skepticism and suspicion;
- (Miall) readers' empathy could produce verifiable results in the beliefs and actions of populations of actual readers;
- (Hoffman) novel reading may participate in the socialization and moral internalization required for the transmutation of empathic guilt into prosocial action;
- though a key ingredient of successful fictional worldmaking, author's empathy does not always transmit to readers without interference;
- (Taylor) novelists as a group may be more empathetic than the general population;
- fiction-writing may cultivate novelists' role-taking skills and make them more habitually empathetic;
- authors' empathy can be devoted to socially undesirable ends;
- empathic distress at feeling with a character whose actions are at odds with a reader's moral code may be a result of successfully exercised authorial empathy;
- empathic inaccuracy may contribute to a reader's strong sense that the author's perspective is simply wrong;
- both authors' empathy and readers' empathy have rhetorical uses, which come more readily to notice when they conflict in instances of empathic inaccuracy;
- concord in authors' empathy and readers' empathy could be a motivating force to move beyond literary response to prosocial action;
- *bounded strategic empathy* operates with an in-group, stemming from experiences of mutuality, and leading to feeling with familiar others;
- *ambassadorial strategic empathy* addresses chosen others with the aim of cultivating their empathy for the in-group, often to a specific end;
- *broadcast strategic empathy* calls upon every reader to feel with members of a group, by emphasizing common vulnerabilities and hopes (universalizing);
- (Hogan) empathy for group-members emerging from categorical identity with a group does not, on its own, lead to an ethics of compassion.

(*Empathy and the Novel* 169–71)

In addition to work that was already underway at the time, acknowledged in parentheses, many of these propositions have since been investigated, sometimes with supporting empirical study. For example, the idea that "concord in authors' empathy and readers' empathy could be a motivating force to move beyond literary response to prosocial action" has been demonstrated in clever studies by Dan R. Johnson, and Markus Appel and Barbara Malečkar have made inroads on the question of whether "readers' perception of a text's fictionality plays a role in subsequent empathetic response," focusing on narrative persuasion.

Fascinating puzzles about narrative techniques (such as the potential impact of free indirect discourse) have been studied by collaborative teams, such as the experimental work of Angus Fletcher and John Monterosso. This is just to name a few of the numerous studies that have contributed to a deeper and more textured understanding of narrative empathy, and upon whom I have relied myself in subsequent work. My own efforts focused on just a few of the hypotheses, particularly the proposals about empathic inaccuracy, immersion reading, and modes of authorial strategic narrative empathy. In the following 15 years or so, I pursued questions that I had left unanswered in *Empathy and the Novel*, some of which I had laid out in the hypotheses; others I had given short shrift or summarily dismissed, such as narrative personal distress.

This volume makes accessible a substantial selection of that subsequent work, which has crossed disciplines to connect them, and has elaborated a theory of narrative empathy first broached in 2006. The version of empathy that I have theorized and studied involves a variety of phenomena, as stimulated by representations in fictional and (to a lesser degree) nonfictional narrative. As I have previously defined it, *narrative empathy* involves

> the sharing of feeling and perspective-taking induced by reading, viewing, hearing, or imagining narratives of another's situation and condition. Narrative empathy plays a role in the aesthetics of production when authors experience it, in mental simulation during reading, in the aesthetics of reception when readers experience it, and in the narrative poetics of texts when formal strategies invite it. Narrative empathy overarches narratological categories, involving actants, narrative situation, matters of pace and duration, and storyworld features such as settings. …
>
> (Keen, "Narrative Empathy" 521)

Narrative empathy is a phenomenon both cognitive and emotional, and because it is stimulated by literary works, it has interested literary scholars and creative writers, teachers, philosophers, psychologists and cognitive scientists, and researchers in many fields. Interdisciplinary and cross-disciplinary conversations about the role of reading in cultivating or harnessing the power of empathic response, about the limits and dangers of reliance on empathy as a moral guide to right action, and about the role of empathy in developing inclusive classrooms and workplaces are now commonplace.

In my home field of literary studies, which has become much more welcoming to work engaging with affective and cognitive science, my work is situated among cognitive/affective narrative theory and feminist criticism of the novel. However, applications and extensions of my theory of narrative empathy have escaped the bounds of my discipline. Indeed, several of the pieces collected here first appeared in journals and collections about law or philosophy. Scholars and researchers in diverse fields have engaged with elements of this work, in cognitive studies, linguistics, and stylistics; philosophy and aesthetics; psychological science and social neuroscience; narrative medicine, the health professions, and medical humanities; legal studies; organizational behavior; computer science (human-computer interaction and robotics); environmental studies; food studies; the science of teaching and learning; art, music, theatre, and dance studies; screenwriting, film and media studies; and gender studies, to name just the most common. Cognitive and emotion scientists, psychologists studying reading and narrative impact, and experts in discourse processing have joined empirically-minded literary scholars in furthering empathy research and developing its applications, for example in medical education. Since my original work in the early 2000s, scholars in many different fields have advanced our understanding of the relations among reading, empathy, attitude-change, and prosocial behavior.

Literary scholars who have contributed to a richer understanding of narrative empathy include: Lisa Blankenship, in *Changing the Subject: A Theory of Rhetorical Empathy* (2019); Fritz Breithaupt, in *The Dark Sides of Empathy* (trans. 2019); Meghan Marie Hammond, in *Empathy and the Psychology of Literary Modernism* (2014); Patrick Hogan, in *Literature and Emotion* (2018) among many works; and Blakey Vermeule, in *Why do We Care About Literary Characters?* (2010). Two forthcoming works, Lisa Zunshine's *The Secret Life of Literature* and Emily Johanssen and Alissa Karl's *Rereading Empathy* are eagerly anticipated by scholars in the field. Approaching the topic of affect from a different angle, the subject has been bracingly studied in Sara Ahmed's fine books and in Carolyn Pedwell's *Affective Relations: The Transnational Politics of Empathy* (2014). Philosophers have significantly advanced our understanding of empathy, especially Amy Coplan and Peter Goldie's *Empathy, Philosophical and Psychological Perspectives* (2011); Jenefer Robinson's *Deeper than Reason: Emotion and its Role in Literature, Music, and Art* (2005), and Heidi Maibom's *Routledge Handbook of Philosophy of Empathy* (2017), which has a section on empathy's role in aesthetics (responses to art). Scientific readers will have been eagerly following the ingenious empathy/reading research of psychologists Dan R. Johnson, Melanie Green, and Philip Mazzocco, David Kidd, Raymond Mar, Keith Oatley, and Diana Tamir, among others. My work is sometimes placed in conversation with that of prominent empathy skeptics such as psychologist Paul Bloom and philosopher Jesse Prinz. Their respective book and article, *Against Empathy* (2016) and "Against Empathy" (2011) suggest their difference from my approach. For better or worse, empathy has become an industry, with prominent applications in statecraft, marketing, medicine, education, and communications. Interest in its uses and concern about its limitations will continue to animate interdisciplinary inquiry, as empathy is criticized and defended.

I am not against empathy. I am primarily interested in countering exaggerated claims for the efficacy of empathy evoked by fiction reading, figuring out how narrative empathy actually works (and why and when it doesn't), and harnessing its potential. My approach—open to empirical evidence, careful about confirmation bias and reasoning from desired results, and curious about applications of ideas across disciplinary boundaries—continues to stimulate interdisciplinary conversation. Many of the authors named in the paragraph above are my interlocuters and colleagues in the burgeoning field of Empathy Studies. Our work is often juxtaposed on syllabi and at scholarly gatherings. Among them, I am known for advancing our understanding of narrative empathy, the kind of empathy that readers experience while reading novels, involving emotion-sharing with fictional characters and other intensities of immersion in fiction. The influence and staying power of my work on narrative empathy has been both a surprise and a source of wonderful opportunities for out-of-field conversations with experts in diverse areas. I hope that this consolidated volume will stimulate fresh discussion among scholars in many fields, both by making my contributions accessible and by pointing out areas of research that are still, over a decade later, ripe for further development. To that end, in the conclusion to this volume, where I emphasize some of what still remains to be discovered about narrative empathy, I have created an updated set of hypotheses.

The volume is not arranged chronologically, though the first essay reproduced is my earliest publication on the topic, "A Theory of Narrative Empathy" from 2006. Instead, the organization reflects how my thinking has developed in three directions: further theorizing, in I. Theories of Narrative Empathy; investigations of readers' identities and experiences on narrative impact, in II. Empathetic Readers; and broader studies and demonstrations, in III. Interdisciplinary Applications of Empathy, Affect, and Cognition. A reader consulting this volume will find in close proximity related essays and chapters that were originally published in scattered locations.

A note on formatting and principles of omission

Throughout the volume, I have regularized references into a uniform author and short-title system. Referential footnotes or endnotes have been incorporated into the body text in parenthetical references. Some substantive footnotes or endnotes have been integrated into the main text: square brackets indicate these interpolations. References appear in a consolidated Works Cited at the end of the volume. Repetitious notes have been elided. In the body text, ellipses indicate cuts, with cross-references within the volume pointing to the substantive source. For example, I typically employ the definition on narrative empathy published in the *Handbook of Narratology* as my standard definition. It is accessible online through the website, *the living handbook of narratology* (www.lhn.uni-hamburg.de/). I also quote it above, and refer the reader of the essays within this volume back to its appearance within this introduction, on page 8. While inevitably this approach requires a bit of flipping back and forth, my excerpting and cross-referencing strategy has enabled me to reproduce theoretical arguments intact, reducing the inevitable repetitions that occur as I set out my stall, before broaching the new ideas or applications that follow. It has made space for the inclusion of several excerpted chapters that would have otherwise not have made the cut.

Each of the pieces reproduced here extends the ideas first treated in depth in *Empathy and the Novel*, applies them, or revisits them for critical reconsideration. The volume thus serves as a companion to *Empathy and the Novel*, but it cannot recapitulate all of that book's arguments. It is widely available in libraries, and still in print at the time of this writing. The only other missing bits constitute a set of web publications, which remain accessible online. They include the aforementioned definition of narrative empathy in *the living handbook of narratology* (www.lhn.uni-hamburg.de/node/42.html). A contribution to the timeline on Dino Felluga's *BRANCH: Britain, Representation and Nineteenth-Century History*, "'Altruism' Makes a Space for Empathy, 1852," indicates the Victorian precursors to the early twentieth-century concept of empathy, and the root of its link to altruism. It can be found here: www.branchcollective.org/?ps_articles=suzanne-keen-altruism-makes-a-space-for-empathy-1852. Finally, my dialogue with Patrick Colm Hogan on narrative empathy as a literary universal, at https://literary-universals.uconn.edu/2017/10/07/narrative-empathy-a-universal-response-to-fiction/ and https://literary-universals.uconn.edu/2017/10/08/universal-principles-do-not-entail-uniformity-of-individual- can be freely accessed on Hogan's Literary Universals Project website.

PART I

Theories of Narrative Empathy

Theories of Narrative Empathy

This section opens with the first essay I published on the subject of empathy and reading, "A Theory of Narrative Empathy," reproduced unabridged. I am forever indebted to James Phelan, who heard me deliver a conference paper on the subject, encouraged me to submit it to *Narrative*, and then cajoled me into doubling and then tripling the original submission. The remaining four pieces excerpted in this theoretical section extend beyond the ideas explored in *Empathy and the Novel*. For example, "Strategic Empathizing: Techniques of Bounded, Ambassadorial, and Broadcast Narrative Empathy" explores how and to what ends authors deliberately exploit the affordances of narrative empathy to reach audiences nearer and further away, developing with analysis of sample texts an aspect of my theory only briefly broached in "A Theory of Narrative Empathy" and in *Empathy and the Novel*. Both my 2018 chapter, "Narrative and the Embodied Reader" and my 2020 essay, "Empathic Inaccuracy in Narrative Fiction," extend my thinking, augmenting my earlier, cursory discussions in *Empathy and the Novel* with deeper investigations of empathic phenomena.

"Narrative and the Embodied Reader" discusses narrative personal distress, or NPD, an aversive empathic response I had earlier reasoned had no place in a theory of narrative empathy. It corrects that decision, offering hypotheses about NPD and linking these legitimately empathic reading responses to the contemporary discussion of trigger warnings. Similarly, in "Empathic Inaccuracy in Narrative Fiction," I revise my earlier, somewhat dismissive thinking about readers' errant experiences of narrative empathy, which I call (narrative) empathic inaccuracy. Just because it is not what the author was going for doesn't render a reader's errant empathic response irrelevant. Indeed, both these corrective elaborations contribute to a

DOI: 10.4324/9781003264071-2

view of narrative communication that genuinely respects readers' contributions to textual co-creation, a topic explored in more detail in the selections in the second section, "Empathetic Readers."

Conversations with audience-members over the years persuaded me that these and other aspects of my original theorizing deserved extension. For example, I have frequently been challenged by passionate advocates who related their empathic responses to different forms of nonfiction lifewriting, including memoirs, person-centered narrative history, biographies, prosopographies (group biographies), and *testimonio*; they insisted that these works evoked empathy as intensely as the novels and works of fiction I originally theorized. "Lifewriting and the Empathetic Circle" follows the path of further elaboration, broadening a theory that was based solely on fictional narrative to one specific variety of nonfiction, lifewriting. In *Empathy and the Novel,* I argued that writing perceived as *fictional* is especially effective at evoking readers' empathy. Building on my discussion of narrative nonfiction in *Narrative Form* (2015) I proposed in this later work that lifewriting should be regarded as a special category of nonfiction that shares with fictional narratives the capacity to invite feeling responses and to evoke readers' empathy.

1

A THEORY OF NARRATIVE EMPATHY

We are living in a time when the activation of mirror neurons in the brains of onlookers can be recorded as they witness another's actions and emotional reactions (Keysers, et al. 501; Gallese, et al. 396). Contemporary neuroscience has brought us much closer to an understanding of the neural basis for human mind reading and emotion sharing abilities—the mechanisms underlying empathy. The activation of onlookers' mirror neurons by a coach's demonstration of technique or an internal visualization of proper form and by representations in television, film, visual art, and pornography has already been recorded (Gallese, "Self-Other"). Simply hearing a description of an absent other's actions lights up mirror neuron areas during fMRI imaging of the human brain (Tettamanti et al. 273). (Though most neuroscientists working on mirror neurons agree that the effects are strongest in real life, face-to-face interactions, what Gallese calls the "shared manifold for intersubjectivity" still operates when subjects see videos, experience virtual reality through computer interfaces, and simply hear narration about others [Blakeslee F1, F4]). The possibility that novel reading stimulates mirror neurons' activation can now, as never before, undergo neuroscientific investigation. Neuroscientists have already declared that people scoring high on empathy tests have especially busy mirror neuron systems in their brains (Keysers, qtd. in Blakeslee F1, F4). Fiction writers are likely to be among these high empathy individuals. For the first time we might investigate whether human differences in mirror neuron activity can be altered by exposure to art, to teaching, to literature.

This newly enabled capacity to study empathy at the cellular level encourages speculation about human empathy's positive consequences. These speculations are not new, as any student of eighteenth-century moral sentimentalism will affirm, but they dovetail with efforts on the part of contemporary virtue ethicists, political philosophers, educators, theologians, librarians, and interested parties such as

DOI: 10.4324/9781003264071-3

authors and publishers to connect the experience of empathy, including its literary form, with outcomes of changed attitudes, improved motives, and better care and justice. Thus a very specific, limited version of empathy located in the neural substrate meets in the contemporary moment a more broadly and loosely defined, fuzzier sense of empathy as the feeling precursor to and prerequisite for liberal aspirations to greater humanitarianism. [Social and developmental psychologists, philosophers of virtue ethics, feminist advocates of an ethic of caring, and many defenders of the humanities believe that empathic emotion motivates altruistic action, resulting in less aggression, less fickle helping, less blaming of victims for their misfortunes, increased cooperation in conflict situations, and improved actions on behalf of needy individuals and members of stigmatized groups (Batson et al., "Benefits" 360–70; Slote, *Morals from Motives* 109–10).] The sense of crisis stirred up by reports of stark declines in reading goes into this mix, catalyzing fears that the evaporation of a reading public leaves behind a population incapable of feeling with others. Yet the apparently threatened set of links between novel reading, experiences of narrative empathy, and altruism has not yet been proven to exist.

This essay undertakes three tasks preliminary to the scrutiny of the empathy-altruism hypothesis as it might apply to experiences of narrative empathy. These tasks include: a discussion of empathy as psychologists understand and study it; a brief introduction to my theory of narrative empathy, including proposals about how narrative empathy works; and a review of the current research on the effects of specific narrative techniques on real readers.

What is Empathy?

Empathy, a vicarious, spontaneous sharing of affect, can be provoked by witnessing another's emotional state, by hearing about another's condition, or even by reading. Mirroring what a person might be expected to feel in that condition or context, empathy is thought to be a precursor to its semantic close relative, *sympathy*. [Although the word *empathy* is a relatively young term, entering English in the early twentieth century as a coined translation of the German word *Einfühlung*, aspects of empathy have been described by philosophers since the days of Adam Smith and David Hume under the older term *sympathy*.] *Personal distress*, an aversive emotional response also characterized by apprehension of another's emotion, differs from empathy in that it focuses on the self and leads not to sympathy but to avoidance. The distinction between empathy and personal distress matters because empathy is associated with the moral emotion *sympathy* (also called *empathic concern*) and thus with prosocial or altruistic action (Batson, *Altruism* 56–7; Eisenberg, "Emotion, Regulation" 671–2; "Development"). Empathy that leads to sympathy is by definition other-directed, whereas an over-aroused empathic response that creates personal distress (self-oriented and aversive) causes a turning-away from the provocative condition of the other. None of the philosophers who put stock in the morally improving experience of narrative empathy include personal distress in their theories. Because novel reading can be so easily stopped or interrupted by an unpleasant emotional reaction to a book, however, personal distress has no place in a literary theory of empathy, though it certainly contributes to aesthetic emotions, such as those Sianne Ngai describes in her important book *Ugly Feelings*.

In empathy, sometimes described as an emotion in its own right, we feel what we believe to be the emotions of others. [Charles Darwin's treatment of sympathy in *The Expression of the Emotions in Man and Animals* clearly includes empathy, though he does not use the term. Paul Ekman, the leading authority on facial expressions as indicators of universal human emotions, does not treat empathy as a core emotion, but as one of the nine starting points for emotional reactions (when we feel what others feel). (Ekman, *Emotions Revealed* 34, 37). Neuroscientist Jaak Panksepp argues that emotional systems in the brain involve central affective programs comprised of neural anatomy, physiology, and chemicals. Panksepp considers empathy one of the higher sentiments (mixing lower, reflexive affects and higher cognitive processes), emerging out of the recent evolutionary expansion of the forebrain (142–3). For philosopher Martha C. Nussbaum, empathy comes into play as a part of compassion, which she treats as a human emotion (*Upheaveals* 327–35). For John Deigh and those working at the intersection of ethics and cognitive science, empathy is one of the moral emotions.]

Empathy is thus agreed to be both affective and cognitive by most psychologists. Empathy is distinguished in both psychology and philosophy (though not in popular usage) from *sympathy*, in which feelings *for* another occur.

So, for instance, one may distinguish empathy from sympathy in this fashion:

Empathy:	*Sympathy:*
I feel what you feel. *I feel your pain.*	I feel a supportive emotion about your feelings. *I feel pity for your pain.*

These examples emphasize negative emotions—pain and pity—but it should be noted from the outset that although psychological and philosophical studies of empathy have tended to gravitate towards the negative, empathy also occurs for positive feelings of happiness, satisfaction, elation, triumph, and sexual arousal. [Positive forms of empathy are drastically underemphasized in the literature (Ainslie and Monterosso)]. All of these positive kinds of empathy play into readers' pleasure, or *jouissance*. [See Barthes for the distinction between the relatively easy pleasure of the readerly text and the bliss that comes when the demanding writerly text helps readers break out of their subject positions.]

Experts on *emotional contagion*, the communication of one's mood to others, have done a better job of studying the full range of emotional states that can be shared through our automatic mimicry of one another. [See for instance the treatment of happiness, joy, and love in Hatfield, et al., *Emotional Contagion.* Theodor Lipps, an important early theorist of empathy, proposed motor mimicry as an automatic response to another's expression of emotion ("Das Wissen von Fremden Ichen").] Indeed, primitive emotional contagion, or "the tendency to automatically mimic and synchronize facial expressions, vocalizations, postures, and movements with those of another person and consequently, to converge emotionally" offers a compelling explanation of a component of our empathy as arising from our physical and social awareness of one another, from birth (Hatfield, et al. 81). Inherited traits play an important role in our disposition to experience emotional contagion, (Zahn-Waxler, et al.), but our personal histories and cultural contexts affect the way we understand automatically shared feelings. [Cultural differences implicate differences in the nature of emotional experience. Our understanding of what it means to be a person in our cultural context affects the way we experience daily emotions of pleasantness and unpleasantness, or whether we feel entitled as individuals to express a particular emotion (Shields).]

So, for instance, emotional contagion comes into play in our reactions to narrative, for we are also story-sharing creatures. The oral storyteller not only takes advantage of our tendency to share feelings socially by doing the voices and facial expressions of characters, but also tacitly trains young children and members of the wider social group to recognize and give priority to culturally valued emotional states. [Oral storytelling is not isolated to preliterate cultures. Children in literate cultures also absorb cultural values and narrative styles through collaborative storytelling (Minami and McCabe).] This education does not create our feelings, but renders emotional states legible through their labels, and activates our expectations about what emotions mean. Narratives in prose and film infamously manipulate our feelings and call upon our built-in capacity to feel with others. Indeed, the early history of empathy as a subject of study emphasized both emotional contagion and aesthetic responses.

The word empathy appeared as a translation of *Einfühlung* in the early twentieth century. In 1909, the experimental psychologist E. B. Titchener translated as "empathy" aesthetician Theodor Lipps' term *Einfühlung*, which meant the process of "feeling one's way into" an art object or another person (Titchener 181–5; Lipps, *Zur Einfühlung*). Notably, Titchener's 1915 elaboration of the concept in *A Beginner's Psychology* exemplifies empathy through a description of a reading experience: "We have a natural tendency to feel ourselves into what we perceive or imagine. As we read about the forest, we may, as it were, become the explorer; we feel for ourselves the gloom, the silence, the humidity, the oppression, the sense of lurking danger; everything is strange, but it is to us that strange experience has come" (198). In the beginning of the twentieth century, the English novelist Vernon Lee brought *Einfühlung* and empathy to a broader literary audience. In a public lecture followed by a [co-authored] magazine piece in a popular journal (Lee and Anstruther-Thomson), Lee advanced a theory of aesthetic perception of form involving empathy, though not (at first) so named. Originally Lee's aesthetics focused on bodily sensations and muscular adjustments made by beholders of works of art and architecture and downplayed emotional responsiveness. By the time she revised and expanded her ideas for presentation in book form, however, Lee had adapted Lipps' understanding of empathy, a parallel development from common sources in German aesthetics.

Defining the purpose of art as, in part, "the awakening, intensifying, or maintaining of definite emotional states" (Lee 99–100), Lee makes empathy a central feature of our collaborative responsiveness (128). In an account that combines motor mimicry, memory, and psychological responsiveness to inanimate objects, Lee argues that empathy enters into

> imagination, sympathy, and also into that inference from our own inner experience which has shaped all our conceptions of an outer world, and given to the intermittent and heterogeneous sensations received from without the framework of our constant and highly unified inner experience, that is to say, of our own activities and aims.
>
> (68)

No sooner had the term been announced and situated so centrally in aesthetic theory for an English-language audience, however, than it received brisk challenge from high modernist quarters. The disdain of Bertolt Brecht for empathy (and his advocacy of so-called alienation effects), the embrace of difficulty by modernist poets, and the dominance of New Criticism, which taught students to avoid the affective fallacy all interfered with the integration of empathy into literary theory until recently. Novelists and novel readers who prized experiences of emotional fusion cultivated narrative empathy throughout periods when the term was in eclipse.

How is Empathy Studied?

The focus on our embodied experience in feminist criticism, disability studies, cognitive approaches to narrative, and some ecocriticism, draws literary studies closer to disciplines that accept the use of making measurements, doing tests and experiments, and interpreting empirical evidence. This section explains some of the methods being used by neuroscientists and developmental and social psychologists to study empathy. Developing the conversation between literature and psychology ought to benefit both disciplines, however, and the subsequent comments on what is known and especially what has not yet been tested about the effects of narrative techniques contributes to a more nuanced application of psychonarratology to questions of interest to social and developmental psychologists.

Psychologists test and record empathy in a variety of ways. Physiological measures, sometimes combined with self-reports, can show the strength or weakness (or presence and absence) of empathic responses. [Evaluation of patients who show changes in behavior as a result of brain injuries, ailments, or surgery contributes to the understanding of empathy (Gratton and Elsinger).] Psychologists measure changes in heart rate and skin conductance (palm sweat). They collect data on perceptible and imperceptible facial reactions, the latter captured by EMG (electromyographic) procedures. [Physiological measures have the advantage of being unaffected by the subjects' desire to present themselves favorably, as may occur in surveys, interviews, or self-reports (Eisenberg, et al., "Physiological"). On deceleration of heart rate in response to negative experiences of others, see K. D. Craig. On the measurement of palmar skin conductance and heart rate in response to images of people in pain, see R. S. Lazarus. For a skin conductance study suggesting that empathetic arousal occurs when subjects believe a person is receiving a painful shock, see Geer and Jarmecky. On facial or gestural responses as indications of empathy, see Marcus. See also Hoffman, "The Measurement of Empathy." On EMG and other physiological measurements of emotional responses, see Cacioppo and Petty.]

[Psychologists] ask subjects how they feel or how they would act in certain situations, gathering responses through self-reports during or immediately after experiments and through surveys. Specialized surveys known as "empathy scales" are used to assess subjects' strength of empathic feeling. [A number of empathy scales developed since the 1950s are still in use by psychologists. The Sherman-Stotland scale includes a factor (VI) measuring "fantasy empathy" for fictional characters in stories, plays, and films (Stotland 135–56). More recent tests of emotional intelligence include the Balanced Emotional Empathy Scale (BEES) (Mehrabian) and Davis's Interpersonal Reactivity Index (IRI). For the IRI, which has subscales in Empathic Concern, Perspective Taking, Fantasy (including narrative empathy), and Personal Distress, see Davis, "A Multidimensional Approach" and "Measuring Individual Differences." Survey methodology has its limitations, as psychologists acknowledge. Eisenberg has repeatedly observed that cultural influences such as sex-role differentiation show up more in the kinds of tests that rely on surveys and interviews and much less (or not at all) in tests using physiological methods (Lennon and Eisenberg).]

Recently, Functional Magnetic Resonance Imaging (fMRI) has had a profound impact on brain science, including the study of empathy. [For a salutary caution on the interpretation of these fMRI studies, which feature such dazzling pictures and often receive quite credulous promotion in the press, see Cacioppo, et al.]. Tania Singer and her colleagues have … document[ed] empathetic responses to witnessing another's pain, supported by fMRI data. This study broke new ground in demonstrating why a person perceives that she feels another's pain, while not literally experiencing the identical sensations. Singer compared what happened in a subject's brain when she was actually shocked, when pain regions in the limbic system (the anterior cingulate cortex, the insula, the thalamus, and the somatosensory cortices) lit up on the fMRI, with what the brain looked like during observation of another's pain. When watching a loved one in the same room receiving a sharp shock, subjects showed active responses in the *affective* parts of the brain's pain matrix (in the anterior insula and anterior cingulate cortex, the lateral cerebellum, and the brainstem), but not in the somatosensory cortices of the brain. The affective brain areas responded to both real and imagined pain. A person not actually experiencing pain but observing a loved one being shocked showed brain activation of matching emotional areas, though not the sensory areas. Empathy alone did not light up the sensory areas for pain. Singer and her colleagues conclude that empathy is mediated by the part of the pain network associated with pain's affective qualities, but not its sensory qualities (Singer et al. 1157). [Singer and her colleagues employed two empathy scales, Mehrabian's Balanced Emotional Empathy Scale and Davis's Empathic Concern Scale (1159).] They observed that subjects with higher scores on general empathy scales "showed stronger activations in areas significantly activated when the subjects perceived their partner as being in pain" (1159). They also discovered that the same empathetic effects could be elicited without an emotional cue—in other words, subjects did not need to see their partners grimacing in pain in order to show empathic responses. An "arbitrary cue" signaling the feeling state of another was sufficient to elicit empathy (1158). This set of results affirms what neuroscientists working on mirror neurons on monkeys have theorized and what philosophers since David Hume have been saying about empathy for centuries. For the first time, brain images supporting the long-standing introspective account of empathy have been recorded.

The questions of how and why empathy works in the bodies and brains of human beings can still only be answered with theoretical speculations about the physiological substrate, though the fMRI-based research described above and recent neuroscience on the shared manifold for intersubjectivity gets researchers closer than they have been before. [The amygdala, anterior temporal cortex, and orbital frontal cortex (as well as physiological synchrony of the autonomic nervous system) are probably involved in empathy, as the evidence of emotional impairment in brain-damaged or diseased patients suggests (Brothers; Levenson and Ruef; and Rosen)]. Stephanie Preston and Frans de Waal propose that witnessing or imagining another in an emotional state activates automatic representations of that same state in the onlooker, including responses in the nervous system and the body. They write that "empathy processes likely contain fast reflexive sub-cortical processes (directly from sensory cortices to thalamus to amygdala to response) and slower cortical processes (from thalamus to cortex to amygdala to response). These roughly map onto contagious and cognitive forms of empathy, respectively" (Preston and de Waal 12). The advantages of automatic responses lie in their speediness. Joseph LeDoux has written about how fear responses in the amygdala provide a quick and dirty, possibly life-saving response to environmental threats, which can then be evaluated as the slightly slower cognitive evaluation of a threat kick in (LeDoux 168–78). What is sometimes called "primitive empathy" may work in the same way, provided a first, fast, feeling response to seeing or learning about another's emotional state, before cognitive evaluation through deliberate role taking occurs. [This account is consistent with the emotion theory of neuroscientist Edmund T. Rolls, who hypothesizes that human brain mechanisms provide two routes to action, one a quick, unconscious prompt for a behavioral response (which we share with other mammals) and the other a slower, language mediated, rational planning faculty. The two routes can produce conflicting results.]

The human capacity for primitive empathy, or the phenomenon of spontaneously matching feelings, suggests that human beings are basically similar to one another, with a limited range of variations. Psychologist Martin Hoffman, for instance, believes that the structural similarities in people's physiological and cognitive response systems cause similar feelings to be evoked by similar events (Hoffman, *Moral Development* 62). However, Hoffman would be the first to concede that similarity itself is not enough to guarantee an empathic response. Singer and her colleagues believe that our survival depends on effective functioning in social contexts, and that feeling what others feel, empathizing, contributes to that success. They suggest that "our ability to empathize has evolved from a system for representing our internal bodily states and subjective feeling states" to ourselves (Singer et al. 1161). In other words, empathy as Singer's group understands it participates in a theory of mind that links second order re-representations of others to the system that allows us to predict the results of emotional stimuli for ourselves. Recent research suggests a mechanism at the neural level that would enable such representations of others' actions, including facial expressions and bodily postures that may convey emotional states. [Mirror neurons fire not only when carrying out an action but also when observing another carrying out the same action. They provide a basis for understanding primates' mind-reading, including human empathy (Gallese et al., "The Mirror Matching"; also Iacoboni).] Contemporary neuroscience theorizes a system for representation of others' feelings that participates in the task of enabling us to understand the motives, beliefs, and thoughts of others. This work on empathy thus supports the theories of evolutionary psychology that emphasize the adaptive function of our social relations (Cosmides and Tooby, "Cognitive"). Given this basis in human shared intersubjectivity, empathy thus appears to many to be a key element in our responsiveness to others.

My work seeks to clarify why the link between narrative empathy and altruism is nonetheless so tenuous. For a novel reader who experiences either empathy or personal distress, there can be no expectancy of reciprocation involved in the aesthetic response. [For working definitions of different vicariously induced emotional states, see Eisenberg and Fabes 111). I follow Nancy Eisenberg in differentiating empathy, aversive personal distress, and sympathy. Empathic response includes the possibility of personal distress, but personal distress (unlike empathy) is less likely to lead to sympathy, if it proceeds beyond evanescent shared feeling.] The very nature of fictionality renders social contracts between people and person-like characters null and void. Unlike the hostage children in Beslan who wished that Harry Potter would come to their rescue, adult readers know that fictional characters cannot offer us aid. Similarly, we accept that we cannot help them out, much as we may wish to intervene: Don't marry him, Dorothea! We may feel intense interest in characters, but incurring obligations towards them violates the terms of fictionality. That is, an empathetic response can be diverted from a pro-social outcome through interfering cognition.

The treatment of emotions and rationality as separate and dichotomous features of our experience has been challenged in recent decades. Thinking and feeling, for Antonio R. Damasio, are part of the same package (Damasio et al., "Somatic." [Damasio's works for general readers (*Descartes' Error*, *The Feeling of What Happens*, and *Looking for Spinoza*) have resulted in wide dissemination of his theories.] In a series of academic articles and popular books, [Damasio] has shown that clinical patients suffering from emotional disorders have cognitive difficulties: Ronald DeSousa has advocated recognition of the rationality of emotions and Joseph LeDoux's cognitive neuroscience focuses on *The Emotional Brain*. Evolutionary psychologists Leda Cosmides and John Tooby speak for a growing group of scientists who believe that "one cannot sensibly talk about emotion affecting cognition because 'cognition' refers to a language for describing all of the brain's operations, including emotions and reasoning (whether deliberative or nonconscious), and not to any particular subset of operations" ("Evolutionary" 98). [Some neuroscientists informally refer to "cogmotions" to emphasize the fusion of the two concepts in their research. (My informant is neuroscientist Dr. Tyler S. Lorig.) Nonetheless, many experts in cognition carry out their work without regard to the emotions, and basic textbooks on cognition rarely refer to emotions. See for instance Reed's introductory college text, *Cognition: Theory and Applications*, 6th ed. Emotional states receive fleeting mention on just three pages of this text. The younger hybrid discipline of Social Cognition is more likely to reflect the understandings of affect and cognition as intertwined (Forgas).] In the relatively recent field known as Cognitive Approaches to Literary Studies, where the work of LeDoux and Damasio has virtually canonical status, matters of affect are generally considered to fall under the umbrella of the term "cognitive." Few literary cognitivists acknowledge that a psychologist might not readily accede to the centrality of emotions to cognition. The sub-disciplinary boundaries within the extremely diverse field of psychology result in different emphases and perspectives on the place of the emotions. Empathy studies have from the start challenged the division of emotion and cognition, but they have also been altered by the convictions and disciplinary affiliations of those who study empathy.

I set aside for the moment the view that emotions and cognition describe different processes of the central nervous system, for empathy itself clearly involves both feeling and thinking. Memory, experience, and the capacity to take another's perspective (all matters traditionally considered cognitive) have roles in empathy. Yet the experience of empathy in the feeling subject involves the emotions, including sensations in the body. In any case, narrative empathy invoked by reading must involve cognition, for reading itself relies upon complex cognitive operations. Yet overall, emotional response to reading is the more neglected aspect of what literary cognitivists refer to under the umbrella term cognition. This does not need to be so. The discipline of aesthetics, which has historical ties both to philosophy and to psychology, as well as to literary studies, has been interested for over a century in empathy as a facet of creativity and an explanation of human response to artworks. [The core elements of the modern concept of empathy in aesthetics can legitimately be traced to Lee, who was also a novelist. As with several key dates in psychology, rival claimants to earliest usage appear. Lipps's 1897 work on *Einfühlung* gets translated in 1909 by experimental psychologist Titchener as *empathy*. Lee drew on Lipps' work for *The Beautiful*. Freud also had Lipps' books in his library and adopted the term *Einfühlung* (Wispé).]

In its strongest form, aesthetics' empathy describes a projective fusing with an object—which may be another person or an animal, but may also be a fictional character made of words, or even, in some accounts, inanimate things such as landscapes, artworks, or geological features. ... The acts of imagination and projection involved in such empathy certainly deserve the label cognitive, but the sensations, however strange, deserve to be registered as feelings. Thus I do not quarantine narrative empathy in the zone of either affect or cognition: as a process, it involves both. When texts invite readers to feel, they also stimulate readers' thinking. [Philosopher Lawrence Blum believes that insofar as emotions of sympathy and empathy promote perspective taking, they may result in better prosocial responses than rationality alone (Blum 122–39).] Whether novel reading comprises a significant enough feature of the environment of literate people to play a critical role in their prosocial development remains to be seen. Even the leap between reading and empathizing can fall short, impeded by inattention, indifference, or personal distress. Readers' cognitive and affective responses do not inevitably lead to empathizing, but fiction does disarm readers of some of the protective layers of cautious reasoning that may inhibit empathy in the real world.

Narrative theorists, novel critics, and reading specialists have already singled out a small set of narrative techniques—such as the use of first person narration and the interior representation of characters' consciousness and emotional states—as devices supporting character identification, contributing to empathetic experiences, opening readers' minds to others, changing attitudes, and even predisposing readers to altruism. In the course of reviewing the available research on this subject, I point out the gaps in our knowledge of potentially empathetic narrative techniques. No specific set of narrative techniques has yet been verified to over-ride the resistance to empathizing often displayed by members of an in-group regarding the emotional states of others marked out as different by their age, race, gender, weight, disabilities, and so forth. [Some studies suggest that people with very empathetic dispositions respond more positively to members of outgroups than less empathetic people do, but for most people, perceived similarity encourages empathy. For a classic study affirming similarity's relationship to higher empathy scores, see Krebs. On outgroups, see Sheehan, et al. On similarity, see the literature review in Davis, *Empathy* (15, 96–9, 105–6, 109, 116–18).] Human beings, like other primates, tend to experience empathy most readily and accurately for those who seem like us, as David Hume and Adam Smith predicted (Kruger; Hoffman, *Empathy* 4, 13, 206).

We may find ourselves regarding the feelings of those who seem outside the tribe with a range of emotions, but without empathy, [as when empathy's replaces egocentrism with ethnocentrism (Sherman)]. If empathetic reading experiences start a chain reaction leading to mature sympathy and altruistic behavior, as advocates of the empathy-altruism hypothesis believe, then discovering the narrative techniques involved matters. It is one thing to discover, however, that high empathizers report empathetic reading experiences, and quite another to show that empathetic reading experiences can contribute to changing a reader's disposition, motivations, and attitudes. If novels could extend readers' sense of shared humanity beyond the predictable limitations, then the narrative techniques involved in such an accomplishment should be especially prized.

A Theory of Narrative Empathy

Character identification often invites empathy, even when the fictional character and reader differ from one another in all sorts of practical and obvious ways, but empathy for fictional characters appears to require only minimal elements of identity, situation, and feeling, not necessarily complex or realistic characterization. Whether a reader's empathy or her identification with a character comes first is an open question: spontaneous empathy for a fictional character's feelings sometimes opens the way for character identification. Not all feeling states of characters evoke empathy; indeed, empathetic responses to fictional characters and situations occur more readily for negative emotions, whether or not a match in details of experience exists. Finally, readers' experiences differ from one another, and empathy with characters doesn't always occur as a result of reading an emotionally evocative fiction.

Several observations help to explain the differences in readers' responses. Most importantly, readers' empathic dispositions are not identical to one another. Some humans are more empathetic to real others and some feel little empathy at all. (Some research suggests that empathizers are better readers, because their role-taking abilities allow them to more readily comprehend causal relations in stories. [On empathy as a precursor to reading comprehension, see Bourg].) The timing and the context of the reading experience matters: the capacity of novels to invoke readers' empathy changes over time, and some novels may only activate the empathy of their first, immediate audience, while others must survive to reach a later generation of readers in order to garner an emotionally resonant reading. Readers' empathy for situations depicted in fiction may be enhanced by chance relevance to particular historical, economic, cultural, or social circumstances, either in the moment of first publication or in later times, fortuitously anticipated or prophetically foreseen by the novelist.

Novelists do not exert complete control over the responses to their fiction. Empathy for a fictional character does not invariably correspond with what the author appears to set up or invite. Situational empathy, which responds primarily to aspects of plot and circumstance, involves less self-extension in imaginative role taking and more recognition of prior (or current) experience. A novelist invoking situational empathy can only hope to reach readers with appropriately correlating experiences. The generic and formal choices made by authors in crafting fictional worlds play a role in inviting (or retarding) readers' empathic responses. This means that for some readers, the author's use of the formulaic conventions of a thriller or a romance novel would increase empathetic resonance, while for other readers (perhaps better educated and attuned to literary effects) unusual or striking representations promote foregrounding and open the way to empathetic reading (Miall and Kuiken, "Literariness?"; Miall, "Beyond").

Novelists themselves often vouch for the centrality of empathy to novel reading and writing and express belief narrative empathy's power to change the minds and lives of readers. This belief of authors mirrors their experiences as ready empathizers. Yet even the most fervent employers of their empathetic imaginations realize that this key ingredient of fictional worldmaking does not always transmit to readers without interference. Author's empathy can be devoted to socially undesirable ends that may be rejected by a disapproving reader. Indeed, empathic distress at feeling with a character whose actions are at odds with a reader's moral code may be a result of successfully exercised authorial empathy. Both authors' empathy and readers' empathy have rhetorical uses, which come more readily to notice when they conflict in instances of empathic inaccuracy (discordance arising from gaps between a author's intention and a reader's experience of narrative empathy). Experiences of empathic inaccuracy may contribute to a reader's outraged sense that the author's perspective is simply wrong, while strong concord in authors' empathy and readers' empathy can be a motivating force to move beyond literary response to prosocial action. The position of the reader with respect to the author's strategic empathizing in fictional worldmaking limits these potential results. I theorize that *bounded strategic empathy* operates with an in-group, stemming from experiences of mutuality and leading to feeling with familiar others. *Ambassadorial strategic empathy* addresses chosen others with the aim of cultivating their empathy for the in-group, often to a specific end. *Broadcast strategic empathy* calls upon every reader to feel with members of a group, by emphasizing common vulnerabilities and hopes through universalizing representations.

Empathetic Narrative Techniques

Consider the commonplace that first person fiction more readily evokes feeling responsiveness than the whole variety of third person narrative situations. Even a college sophomore with a few weeks' training in theoretical terms can report that within the category of first person narratives, empathy may be enhanced or impeded by narrative consonance or dissonance, unreliability, discordance, an excess of narrative levels with multiple narrators, extremes of disorder, or an especially convoluted plot. Genre, setting, and time period may help or hinder readers' empathy. Feeling out of sorts with the implied readership, or fitting it exactly, may make the difference between a dutiful reading and an experience of emotional fusion. [For this catalog of helps and impediments to empathetic reading of first person fiction, I draw upon the in-class essays of the students in English 232, The Novel, composed on 20 February 2006, answering this question: "How does your recent reading experience in this course square with the notion that first person narration is especially productive of empathetic reading? What differences in technique in the variety of first person narrative situations might alter readers' responses?"] Contrasting first person with third person puts the question too broadly, with too many other variables, to reach a valid conclusion. Narrative theorists can contribute specificity and subtlety to the research into narrative empathy.

A variety of narrative techniques have been associated with empathy by narrative theorists and discourse processing experts carrying out empirical research into literary reading. The formal devices themselves are regarded as empathic in nature by some theorists and researchers, while for others the disposition of the reader towards the text can be measured by inquiring about particular consequences of literary reading. The observations made by this latter group often lead to speculations about narrative technique. Mapping these ostensibly empathetic narrative techniques draws attention to the many aspects of narrative form that have *not yet* been associated with readers' empathy, but which ought not to be ruled out without careful consideration.

The most commonly nominated feature of narrative fiction to be associated with empathy is *character identification*. Specific aspects of characterization, such as naming, description, indirect implication of traits, reliance on types, relative flatness or roundness, depicted actions, roles in plot trajectories, quality of attributed speech, and mode of representation of consciousness may be assumed to contribute to the potential for character identification and thus for empathy. [Very little empirical research has been attempted to verify the theoretical speculations about aspects of characterization that operate in readers' character identification. Bortolussi and Dixon's pioneering study *Psychonarratology* reports their findings that character actions contribute to readers' assessments of character traits, while self-evaluations provided by the narrator (description) do not. However, the test stories employed first-person narrators, so narrators' evaluations of characters in third-person fiction cannot be included in this preliminary conclusion (160–5).] The link between readers' reports of character identification and their experiences of narrative empathy has not yet been explained.

A close second for formal quality most often associated with empathy would be *narrative situation* (including point of view and perspective): the nature of the mediation between author and reader, including the person of the narration, the implicit location of the narrator, the relation of the narrator to the characters, and the internal or external perspective on characters, including in some cases the style of representation of characters' consciousness. [Schneider represents narrative situation as a factor in eliciting readers' empathy, and lack of representation of inner life as a likely inhibitor of it.] Many other elements of fiction have been supposed to contribute to readers' empathy. These include the repetitions of works in series (Warhol, *Having* 71–2; Hakemulder, *Moral* 93, 143) and length. [Nussbaum's empathy-inducing novels are invariably long. Writing about the character David Copperfield's reading habits in Dicken's novel of that name (1849–50), Nussbaum comments, "he remains with [books] for hours in an intense, intimate, and loving relationship. As he imagines, dreams, and desires in their company, he becomes a certain sort of person." For Nussbaum the length of the immersion is a vital component of the process, permitting intensity, dreaming, and desiring that develops the reader's loving heart (Nussbaum, *Love's* 230–1).] Genre expectations [may play a role (Jameson); Zwaan … compares readers' behavior when processing texts labeled as "news stories" or "narratives." Bortolussi and Dixon aptly caution that research in discourse processing has focused on broad generic distinctions rather than on narrative fiction's subgenres (253–4). For emotional responses to fictional subgenres in television , see Bryant and Zillmann, eds. Literary genre critics have been reluctant to adopt findings from mass communications research (to the extent that they are aware of them), perhaps because audiovisual (iconic) representations are assumed to be more emotionally stimulating than the verbal representations of prose narrative fiction. This assumption, however, has not been investigated systematically.]. Vivid use of settings [has been proposed: feminist criticism often celebrates the power of women's writing's vividly represented spaces and places, in tandem with identity themes, to work out boundary-crossing potentials for connection, communication, and change (Friedman).] Metanarrative commentary [may invite empathy: See the account of Nünning's remarks on empathy-inducing functions of metanarration, in Fludernik, "Metanarrative and Metafictional Commentary" (39).] Aspects of the discourse that slow readers' pace (foregrounding, uses of disorder, etc.) [have been nominated: Relevant to slower pace as potentially fostering empathy is Zillmann, who hypothesizes that the fast pace of television news stories and dramas may impede empathetic response (160–1). Miall's work on foregrounding and empathy in literary texts correlates a slower reading pace with enhanced empathy.] The confirmation of many of the hypotheses about specific narrative techniques and empathy has yet to be undertaken in most cases, but the work that has been done *as often* fails fully to support the commonplaces of narratology as it authenticates them (van Peer, "Justice"). Whether this has to do with faulty experimental design, insufficient grasp of the nuances of narrative theory, or verifiable confutations of theory has yet to be discovered.

Character Identification

To begin with the necessary clarification, character identification is not a narrative technique (it occurs in the reader, not in the text), but a consequence of reading that may be precipitated by the use of particular techniques of characterization. [Character identification thus exemplifies what Marisa Bortolussi and Peter Dixon identify as readers' mental constructions, as opposed to textual features (28). Bortolussi and Dixon systematically measure how particular readers process specific textual features in narratives, but the experimental results bridging disciplines of discourse processing and narrative theory are still quite scanty (Diengott).] These qualities have not yet been investigated in a comprehensive fashion. . . . In contrast, Jèmeljan Hakemulder suggests that readers experiencing strong admiration of an author's writing style may engage less readily with the fictional world and its inhabitants (*Laboratory* 73–4). Readers' personal involvement with a fictional character may (or may not) be contingent upon the use of a particular technique or the presence of certain representational elements that meet with their approval. [Writing about identification with dramatic characters, Zillman argues that the audience-member's disposition precipitates empathic and counterempathic reactions and suggests that audiences must be made to care about characters one way or another. He believes that enactment of good or evil deeds by protagonists and antagonists, with opportunities for the moral appraisal of their actions, promotes strong emotional reactions ("Mechanisms").] Keith Oatley believes that readers' personal experiences of patterns of emotional response provoke sympathy for characters, especially as readers identify with characters' goals and plans ("Taxonomy"). David S. Miall and Don Kuiken argue that emotional experiences of literature depend upon the engagement of the literary text with the reader's experiences, but they emphasize foregrounding effects at the level of literary style that shake up conventions, slow the pace, and invite more active reading that opens the way for empathy. [In this respect Miall and Kuiken are in accord with earlier work that demonstrates a relationship between a subject's prior similar experiences and empathy felt for another in the same situation (Stotland).] (Miall and Kuiken, "Literariness?" 121–38; Miall, "Beyond"). Don Kuiken's research shows that readers who linked themselves to story characters through personal experiences were more likely to report changes in self-perception, if not actual empathy (Kuiken, et al., "Locating"). Max Louwerse and Kuiken suggest that empathy may work as a gap-filling mechanism, by which a reader supplements given character traits with a fuller psychologically resonant portrait (170). [Their research confirms some of what Iser proposes about active reading as gap-filling (Iser, *Act* 168–9).] Readers' judgments about the realism of the characters are supposed to have an impact on identification (cf. Konijn and Hoorn; Walsh "Why we Wept"), and the similarity of the reader to the character is widely believed to promote identification (Klemenz-Belgardt 368; Jose and Brewer). [Hakemulder reports on recent studies confirming the importance of personal relevance for intensity of reader response (*Moral* 71).] None of these phenomena, however, inhere in particular narrative techniques contributing to character identification.

A few techniques of characterization have actually been tested for their relation to readers' emotional responsiveness or empathy. Characters' involvement in a suspenseful situation provokes physiological responses of arousal in readers even when they disdain the quality of the narrative (Wünsch, cited in Hakemulder, *Moral* 73). Plot-laden action-stories have been shown to promote faster reading than narratives focusing on characters' inner lives (Chupchik and Lázló), which may suggest by contrast greater reflectiveness on the part of character-focused readers, as Hakemulder supposes (*Moral* 74). However, this does not account for the quick, apparently involuntary responses to particular plot situations inspired by trashy novels. Speedy reading may be a token of involvement in a character's fate, identification, and even empathy. With the exception of appraisal of causality, virtually nothing about the role of plot structure has been associated with readers' empathetic responses, or tested in controlled settings. [Research into the empathy evoked by various genres of television advertisements suggests that discontinuous, nonlinear "vignette" ads discourage empathy, whereas classical, character-centered dramatic form in ads evokes viewers' empathy (Stern).] Aspects of plot structure and narration that might have a role in invoking readers' empathy include the control of timing (pace), order (anachronies), the use of nested levels of narrative (stories within stories), serial narrative, strong or weak closure, the use of subsidiary (supplementary, satellite) plot events, repetition, and gaps. [For a good application of cognitive theory on levels of embedding to readers' capacity to comprehend embedded accounts of characters' mental states, see Lisa Zunshine, "Theory of Mind."] Since each one of these structural categories contains an array of possibilities for characterization, their neglect leaves us with an incomplete picture of the devices whose use makes character identification possible.

Many aspects of characterization familiar to narrative theorists have not yet been tested in controlled experiments, despite their nomination by theorists. The naming of characters (including the withholding of a name, the use of an abbreviation or a role-title in place of a full name, or allegorical or symbolic naming, etc.) may play a role in the potential for character identification. The descriptive language through which readers encounter characters is assumed to make a difference (content matters!), but what about grammar and syntax? Does the use of present tense (over the usual past tense) really create effects of immediacy and direct connection, as many contemporary authors believe? The old "show, don't tell" shibboleth of creative writing classes remains to be verified: direct description of a character's emotional state or circumstances by a third-person narrator may produce empathy in readers just as effectively as indirect implication of emotional states through actions and context (Booth, *Rhetoric* 129–33, 243–66, 274–82, 379–91). David S. Miall has suggested in "Affect and Narrative" that characters' motives, rather than their traits, account for the affective engagement and self-projection of readers into characters, though it remains unclear when, and at which cues, readers' emotional self-involvement jump-starts the process of interpretation. Bortolussi and Dixon believe that "transparency," or the judgment of characters' behavior as sensible and practical, contributes to identification (240). This may be too simple: even traditional novels are complex, polyvocal, and various, and Wayne Booth offers this sensible caution: "What we call 'involvement' or 'sympathy' or 'identification', is usually made up of *many reactions* to author, narrators, observers, and other characters" (*Rhetoric* 158, my emphasis). Some way of accounting for the multiplicity of reactions making up a normal novel reading experience needs to be devised in order to study the transition from distributed characterization in narrative fiction and readers' everyday synthesis of their reactions into an experience of character identification.

This may mean setting aside some common value judgments about techniques. For instance, the critical preference for psychological depth expressed by the "roundness" of characters "capable of surprising in a convincing way" (Forster, *Aspects* 78), does not preclude empathetic response to flat characters, minor characters, or stereotyped villains and antagonists. Drawing on the literature of cognitive social psychology, Richard J. Gerrig has suggested that readers are likely to make category-based judgments about fictional characters, and to emphasize attributed dispositions of characters over their actual behavior in situations ("Construction"; *Experiencing*). This theory suggests, as Forster intuited, that flat characters—easily comprehended and recalled—may play a greater role in readers' engagement in novels than is usually understood. Fast and easy character identification suffers in theorists' accounts of the reading process, which often privilege more arduous self-extension and analogical reasoning. Patrick Colm Hogan, for instance, regards categorical empathy (with characters matching a reader's group identity) as the more prevalent form, while situational empathy, the more ethically desirable role taking, depends upon a reader's having a memory of a comparable experience, which is never guaranteed (Hogan, "Epilogue"). [Though this article suggests a preference for the cognitive role-taking Hogan associates with situational empathy, his later very brief treatment of readers' empathy in *Cognitive Science, Literature, and the Arts* improves on his theory by describing how emotion triggers invoke quick-and-dirty responses, as well as imaginative role-taking, neither of which need be denigrated as egocentric (*Cognitive* 186–7). For work confirming the role of lived experience in spontaneous situational empathy with characters on film documentaries, see Sapolsky and Zillmann, "Experience and Empathy." Women who had given birth responded to a medical film of actual childbirth with more intense physiological reactions; otherwise, gender and related experiences had a negligible effect on empathy.] If Hogan's situational empathy alone leads to the ethics of compassion, as he has it, then quick-match categorical empathy looks weaker and more vulnerable to bias through ethnocentrism or exclusionary thinking. We do not know, however, that categorical empathy does *not* lead to compassion, no more than we know the ethical results of situational empathy for fictional characters. Neither hypothesis has yet been tested. While literary critics and professionals value novels that unsettle convictions and contest norms, readers' reactions to familiar situations and formulaic plot trajectories may underlie their genuinely empathetic reactions to predictable plot events and to the stereotyped figures that enact them (Jauss 152–88, esp. 159 figure; Hogan, *Mind*). The fullness and fashion by which speech, thoughts, and feelings of characters reach the reader are very often supposed by narrative theorists to enhance character identification, as I discuss below, but relatively externalized and brief statements about a character's experiences and mental state may be sufficient to invoke empathy in a reader. Novelists do not need to be reminded of the rhetorical power of understatement, or indeed of the peril of revealing too much. Indeed, sometimes the potential for character identification and readers' empathy *decreases* with sustained exposure to a particular figure's thoughts or voice (Andringa, et al. 154–5).

Narrative Situation

It has been a commonplace of narrative theory that an internal perspective, achieved either through first person self-narration, through figural narration (in which the 3rd person narrator stays covert and reports only on a single, focal center of consciousness located in a main character) or through authorial (omniscient) narration that moves inside characters' minds, best promotes character identification and readers' empathy. Wayne Booth, for instance, writes, "*If* an author wants intense sympathy for characters who do not have strong virtues to recommend them, *then* the psychic vividness of prolonged inside views will help him (Booth 377–8, emphasis in original). The technique also works for characters in which readers have a natural rooting interest, such as Jane Austen's heroines. Booth's detailed account of how Austen uses the inside view to promote sympathy for the flawed Emma is a classic of narrative theory (245–56). Booth asserts, "By showing most of the story through Emma's eyes, the author insures that we will travel with Emma rather than stand against her" (245). Austen, one of the early masters of narrated monologue to represent characters' consciousness, crafts smooth transitions between her narrator's generalizations about characters' mental states (psycho-narration) and transcriptions of their inner thoughts, in language that preserves the tense and person of the narration (Cohn, *Transparent* 14). Also called free indirect discourse, narrated monologue presents the character's mental discourse in the grammatical tense and person of the narrator's discourse.

Subsequent theorists have agreed that narrated monologue has a strong effect on readers' responses to characters. David Miall specifically mentions the means of providing "privileged information about a character's mind," free indirect discourse, as especially likely to cue literariness and invite empathic decentering ("Necessity" 54). Sylvia Adamson arrives independently at a similar point, arguing that narrated monologue should be understood as "empathetic narrative." In Adamson's language the representational technique and its ostensible effects fuse. *Quoted monologue* (also called interior monologue, the direct presentation of characters' thoughts in the person and tense of their speech) also has its champions, who regard the move into first person as invariably more authentic and direct than the more mediated or double-voiced narrated monologue. *Psycho-narration*, or the narrator's generalizations about the mental states or thoughts of a character has fewer advocates, perhaps because it is associated with traditional narratives such as epics. However, both Wayne Booth and Dorrit Cohn suggest that psycho-narration can powerfully invoke character identification, and Cohn points out that both poetic analogies and metaphors for feeling states (as Virginia Woolf often employs) require the use of psycho-narration (Booth, *Rhetoric* 3–16; Cohn *Transparent* 46–57). Despite the frequent mention of narrated monologue as the most likely to produce empathy (Palmer, *Fictional* 138), quoted monologue and psycho-narration also give a reader access to the inner life of characters. Most theorists agree that purely externalized narration tends not to invite readers' empathy. [Three good starting points for recent work on the representation of consciousness are Fludernik's magisterial *The Fictions of Language and the Languages of Fiction*; the essays of Zunshine, "Theory of Mind" and "Richardson's Clarissa and a Theory of Mind"; and the phenomenological theory of Butte].

In addition to these speculations about modes of representing inner life, the person of the narration often seems likely to effect readers' responses to narrative fiction and its inhabitants. In particular, first person fiction, in which the narrator self-narrates about his or her own experiences and perceptions, is thought to invite an especially close relationship between reader and narrative voice. For instance, Franz Stanzel believes that the choice of internal representation of the thoughts and feelings of a character in third person fiction and the use of first person self-narration have a particularly strong effect on readers. Novelist and literary theorist David Lodge speculates that historical and philosophical contexts may explain the preference for first person or figural third person narrative voice: "In a world where nothing is certain, in which transcendental belief has been undermined by scientific materialism, and even the objectivity of science is qualified by relativity and uncertainty, the single human voice, telling its own story, can seem the only authentic way of rendering consciousness" (Lodge 87). However, the existing experimental results for such an association of technique and reaction are not robust. In several studies of Dutch teenagers, W. van Peer and H. Pander Maat tested the notion that first person narration creates a "greater illusion of closeness ... allowing the reader a greater and better fusion with the world of the character" ("Perspectivation" 145). [Van Peer and Pander Maat designed experiments using five versions of stories, rewritten to test the relationship between positive internal focalization and readers' allocation of sympathy]. They conclude "it remains unclear why point of view has no more powerful and no more overall effect on readers, given the effort devoted by authors in order to create these devices that produce a point of view" (152). While noting that readers certainly express preferences about point of view and prefer consistency over inconsistency, they found that enhancement of sympathy for protagonists through positive internal focalization actually weakened as teenagers matured (152–4).

Lodge concedes that the first person voice "is just as artful, or artificial, a method as writing about a character in the third person," but he insists that it "creates an illusion of reality, it commands the willing suspension of the reader's disbelief, by modeling itself on the discourses of personal witness: the confession, the diary, autobiography, the memoir, the deposition" (Lodge 87–8). In my book [*Empathy and the Novel*] I argue the opposite, that paratexts cuing readers to understand a work as fictional unleash their emotional responsiveness, in spite of fiction's historical mimicry of non-fictional, testimonial forms. My research suggests that readers' perception of a text's fictionality plays a role in subsequent empathetic response, by releasing readers from the obligations of self-protection through skepticism and suspicion. Thus they may respond with greater empathy to an unreal situation and characters because of the protective fictionality, but still internalize the experience of empathy with possible later real-world responsiveness to others' needs. While a full-fledged political movement, an appropriately inspiring social context, or an emergent structure of feeling promoting change may be necessary for efficacious action to arise out of internalized experiences of narrative empathy, readers may respond in those circumstances as a result of earlier reading.

How Narrative Empathy Works: Authors and Audiences

The dispositions and beliefs of novelists themselves also belong in a thorough study of narrative empathy. Fiction writers report looking at and eavesdropping on their characters, engaging in conversations with them, struggling with them over their actions, bargaining with them, and feeling for them: characters seem to possess independent agency. In a remarkable study of 50 fiction writers, Taylor and her collaborators discovered that 92% of the authors reported some experience of the illusion of independent agency (IIA) and that the more successful fiction writers (those who had published) had more frequent and more intense experiences of it. Taylor hypothesizes that IIA could be related to authors' expertise in fantasy production (Taylor et al. 361, 376–7), suggesting that it occurs more easily and spontaneously with practice, or that writers naturally endowed with creative gifts may experience it more readily. Though clearly novelists still do exercise their authority by choosing the words that end up on the page, they may experience the creative process as akin to involuntarily empathizing with a person out there, separate from themselves. Several tests administered by Taylor to her subjects support this connection. Taylor found that the fiction writers as a group scored higher than the general population empathy (361). Using Davis's Interpersonal Reactivity Index (IRI), a frequently used empathy scale, Taylor measured her subjects' tendency to fantasize, to feel empathic concern for others, to experience personal distress in the face of others' suffering, and to engage in perspective-taking (369–70). Both men and women in her sample of fiction writers scored significantly higher than Davis's reported norms for the general population, with females scoring higher in all four areas than males. Fiction writers of both genders stood out on all four subscales of Davis's IRI, but they were particularly off the charts for fantasy and perspective taking. Taylor speculates that "these two subscales tap the components of empathy that seem most conceptually related to IIA and might be seen as 'grown-up' versions of variables associated with children who have imaginary companions (pretend play and theory of mind skills)" (377).

Taylor's discoveries lead to speculation about the function of narrative empathy from the authors' perspective: *fiction writers as a group may be more empathetic than the general population*. However, we must also consider the difficulty of pinning down the difference between innate dispositions and results of practice and habitual use in groups of people; thus, *the activity of fiction writing may cultivate novelists' role-taking skills and make them more habitually empathetic.* These proposals do not imply that the actual behavior of fiction writers is any better than the population at large. Even the most ardent advocates of narrative ethics hesitate to argue that being a novelist correlates with being a better person, and novelists known to be nice people sometimes also exercise their empathy on behalf of nasty characters.

Most theories of narrative empathy assume that empathy can be transacted accurately from author to reader by way of a literary text (critiques of literary empathy disparage this goal as an unwholesome fantasy or projection). The comments of writers about their craft suggest the formation of a triangulated empathic bond. In this model authors' empathy contributes to the creation of textual beings designed to elicit empathic responses from readers. In fact there is no guarantee that an individual reader will respond empathetically to a particular representation. Because real people—for instance, objects of pity presented by charitable organizations—might find their position in that empathic triangle discomforting, critics of empathy claim it results in misunderstanding or worse.

From the failures of empathetic individuals to question whether their assessments of the other's feelings could be off base comes a great deal of the negative reputation of empathy as a particularly invasive form of selfishness. (I impose my feelings on you and call them your feelings. Your feelings, whatever they were, undergo erasure.) Contrary to this fearful scenario, the research on empathic accuracy records the remarkable degree of correctness in human mind-reading abilities, though to be sure more cross-cultural verification of these findings would be welcome (Ickes, ed. *Empathic Accuracy*). Whether from expert reading of facial cues, body language, tone of voice, context, or effective role taking on the part of the empathizer, ordinary subjects tend to do pretty well in laboratory tests of empathic accuracy. Verification can be achieved readily enough through interviews cross-checked with physical measurements and observations.

When we respond empathetically to a novel, we do not have the luxury of questioning the character: we cannot ask, Is that how you really felt? The text, however, may verify our reactions even as it elicits them. No one narrative technique assures readers that our empathetic reaction precisely catches the feelings embedded in the fictional characters. For this reason, extratextual sources, such as interviews with authors, become important tools in assessing literary empathic accuracy. My term *empathic inaccuracy* describes a potential effect of narrative empathy: *a strong conviction of empathy that incorrectly identifies the feeling of a literary persona.* Empathic inaccuracy occurs when a reader responds empathetically to a fictional character at cross-purposes with an author's intentions. Authors also sometimes evoke empathy unintentionally. This accident contributes to empathic inaccuracy. Unlike in real world, face-to-face circumstances, the novel-reading situation allows empathic inaccuracy to persist because neither author nor fictional character directly confutes it. Indeed, literary studies privileges against-the-grain interpretations of fiction that may be founded on deliberate acts of role taking that subvert the authors' apparent intentions and increase empathic inaccuracy. A reader persuaded that she has felt with a fictional character may defy the stated or implicit intentions of an author. When the author's intention matches the reader's feelings and the agreement resonates with empathic accord, then the introduction of alternative perspectives on the matter at hand may meet with disbelief or outrage. *Empathic inaccuracy,* to craft a proposal out of this circumstance, *may then contribute to a strong sense that the author's perspective is simply wrong.* This is by no means an unproductive critical stance.

For those writers who hope to reach readers with emotionally resonant representations, the struggle against empathic inaccuracy thus has two component liabilities, failure and falsity. On *failure* of narrative empathy, I propose that while *author's empathy may be an intrinsic element of successful fictional worldmaking, its exercise does not always transmit to readers without interference.* A second form of empathic inaccuracy occurs when authors represent a practice or experience that unintentionally evokes empathy in readers, against authors' apparent or proclaimed representational goals. Focus on the *falsity* of narrative empathy expresses the concern that experiencing narrative empathy short-circuits the impulse to act compassionately or to respond with political engagement. In this view, narrative empathy is amoral (Posner 19), a weak form of appeal to humanity in the face of organized hatred (Gourevitch 95), an obstacle to agitation for racial justice (Delgado 4–36), a waste of sentiment and encouragement of withdrawal (Williams 109), and even a pornographic indulgence of sensation acquired at the expense of suffering others (Wood 36). To some feminist and postcolonial critics, empathy loses credence the moment it appears to depend on a notion of universal human emotions, a cost too great to bear even if basic human rights depend upon it. [Indeed, human rights are not exempted from criticism. Some regard "the whole idea of 'universal' human rights" as a "gigantic fraud, where Western imperialist or excolonial powers try to pass off their own, very specific and localized idea of what 'rights' should be as universal, trampling roughly over everyone else's beliefs and traditions." (Howe 3).] The fearful view of author's empathy as corrupting readers by offering them others' feelings for callous consumption leads in some quarters to the depiction of empathy itself as a quality that weakens humans and makes them vulnerable to others' cruelest manipulations. Narrative empathy becomes yet another example of the western imagination's imposition of its own values on cultures and peoples that it scarcely knows, but presumes to feel with, in a cultural imperialism of the emotions. Empathic inaccuracy, in this quarrel with moral sentimentalism, then becomes evidence of the falsity of the whole enterprise of sympathetic representation.

Rather than attempting to eliminate empathic inaccuracy by arguing with or correcting readers' feeling responses, recognizing the conflict between author's empathy and reader's empathy opens the way to an understanding of narrative empathy as rhetorical. *Both authors' empathy and readers' empathy have rhetorical uses, which may be more noticeable when they conflict in instances of empathic inaccuracy.* By using their powers of empathetic projection, authors may attempt to persuade readers to feel with them on politically charged subjects. Readers, in turn, may experience narrative empathy in ways not anticipated or intended by authors. When those readers articulate their differences with a text's or an author's apparent claims, they may call upon their own empathetic responses as a sort of witness to an alternative perspective. Arguments over empathic differences between authors and readers, or among readers with different emotional reactions to a shared text, give feeling responsiveness to fiction a status it has not often been granted in academic analysis of literature. Narrative empathy can impede or assist arguments staged in the public sphere. Indeed, the existence of empathetic novel reading experiences, whether accurate or not, often enters into debates covertly. More self-consciousness about our own experiences of narrative empathy depends in part upon identifying where we stand as members of the diverse audiences reached by authors' empathetic representations.

Narrative empathy intersects with identities in problematic ways. Do we respond because we belong to an in-group, or can narrative empathy call to us across boundaries of difference? Even this formulation could be read as participating in a hierarchical model of empathy. The habit of making the reactions of white, western, educated readers home base for consideration of reader response has not yet been corrected by transnational studies of readers, though narrative theorists such as Peter J. Rabinowitz offer subtle ways of understanding the various audiences narrative fiction may simultaneously address. When the subject positions of empathizer and object of empathetic identification are removed from the suspect arrangement that privileges white western responses to subaltern suffering, the apparent condescension of empathy can be transformed by its strategic use. *Strategic empathy* is a variety of authors' empathy, by which authors attempt to direct an emotional transaction through a fictional work aimed at a particular audience, not necessarily including every reader who happens upon the text.

Three varieties of strategic empathizing may be observed at work in contemporary narrative fiction, though I feel sure they also pertain to the hopes of authors in earlier periods as well. First, *bounded strategic empathy occurs within an in-group, stemming from experiences of mutuality, and leading to feeling with familiar others.* The bards of the in-group call upon bounded empathy, and lack of familiarity may indeed prevent outsiders from joining the empathetic circle. Certainly some experiences of empathic inaccuracy can be accounted for by recognizing that readers do not belong to the group invited to share bounded strategic empathy (not in the implied readership and blocked from aspirations to join the authorial audience). Second, *ambassadorial strategic empathy addresses chosen others with the aim of cultivating their empathy for the in-group, often to a specific end.* Appeals for justice, recognition, and assistance often take this form. Mulk Raj Anand's *Untouchable* (1935) provides a good example of ambassadorial strategic empathy in a novel, written in English for a readership outside the caste system that in the 1930s still governed India. Third, *broadcast strategic empathy calls upon every reader to feel with members of a group, by emphasizing our common vulnerabilities and hopes.* The Kenyan novelist Ngũgĩ wa Thiong'o has deliberately employed broadcast strategic empathy in his fiction, provocatively embracing the universality so often rejected by contemporary champions of difference. The fact that many postcolonial novelists aspire to extend readers' sense of our shared humanity suggests that broadcast strategic empathy deserves attention more nuanced than refusal of empathy as an impossible goal of representation.

Unanswered Questions

In the book from which this essay is derived, I subject to critical scrutiny the literary version of the empathy-altruism hypothesis, which holds that novel reading, by eliciting empathy, encourages prosocial action and good world citizenship. If indeed such a link could be substantiated (it has not yet been verified), then investigation of the effects of narrative techniques on real readers would have to extend beyond generalizations about character identification and a small subset of narrative situations. To the questions currently under investigation many more may be added.

What effect (if any) does consonance (relative closeness to the related events) and dissonance (greater distance between the happening and the telling) have on readers of first person, self-narrated fictions? Does a plural, communal narrative voice, a "we" narration, bring the reader into a perceptive circle where empathetic reactions are more readily available? Does the use of second person "you" narration enhance the intimacy of the reading experience by drawing the reader and narrator close, or does it emphasize dissonance as it becomes clear that "you" can't include the reader? In third person fiction, does the use of a figural reflector, rather than an authorial (omniscient) narrator make any difference in readers' emotional responsiveness to situations and character? [Bortolussi and Dixon have done the best work on this subject, though they phrase the question differently: to what degree do readers fuse narrators and characters as a result of perceptual access to a particular character's perspective, thus develop a rooting interest in that character and making assumptions about the narrator's and author's gender (166–99).] Does the location of the narrator inside (or outside) the story-world effect readers' reactions to the content of the narration? Does a covert narrator, who scarcely does more than provide cues about characters' movements and speech, disinvite empathy for those characters, or invite readers to see the action with a greater sense of immediacy, as if it were a play, as Bortolussi and Dixon suggest (202)? In the most fully polyphonic novels, in which a single narrative perspective is simply not available to the reader, does readers' empathy increase, dwindle, or vary according to the page they are on?

Finally, to bring the questions back to what happens in actual readers, if a narrative situation devised to evoke empathy fails to do so, does the fault lie in the reader, or in the overestimation of the efficacy of the technique? While I am inclined to agree with Wayne Booth that no one ethical effect inheres in a single narrative device, the commentary on narrative form often asserts (or assumes) that a specific technique inevitably results in particular effects—political, ethical, emotional—in readers. These views, in my opinion, should be subjected to careful empirical testing before any aspect of narrative technique earns the label of "empathetic." To persist in the nomination of favored techniques as empathetic without attention to the full range of techniques that may be contributing to empathetic effects renders the study of narrative empathy an impressionistic endeavor at best.

2

FROM STRATEGIC EMPATHIZING

Techniques of Bounded, Ambassadorial, and Broadcast Narrative Empathy

This essay presents an exercise in narratological model-building, whose purpose is to add to the theoretical understanding of the relationship among authorial audiences (comprised of those ideal readers imagined and hoped for by authors) and actual, historic audiences made up of a variety of real readers. It participates in a rhetorical narratology (Booth, Phelan, Rabinowitz), bringing questions about the transactions between authors and readers through novels to an ongoing discussion of the role of narrative empathy. The resources of rhetoric, with its traditional emphases on authorial tactics, textual strategies, and audience responses, appropriately match the critical needs of a theory of narrative empathy, which must account for the empathy of both authors and readers, as well as the potentially empathetic tropes and techniques of narrative texts .... [T]he methodological challenge of theorizing narrative empathy at work in fictional texts, in authors, and in audiences includes reference to a variety of disciplines, from cognitive science to the sociology of reading. The term *strategic empathizing*, devised to slant rhyme with Gayatri Chakravorty Spivak's *strategic essentializing* points to the intentional, though not invariably efficacious, work of authors to sway the feelings of their readers in audiences closer and further from the authors of and subjects of representation. Like strategic essentializing, strategic empathizing occurs when an author employs empathy in the crafting of fictional texts, in service of "a scrupulously visible political interest" (Spivak 214). That these interests make different demands on the various audiences that may read and respond to the invitation to emotional resonance provides the starting question for this essay: How does strategic empathy reach readers in immediate, more distant, and totally remote audiences, where the metaphor of nearness/distance also correlates with familiarity/strangeness and sameness/otherness.

DOI: 10.4324/9781003264071-4

... I embrace the metaphorical resonances of critical and theoretical terms and do not attempt to achieve figurative neutrality. In proposing three new terms, I attempt to avoid the mixed metaphors that often complicate the underdepths of theoretical jargon. To choose my three categories of bounded, ambassadorial, and broadcast narrative empathy I imagined a metaphor world we can call the medieval village. Circumscribed by traditional boundary-lines, the village is small enough to be a known community, perhaps consisting of only 200 souls. Yet even in this small world time passes and the younger generation needs to be reminded of the common struggles, the cherished past, the historic traumas, the idealized and possibly unrealizable dreams, the social rules and codes of those who belong there. The bard of the in-group addresses these villagers as villagers. Once in a while the villagers send the children out to beat the bounds of their little parish, so that everyone will remember forever where the line that separates inside from outside lies. In that outside other villages exist: missions of embassy sometimes send a representative villager as an ambassador to treat with or make common cause with distant strangers. More often, though, the villagers meet strangers and foreigner in the marketplace. This village's survival depends upon agriculture, and from that work comes my last metaphor, that of broadcast empathy. Our modern sense of electronic broadcasting over the airwaves also relies on an original sense of seed-planting: a sower dips his hand into the grain and casts it in a broad sweep so that the seeds may be scattered across the field. These three senses undergird my categories of strategic empathizing, which model an author's potential attitude towards readerships right at home, in a neighboring but distant village, or out in the wide world, as far as a bird with a seed in its beak, or its belly, might choose to fly.

As a part of what forms our membership in a novel's audience, empathy intersects with our identities and experiences in complicated ways. I have argued ... that readers' empathy is considerably more difficult to predict and assess than has usually been assumed (*Empathy and the Novel* 65–84). No one prose narrative fiction evokes empathy from all its readers. Readers differ in their emotional dispositions, some more likely to respond with shared feeling and others not likely to experience emotional fusion with a fictional text at all (xi, 72–3). This suggests that fiction writers do not entirely control the degree to which their emotionally evocative fictions actually stimulate readers' empathy .... [S]ome fiction writers eschew the goal of evoking narrative empathy, going instead for effects of estrangement, shock, or disgust (Ngai, *Ugly*): Monika Fludernik has suggested that heavily ironic fiction, as for example some of Nadine Gordimer's work, deliberately rebuffs readers' empathetic responsiveness (*Fictions* 5–6, 291, 312) .... [T]his essay concentrates on the rhetorical situation that pertains when a novelist or writer of short fiction sets about to evoke readers' empathy, in narratives that may have more than one built-in audience, as Peter J. Rabinowitz and Brian Richardson have argued. [Rabinowitz and Richardson offer subtle ways of understanding the various audiences narrative fiction may simultaneously address, and the conditions that pertain when we choose to join them].

I call this effort on writers' part *strategic empathizing*, a variety of authors' empathy, by which authors attempt to direct an emotional transaction through a fictional work aimed at a particular audience, not necessarily including every reader who happens upon the text. For if we experience narrative empathy as readers, we should inquire if we respond because we belong to an in-group, or because narrative empathy calls to us across boundaries of difference. Might a reading experience that leaves us cold reach another reader in part because the strategic empathy of the author meets in that other reader a member of a sought-for audience? Might a single narrative text evoke empathy that draws on our group belonging in one instance, our shared humanity in another; our situational familiarity with similar circumstances in one scene, our self-recognition in another, our imaginative extension to embrace the totally unfamiliar in yet another? Might a narrative evoke empathy from its immediate, contemporaneous audience and quizzical puzzlement from the posterity audience, reading 100 or 200 years later? Alternatively, a posterity audience may respond with more skepticism or coolness than the earliest readership. To identify, as Raymond Williams incisively does, the sentimental "structure of feeling" called up by the mid nineteenth-century industrial novelists, suggests that he stands outside that structure of feeling, detecting its emergence, but invulnerable to and indeed critical of its rhetoric of Christian charity and obligation to the voiceless poor (*Marxism* 132–4). Time passes and new readers respond to texts that have previously been considered intensely emotionally evocative with indifference, disapproval, indignation, perhaps even with a deliberately cultivated objectivity (critical distance). Contrarily, some novelists reach readers most susceptible to emotional fusion with their creations in their texts' after-years—think of the reception history of Joyce's *Ulysses* (1922). Arguably, Joyce's sympathetic imagination, exercised in the character creation of Leopold Bloom, meets its significant empathetic readership much later in the twentieth century. While some novelists write with that posterity audience in mind, many more direct their acts of imaginative communication laterally—out into a wider global but contemporary world, containing living readers. The effort to reach specific audiences to evoke fellow-feeling, compassion, and even political or economic responses often bears the traces of authorial strategic empathizing.

... I propose a preliminary model of three varieties of strategic empathizing. First, *bounded strategic empathy occurs within an in-group, stemming from experiences of mutuality, and leading to feeling with familiar others*. This kind of empathy can be called upon by the bards of the in-group, and it may indeed prevent outsiders from joining the empathetic circle. I have written in *Empathy and the Novel* (137–8) about the difficulty my male students have in responding at all—let alone empathetically—to a scene of vengeance in Opal Palmer Adisa's 1997 novel *It Begins with Tears* (137–8). The hot-chili-pepper punishment, in which a misbehaving woman has chopped chilis stuffed into her orifices (Adisa 131–7) stimulates physical flinching and protective body language from female readers. It seems not to reach male readers in the same way: those willing to speak mention embarrassment, disapproval, and discomfort, but not the empathy and even motor mimicry female readers report. Though we are prone to notice the delineations of class, gender, sexuality, and ethnicity that mark a text as "for" one audience and "not so much for" another, an effort of strategic empathizing may also be bounded by the toggle switch of experience. Either you have lost a child, or you have not; either you have battled a fatal disease, or not; either you have been raped, or you have not. The gate swings open to invite you in, or it stays closed. Now nothing prevents a reader who "has not" from clambering over the gate and reading a work exercising bounded strategic empathy, and the persistent reader (curious? voyeuristic? reading for an assignment?) may or may not become part of the authorial audience, in Rabinowitz's term. The disinvited reader may not choose to, or be able to, live up to the terms of the ideal audience projected by a narrative. Certainly some common experiences of readerly antipathy and of empathic inaccuracy (the incorrect attribution of a shared feeling at cross purposes to the author's documented representational aims) can be accounted for by acknowledging the existence of readers outside the special group invited to share bounded strategic empathy.

Any serious discussion of character identification in narrative fiction should acknowledge the prevalence of empathic inaccuracy. Not only do readers choose variously to "travel with" characters whose perspectives do not seem, to teachers or critics, to be the central figures in narratives, but they (we!) also often mistakenly attribute feelings and motives to characters. It happens all the time, and no wonder. Our gap-filling reading habits encourage us to intuit, to correct discordant details by misremembering, to confabulate in the absence of evidence. Just as we wallpaper over the blind spots in our visual field, we imagine what makes sense to us to imagine with respect to characters' behavior, motives, feelings, and effects on others in the fictional world. When we respond empathetically to a novel, we do not have the luxury of questioning the character: we cannot ask, Is that how you really felt? Empathic inaccuracy thus describes a potential effect of character identification and narrative empathy: a strong conviction of empathy that *incorrectly* identifies the feeling of a literary persona. Empathic inaccuracy occurs when a reader responds empathetically to a fictional character at cross-purposes with an author's intentions. Authors also sometimes evoke empathy unintentionally. This accident contributes to empathic inaccuracy. Unlike in real-world, face-to-face circumstances, the novel-reading situation allows empathic inaccuracy to persist because neither author nor fictional character directly confutes it. This is not necessarily to be lamented. Out of our differences and misreadings our interpretations come, for literary study privileges against-the-grain interpretations of fiction that may be founded on deliberate acts of role taking that subvert the authors' apparent intentions.

More often than not, critical readers excluded from the target audience of a novel dismiss or disparage the work for not living up to their expectations. Even readers who feel that a novel speaks to them may discover other real readers who see something else entirely in the work. Indeed, as Brian Richardson observes, "divergent audiences are regularly addressed in a literary work, and in many cases the disparate groups fail to mesh" ("Multiple" 38). Sometimes a novelist writes to more than one audience simultaneously, with a hope of bridging the gap between them. Novelists with a purpose may set out to reach—and change—a target audience. These situations may encourage the use of the second kind of strategic empathizing, *ambassadorial strategic empathy*. Ambassadorial strategic empathy, a second variety of authors' empathy, also directs an emotional transaction through a fictional work aimed at a particular audience, not necessarily including every reader who happens upon the text. While all readers are vulnerable to experiences of empathic inaccuracy, successfully exercised ambassadorial strategic empathy can be a powerful rhetorical tool in reaching and swaying the feelings of audiences. It may teach readers to feel with otherwise alien fictional others. [Feeling with fictional others does not guarantee changes in the capacity to feel with real others and does not predict altruistic behavior on real others' behalf. For my argument that the transposition of the "empathy-altruism" hypothesis to experiences of narrative empathy lacks experimental support, see *Empathy and the Novel* (90–2, 99, 116, 145)]. *Ambassadorial strategic empathy addresses chosen others with the aim of cultivating their empathy for the in-group, often to a specific end.* Appeals for justice, recognition, and assistance often take this form.

Mulk Raj Anand's *Untouchable* (1935) provides a good example of ambassadorial strategic empathy in a novel. Anand, a disciple of Nehru and Gandhi, and acquaintance of Bloomsbury Group figures, writes for an international audience in a humanist spirit, seeking to eliminate social injustice [on Anand's life, see M. Fisher, *Wisdom*]. *Untouchable* tells the story of a latrine sweeper, Bakha, a lovely young man of a traditionally untouchable caste. Regarded as polluted through traditional association with the "dirt" that he removes from latrines, the contaminated Bakha comes to catastrophe when a rich Hindu merchant accidentally brushes against him. Repeatedly abused through violent shouting and cursing, with which a crowd enthusiastically joins, Bakha reacts with paralysis, fear, dumb humility, and perspiring inaction. Simple phrases of psycho-narration describe Bakha's evolving feelings in six intervals to a scene otherwise comprised of the shouts and insults of the sweeper's tormentors (Anand 46–9). When he finally breaks his silence to deny a child's wild accusation, Bakha experiences the crowd's oppressive force:

> To Bakha, every second seemed an endless age of woe and suffering. His whole demeanour was concentrated in humility, and in his heart there was a queer stirring. His legs trembled and shook under him. He felt they would fail him. He was really sorry and tried hard to convey his repentance to his tormentors. But the barrier of space that the crowd had placed between themselves and him seemed to prevent his feeling from getting across.
>
> (49)

This simple description of the physical symptoms of fear, regret, and mute appeals to a sadistic audience garners an empathetic response from many readers that I have surveyed (college aged students, reading the novel in a Postcolonial Literature class). They point out that Anand steers the reader towards empathy with Bakha, despite his disturbing abjectness, by making the crowd's malign emotionality so terrifying. They recognize his response to a mob. Even sheltered American students with relatively little foreign travel experience and no first-hand familiarity with poverty recognize and empathize with the feelings of a victim of bullying.

Based on my students' reactions, I hypothesize that this passage presents an instance where readers' empathy precedes character identification, perhaps because they can generalize from Bakha's experiences to a more familiar one. Anand employs description of bodily states and simple psycho-narration, in combination with the alternating passages of dialogue (abusive taunts), to evoke the empathetic reaction. But the author's effort to transfer readers' empathy into an empathetic conviction of injustice falters, in part because of a shift in narrative technique. In a subsequent passage, Bakha reflects on the injustice of his experiences and finally becomes hurt and enraged. Anand begins with psycho-narration, presenting an analogy for Bakha's feelings: "His feelings would rise like spurts of smoke from a half-smothered fire, in fitful, unbalanced jerks when the recollection of some abuse or rebuke he had suffered kindled a spark in the ashes of remorse inside him" (51). The passage then yields to a long interior monologue, tagged apologetically in partial explanation of Bakha's abject silence during the prior scene: "he asked himself in the soundless speech of cells receiving and transmitting emotions, which was his usual way of communicating with himself." Bakha's inner voice rehearses his experience in quoted monologue, but Anand fails to elicit my students' empathy using this technique. Distress and distaste replace empathy. Further, students report pushing away from the character as he rants inwardly,

> Why was all this fuss? Why was I so humble? I could have struck him! And to think I was so eager to come to town this morning. Why didn't I shout to warn the people of my approach? .... Not one of them spoke for me! The cruel crowd! All of them abused, abused, abused. Why are we always abused? ...For them I am a sweeper, sweeper—untouchable! Untouchable! Untouchable! That's the word! Untouchable! I am an Untouchable!
>
> (51–2)

Paradoxically, the copious representation of the inner speech of the subaltern character backfires, resulting in the decoupling of character identification and an abrupt transition from empathy to distance, frustration, or even uneasy snickering at the over-the-top interior monologue. Arguably, these twenty-first-century teenaged American readers were not the readers Anand had in mind as he deployed Bakha's thought-transcript.

Anand wrote *Untouchable* in English in 1930 both for an educated revolutionary Indian elite and for an audience of British intellectuals (including Marxists and anti-imperialists) who might be imagined to influence public opinion on the matter of caste prejudice. Reading the novel 75 years after its first publication, as a member of its posterity audience, one may react to its affective tenor as "hysterical emotionalism" (H. Williams 412), or as a still moving depiction of the traumatic events in one day in a stunted life. My students' reports suggest that separate pages evoke different intensities of emotional responsiveness, not all of them supportive of Anand's aims. They sense the gap between their subject positions and Bakha's, but also between their identities as real readers and the (historical) authorial audience Anand implies through his ardent rhetoric. The very labels that we apply to novels—Marxist propaganda, aspirant modernism, Indian patriotism, postcolonial fiction—bespeak attitudes that label us as members of particular audiences, who may or may not be reached by ambassadorial empathy. The identity and experience of the novelist may also figure into the potential of ambassadorial strategic empathy. As E. M. Forster comments in his introduction to *Untouchable*, "No European, however sympathetic, could have created the character of Bakha, because he would not have known enough of his troubles. And no Untouchable could have written the book, because he would have been involved in indignation and self pity" (Forster, "Introduction" vi–vii). Anand came from the martial Kshatriya caste and he wrote in European exile, factors of distance that seemed to Forster intrinsic to the success of Anand's polemical representations. But too much distance can interfere with narrative empathy. If we consider irony, the figure exploiting gaps, as the rhetorical opposite of empathy, then distances of time and location, as well as gaps in experience, might well weaken the potential for strategic empathizing out of its own time to evoke an appropriate response. It would be interesting to discover if contemporary Indian readers the same age as my students still feel the evocative power of Anand's ambassadorial strategic empathy.

If matters of identity and experience most obviously delimit the audience of texts employing bounded strategic empathy, ambassadorial empathy is most marked by the relationship between the time of reading and the historical moment of publication, when the text gets sent out in the world to perform its ambassadorial duty by recruiting particular readers to a present cause through emotional fusion. [A]mbassadorial strategic empathy is time sensitive, context- and issue-dependent. Accompanying paratextual statements of intention on the part of writers and organizations render an effort to effect ambassadorial strategic empathy more recognizable. For instance, Alice Walker leaves her readers in no doubt as to the purpose of *Possessing the Secret of Joy* (1992): the novel concludes with an afterword advising readers about sources of more information and announces that a portion of the novel's royalties will be dedicated to educational programs about Female Genital Mutilation (281–3). The specifically *ambassadorial* quality of Walker's strategic empathizing comes through as she relates how Tashi, a fictional character who makes brief appearances in two earlier novels, demands her own novel (282) and how the actress, a Kenyan, who plays the character in a film, reminds Walker of the actual Kenyan girls dying from FGM. Note the imagery of modern travel in Walker's account, as her empathetic ambassador arrives in the West, carrying in her person the reminder of suffering far away: "I was reminded that in Kenya, even as this young woman was being flown to Los Angeles to act in the film, little girls were being forced under the shards of unwashed glass, tin-can tops, rusty razors and dull knives of traditional circumcisers" (282). The use of a bridge character (at least part-way familiar to the more distant target audience), in this case the educated Tashi or the film actress who represents her, is a technique commonly employed to achieve effects of ambassadorial strategic empathy.

A text's reception, including hostile responses as well as enthusiastic accounts of rapport and conversion to the cause, also preserves the traces of ambassadorial strategic empathy at work. In no case would a scholar expect to find a uniformly positive record. Polemical, didactic, biased, purposeful: novels employing ambassadorial strategic empathy in order to reach and even change target audiences also meet resistance .... Hostile responses in the immediate aftermath of publication indicate a contentious issue; dismissive responses from audiences in posterity may suggest either a continuation of the original argument or undervaluing of the original motivation. For instance, according to Gregory S. Jackson, the biggest selling novels in late nineteenth-century America "aimed to facilitate private devotion, strengthen moral autonomy, and foster social engagement" of Protestant readers (642). A secular twenty-first-century reader of Charles Sheldon's *In His Steps* (1896) may not respond with the religious conversion invited by the novel, but in its own time, readers of *In His Steps* testified to the way the novel influenced them and their practical Christianity (643). Writing about the late nineteenth-century subgenre of the American novel that he names "homiletic" fiction, Jackson observes that critical understanding of the function of novels that seem trashy to us now eludes us "because prevailing theories of genre lack a nuanced understanding of the psychology of highly specialized readerships" (643). Indeed, when literary history records huge sales figures and the critical history indicates only how dreadful, forgettable, or low quality a novel seems, then it's a fair assumption that the original audience for an author's ambassadorial strategic empathizing has disappeared.

The judgments of literary merit critics make about narrative fiction do not reliably correspond with evidence of a text's transaction of strategic empathy from author to target audience(s). Indeed, a novel's bestseller status may simultaneously interfere with its reputation among tastemakers and vouch for its empathetic intensity for its readership. This may especially be the case in fictions that deploy *broadcast strategic empathizing* in an attempt to reach the widest possible audience .... Popular and middlebrow fiction often succeeds because it evokes readers' empathy more effectively than more demanding, experimental or deliberately difficult texts (Keen, *Empathy and the Novel* 101–09). This effect extends to the popular subgenres of contemporary fiction, including fantasy, thrillers, detective fiction, and romance novels (realism is not a pre-requisite for readers' empathy). Wherever immersion reading takes place, by readers conscious of the fictionality of the novels in which they submerge themselves, opportunities for intense emotional fusion exist, and some novelists (especially bestselling authors) exploit their worldmaking powers to reach the widest range of readers (xii–xiv, 4, 69, 168). [For a theoretical elaboration of the nature of fictionality as an interpretive frame conditioning readers' comprehension, see Richard Walsh, *The Rhetoric of Fictionality* 44–45].

Broadcast strategic empathy calls upon every reader to feel with members of a group, by emphasizing our common human experiences, feelings, hopes, and vulnerabilities. Narrative empathy in the form of an author's broadcast strategic empathizing employs a universal tool (language) to reach distant others and transmit the particularities that connect a far-away subject to a feeling reader. While not all novelists seek to influence as many and as various a set of readers as their books can reach, some do, and we reliably find in their fiction opportunities for character identification emphasizing the commonalities of our embodied experiences, our psychological dispositions, and our social circumstances. For example, Ernest J. Gaines' representation of meals cooked in love, traumatically rejected, and (finally) eaten in healing communion in his novel *A Lesson Before Dying* (1993) calls upon our near universal understandings of the significance of food and of what it means to be human. In a novel that takes as its subject the recuperation of an unjustly convicted death row inmate's humanity, scenes of eating chart Jefferson's progress from dehumanized "hog," who eats from a bag on the floor like an animal (83), to a fully human man who meets his death in the electric chair with dignity. A reader does not need to know the taste of the particular dishes cooked by his aunt for the condemned prisoner, Jefferson, to recognize and respond to Gaines' exercise of broadcast strategic empathizing. Though scarcely literate, Jefferson records his last meal, cooked by his aunt (nanan) before his execution:

> shef guiry ax me what I want for my super an I tol him I want nanan to cook me som okra an rice an som pok chop an a conbred an some claba an he say he gon see what he can do an say what I want for desert an I tol him jus a little ice crme in a cup an a moon pie
>
> they took me an let me stan under the shoer wit a new bar a sope an they giv me a big wite clen tower an brot me back an I put on some clen close an set down cause my foor was yer an I et it ever bit an it was the bes meal I kno my nanan ever cook
>
> (232)

Widely adopted as a novel to be read by whole cities of readers, across age groups, genders, races, and social classes, *A Lesson Before Dying* happens to have been favorably reviewed by literary critics, but it has also passed the more difficult test of becoming a word-of-mouth classic (frequently compared to and paired with Harper Lee's *To Kill a Mockingbird* [1960]). In this case, large numbers of readers have responded empathetically to Ernest Gaines's broadcast strategic empathizing. Despite their manifest differences and distance from Jefferson, many readers respond with spontaneous emotional fusion—empathy—and with mature concern—sympathy—for Gaines's character.

I have argued in *Empathy and the Novel* that despite the disrepute of human universals among theorists and skepticism about the representation of coherent selves, novelists persist in inviting readers into intense experiences of character identification. Evoking readers' empathy with fictional characters, while not identical with character identification (one can empathize with a disliked character, for example), remains a goal of many contemporary novelists. This phenomenon is so ubiquitous as hardly to deserve demonstration, except that one might get the impression from literary criticism that trading on shared feelings had long since been discredited as a goal of novelistic representation. The runaway success of books like Gaines's *A Lesson Before Dying* confutes this belief of contemporary critical discourse on the novel. Middlebrow novels that can cultivate readers' empathy and deliver intense experiences of immersion and character identification are more likely to succeed in the marketplace. Postcolonial novelists often deliberately employ broadcast strategic empathy in their fiction, provocatively embracing the universality so often rejected by contemporary champions of difference, including many postcolonial theorists.

For postcolonial novelists seeking a world readership, the techniques that offer opportunities for character identification include the use of bridge characters (sharing some traits with target audiences) and the construction of an array of character types, to maximize the chances that a reader can "travel with" one of the characters. For instance, Rohinton Mistry's *A Fine Balance* (1995) uses a bridge character (a student) and also depicts a cluster of characters with different ages, genders, religions, and social positions, in an effort to reach a wide range of readers through broadcast character identification. I call this the *Little Women* effect, where there's a different sister for every kind of girl reader. Mistry's representational efforts are both painstakingly documentary and unapologetically universalizing. Mistry, a Canadian citizen of subcontinental Indian origin, writes in English, as do many of the most famous of the postcolonial novelists who reach a world readership. Yet writing in the global *lingua franca* is not a requirement for the exercise of authorial strategic empathizing. The Kenyan novelist Ngũgĩ wa Thiong'o, who has written in Gikuyu since the early 1980s (after publishing English novels as James Ngũgĩ), also deliberately employs broadcast strategic empathy in his fiction. Criticizing the use of language as a tool of colonialism, and rejecting the accommodation made by what he terms Afro-European literature, Ngũgĩ makes a point of claiming a world audience for small languages such as Gikuyu.

The particularity of experience inside a specific language and culture transmits to a wider world, and this culture-crossing effect is made possible, according to Ngũgĩ, by the universal linguistic capacities of human beings:

> The capacity to speak, the capacity to order sounds in a manner that makes for mutual comprehension between human beings is universal. This is the universality of language, a quality specific to human beings. It corresponds to the universality of the struggle against nature and that between human beings.
>
> ("Language" 15)

Acknowledging universality among humans (not just their language, but their struggles to survive) does not mean, for Ngũgĩ and other postcolonial writers, losing the particularity of their experiences and representations. Differences survive the process of communication. Ngũgĩ writes:

> the particularity of sounds, the words, the word order into phrases and sentences, and the specific manner, or laws, of their ordering is what distinguishes one language from another. Thus a specific culture is not transmitted through language in its universality but in its particularity as the language of a specific community with a specific history. Written literature and orature are the main means by which a particular language transmits the images of the world contained in the culture it carries.
>
> (15)

Ngũgĩ's criticism of colonialist uses of language not only diagnose the "dissociation of sensibility" in children linguistically separated from their natural and social environment (17), but also announces a political goal of reconnection with national languages and experiences, in order to defeat imperialism and make alliances with "the other peoples of the world." Thus the cure for the Eliotian dissociation of sensibility offers hope: "unity in that struggle would ensure unity in our multilingual diversity" (30). Ngũgĩ's local and particularist interests in the wellbeing of Kenyans and the thriving of African cultures reaches out in an affirmation of global social bonds: "Unity in that struggle… would also reveal the real links that bind the people of Africa to the peoples of Asia, South America, Europe, Australia and New Zealand, Canada and the U. S. A." (30).

For Ngũgĩ as a novelist, now writing only in Gikuyu and translating his own work into English for his world readership, human commonalities deriving from our embodied experiences undergird even his most ironic and fantastic representations. A soul temporarily in bird form considers leaving its body behind on the garbage dump:

> Yes, to go wherever it wishes without the endless restraining demands of the body: I am thirsty, I want water to drink; I am hungry, I want food to eat; I am naked, I need some clothes; I am out in the rain, I need some shelter; I am ill, I must find a doctor. I must catch a bus but I have no money. I must pay school fees, taxes …
>
> (*Wizard* 40)

Restored to his body, this everyman character discovers healing gifts that serve as an antidote to the ailments of a corrupt (fictional) African nation. Though *Wizard of the Crow* is harshly satirical, often ironic, and frequently humorous, the healer's story depends upon a kind of mind-and-body reading that can fairly be described as empathetic (though it is also magical). Ngũgĩ employs broadcast strategic empathizing to marshal readers' sympathy for Africans even as he excoriates the corruption of a totalitarian state. Even in a heavily ironic and satirical novel, effects of strategic empathizing can gleam through the verbally distancing overlay of caricature and critique. Thus empathetic and ironic effects, evidently opposite in their rhetorical strategies, can enhance the piquancy of each other's coexistence in a single fictional world. The different tones employed by Ngũgĩ may imply different audiences or they may signal the construction of a more fluid authorial audience, whose capacity to shift from sardonic appreciation of satire, to laughter, to empathetic engagement is a constituent characteristic. Taking pleasure in juxtapositions of tone and rhetorical position, including the evident extremes of irony and empathy, may be a quality of a contemporary world readership of considerable diversity. The habit of making the reactions of white, western, educated readers "home base" for consideration of reader response has not yet been corrected; certainly better transnational studies of readers and audiences would assist in understanding how a novel can be alternately ironical and empathetic, or a novel for knowledgeable Africans and a less experienced world readership simultaneously. Irony and satire function to win an audience's trust ("this author is no dummy; he sees the world with all its warts and wrinkles") and then rewards the initiates with opportunities for intense emotional fusion through character identification.

Throughout this essay, I have attempted to think through three modes novelists employ when they direct their authorial empathy (so vital to fictional world-making and character creation) towards target audiences. Despite the difficulty of predicting which narrative texts will consistently evoke empathy from readers, many novelists still work with the aim of cultivating their audience's empathetic imaginations. Recognizing bounded, ambassadorial, and broadcast strategic empathy in the narrative techniques, implied audiences, and reception histories of contemporary world fiction makes a preliminary step in the process of understanding how narrative texts themselves practice and theorize identification. We also ought to give credence to authors' statements of intention, especially when sales records, reception histories, and literary influence suggest that they succeed in reaching the audiences they target with their strategic empathizing. But as I have argued in *Empathy and the Novel*, we should take care not to attribute certain ethical effects to particular narrative techniques, lest we underestimate the challenges inherent in bridging the gap between feeling author and feeling reader.

3

FROM EMPATHIC INACCURACY IN NARRATIVE FICTION

In this essay, I expand upon my previous proposals about *empathic inaccuracy*: "A reader persuaded that she has felt with a fictional character may defy the stated or implicit intentions of an author .... *Empathic inaccuracy*, to craft a hypothesis out of this circumstance, *may then contribute to a strong sense that the author's perspective is simply wrong*" (Keen, *Empathy and the Novel* 139–40, emphasis in original). I base my definition of empathic inaccuracy on the psychological concept of empathic accuracy, studied by William Ickes and others. This cognitive capacity involves the relative abilities of people correctly to infer others' dispositions, personality traits, and psychological states, including their thoughts and feelings (Ickes "Empathic"). Empathic accuracy can be stronger or weaker in an individual, and it is usually measured after interviewing subjects and target individuals. Ickes makes the recommendation that "the most straightforward way to measure empathic accuracy is to compare the content of a target person's actual thoughts and feelings with the content of the corresponding inferred thoughts and feelings reported by the perceiver" (Ickes 591). The ensuing psychological research program into empathic accuracy includes the recognition that even though most humans are adept at making these inferences, we also consistently overestimate our own empathic abilities (as cross-referenced with results on Mark Davis's Interpersonal Reactivity Index, or IRI [Davis "Multidimensional"]). Ickes states, "various self-report measures of empathic skills and empathic accuracy proved to be disappointingly poor predictors of actual empathic accuracy" (Ickes, "Empathic" 603) and concludes, "in general, people lack meta-knowledge regarding their own empathic accuracy" (603). Ickes cautions that in some circumstances, people may actually be motivated to misinterpret others' thoughts and feelings by making inaccurate inferences about their dispositions (607).

DOI: 10.4324/9781003264071-5

Considering the unusual circumstance of fiction reading, in which the empathic transaction occurs between a real human being (a reader) and inanimate creations made up of marks on the page (characters and other actants), in my earlier work I reasoned that empathic accuracy in fiction reading is both common and unverifiable: one cannot interview a fictional character about her mind-content and emotions. However, I also intuited that most fiction readers simply accept the narrator's reports about characters' mental representations, bodily sensations, and fleeting thoughts and feelings. This kind of empathic accuracy could be regarded as a default setting in fiction, akin to the assumption that details of setting refer to the natural physical world unless otherwise noted. Readers readily extrapolate from dialogue, reported actions, and scenes with other things and persons of the fictional world to reach quick-and-dirty assessments supporting their empathy with characters. That is, empathic accuracy is a *de facto* expectation of a comprehending reading of fiction. I also previously observed readers empathizing at cross-purposes with the text's cues (against authors' intentions), and those I spoke to denied authors' perspective on the matter of their fictional creations any special status. The inaccurate empathizers were on solid theoretical ground in disregarding authorial intentions, but when it comes to interpretation, it's not quite the case that anything goes. Experiences of empathic inaccuracy can also lead to the negative judgment that *readers'* empathic feelings are wrong.

This essay extends my earlier theorizing by grappling with the problem of empathic inaccuracy as a phenomenon of fiction reading, recognizing its defining quality of errancy (or at the very least idiosyncrasy) in divergent emotional reactions to fiction, without veering into normative prescriptivism supporting judgments of either authors or readers. I seek instead to understand better the phenomenon of empathic inaccuracy as an undeniable though hardly universal impact of narrative fictional texts. Literary education often masks a tacit prescriptivism under its cultivation of critical tact, but paradoxically, the same teachers who guide students to interpretations that stay within acceptable bounds also celebrate resistant, cross-grain, and revisionist readings advanced by literary professionals. I take as a given that empathic inaccuracy exists among both ordinary and trained readers. It is related to what feminist narratologist Susan Lanser describes as negative plotting, in which "particular events or full stories take on (primary or enhanced) meaning in relation to their textually triggered, *though not necessarily textually inscribed*, antitheses" (Lanser, "Negative," emphasis in original). I follow Lanser's lead in taking seriously the evidence of divergent, even antithetical, responses from trained resistant readers and self-taught ordinary readers.

The existence of a large, unruly audience of pleasure readers (whose emotional experiences with fiction have become increasingly legible due to online reading communities of nonprofessionals) has stimulated academic literary studies to generate its own rarified mode of response. This mode, as Rita Felski argues, suppresses evidence of its affective drives even as it cultivates the pleasures of unmasking concealed meanings (Felski, "Suspicious"). It differentiates itself from the activities of ordinary readers, often by making sweeping gestures dismissive of popular fiction or genres especially associated with large female readerships (Keen, *Empathy* 82–4). It prizes uniqueness and difference in interpretation, extending the value of distinctive interpretations into the training ground of the undergraduate literature classroom. There in the classroom, a regime of more-or-less right reading coaches students to channel their responses to fiction in appropriately critical directions, through focus on form, theme, or theory, and discourages sharing of reports of emotional responses—aside from previously sanctioned sensations dignified by prior reception history. To resonate with Elizabeth Bennet's initial scorn or dawning admiration of Mr. Darcy is to join a company of millions. To feel curiosity, surprise, and suspense, the core affects of narrativity, is to be a competent reader responding to the promptings of narrative form. When it comes to content, especially the represented persons of fiction, to empathize with an orphan, a helpless animal, a member of a despised outgroup, or a charismatic anti-hero is allowed, but it is embarrassing to find oneself alone in empathizing with Lee Harvey Oswald, Mr. Causabon, Dolores Umbridge, or Jar-Jar Binks. It turns out that your peers can and do find you wrong about that. From their professors students learn how to convert ordinary reading into literary "readings," but as they develop the skills to create original analyses, they also learn from their classmates and their teachers to suppress evidence of empathic inaccuracy. This makes empathic inaccuracy very difficult to study, because the collection of examples involves the risk of shaming readers, or in participating indirectly in the unfortunate social media genre, ridicule of student idiocy. Attentive literature teachers reckon with empathic inaccuracy when they skillfully avoid allowing divagations spurred by rogue emotional responses to take classroom discussions off course.

The context of my original observations about empathic inaccuracy was a rhetorical narratological exploration of narrative empathy. There I dodged making prescriptions to cure this inaccuracy, and emphasized the unruly experiences of reading fiction feelingly:

> Rather than attempting to eliminate empathic inaccuracy by arguing with readers' feeling responses, recognizing the conflict between author's empathy and reader's empathy opens the way to an understanding of narrative empathy as rhetorical: *both authors' empathy and readers' empathy have rhetorical uses, which may be more noticeable when they conflict in instances of empathic inaccuracy*
>
> (Keen, *Empathy and the Novel* 140, *emphasis in original*)

The co-creation of fictional worlds through the imaginative collaboration of readers and authors can involve responding to evoked emotion (Rosenblatt 1938), but as I wrote in 2007, readers "may experience narrative empathy in ways not anticipated or intended by authors" (Keen *Empathy* 140). (See the definition of narrative empathy above, 8).... [N]arrative empathy consists of phenomena that operate in and on creation and reception (See Keen, *Empathy* 65–99, 121–43). Though formal strategies of representation invite empathy, as narrative theorists following Sternberg believe, a many-to-many correspondence between techniques and effects, rather than a one-to-one relation is likely to evoke many feelings from different readers (Sternberg, "Proteus").

Extrapolating from my earlier theorizing about narrative empathy in light of empathic inaccuracy, I offer here some related observations, stemming from readers' contributions (conscious or unconscious) to the fictional world they co-create with authors:

1. Empathic readers share feelings with characters and other actants in fictional worlds created by authors, but the feelings are not controlled by authors.
2. Without authors or texts, the specific emotions evoked by narrative fictions would have no occasion (differentiating the phenomenon from feelings evoked by remembering or daydreaming).
3. Readers' empathy vouches for the empathy-inducing capacity of a fictional text.
4. Fictional texts evoke empathy unevenly, unpredictably, inaccurately, and in some cases not at all.
5. Without readers, fictional texts are emotionally inert; readers activate the emotional potentiality of fictional worlds.
6. Authors and texts may attempt to script but do not control the emotional experience of high- or low-empathy readers.
7. Narrative empathy is not limited to feelings mirroring the represented emotions of fictional characters. Some readers resonate strongly to moods associated with settings and others are highly attuned to the in-built affects of narrativity, curiosity, surprise, and suspense.

Points 4, 5, and 6 receive emphasis in the pages that follow, for narrative empathy for fictions sometimes results in empathic inaccuracy, when readers respond empathetically at cross-purposes with the intentions of the work, or when authors evoke empathy accidentally.

The elements that pertain to a theory of empathic inaccuracy point to narrative empathy's role in a rhetorical communication model of narrative, one that admits and indeed depends upon acknowledgment of *a gap* between authors' actions, as instantiated in the text, and readers' behavior and experience when confronted with textual prompts. Gaps are not a flaw in the communication model of narrative: far from it. Without elision narratives would be impossibly long: all narratives have some gaps in the story, and not all plot events are directly narrated. The demands of narrative temporality and pace demand gaps, or elision, where a text contains no discourse but story events are implied to have occurred. Fictional characters and the story-worlds they navigate may be described, but never completely: whole zones of embodied experience are routinely omitted. Gap-filling imagining, as reception theorists from Louise Rosenblatt to Wolfgang Iser have perceived, must be contributed by readers in their active co-creation of narrative fiction. Empathic inaccuracy can be regarded as a built-in risk of what Iser theorizes as the gap-filling imagining of all literary reading (Iser, "Reading Process"). Invited by the unrepresented story implied to occur during elisions in the discourse, by temporal leaps (not always filled in through later analepses), and by techniques of summary that leave out more than they can ever contain, readers routinely supply imaginative material, by no means always sourced from textual cues, to their reading. Fictional character-creation tacitly commands the embodied consciousness of readers to fill in much of what is conventionally omitted from descriptions of textual entities, for narrative calls up an illusion of bodily materiality with as small a gesture as a name or a role (Elizabeth Bennet; the pawnbroker). Catherine Gallagher calls fictional characters "nobodies" (*Nobody's Story*). There is a long tradition of insisting on their fundamentally textual nature, but as E. M. Forster observed, readers give bodies to Homo Fictus even when social convention prevents authors from describing most of their embodied experience (*Aspects* 48–50). This opens the way for all sorts of unique, quirky, and even outlandish contributions to fictional world-making.

A capable co-creating reader responds to textual prompts embedded in narrative to fill the lattice-work of discourse with story-enhancing substance drawn from memory, dreams, prior reading, and personal experience. This contribution of the reader is routine, if rarely acknowledged, and we can no more stop it than we can willfully cease to paint over the blind spots in our visual fields. Novelists count on this facility of readers and they manipulate it. Narrative enigmas positively instruct readers to spin out potential turns of event, some of which never come to pass, but still exist as a counterfactual imagining called up (often for purposes of suspense) and never wholly eradicated from readers' memories. Co-creation becomes especially legible when a reader contributes something so unusual to the fictional communication that other readers balk or authors object. The gap-filling imperative of fiction reading virtually guarantees that quite a lot of the time, readers will supply extraneous or erroneous elements to their reading. This raises questions about the interrelation of readers' and authors' empathy. If we had reliable access to authors' intentions for their creations, would we gain insight into readers' empathy? Does readers' empathy illuminate the empathy of the text's creator(s)?

Readers' empathy refers to the phenomenon of readers', listeners', or viewers' catching and sharing feelings with narrated representations. (Strong emotions felt *about* a narration, including reactions to content or feelings that inform aesthetic judgments, should be regarded as distinct from readers' empathy, though the two kinds of response may occur nearly simultaneously or intermittently.) Readers' empathy usually entails a match in one's bodily sensations, mood, and motivations to a character's, and can contribute to character identification, though not inevitably. Sensations of reader's empathy can be brief, fleeting, and soon forgotten, although they can also be recurrent, sustained, and memorable, and may sustain a sense of relationship with a fictional character. However, readers' empathy is not limited to emotion-sharing with characters. One may also feel sensations of motor mimicry such as spatial orientation resulting from directional cues embedded in an immersive fictional world. The location of those cues, like other prompts to narrative empathy and readerly co-creation, is textual. Texts may thus be regarded as scripts for narrative empathy, but by themselves they are inert, requiring the meeting of readers' and authors' minds to come to imaginative life. I hypothesize that *authors' empathy* plays a role in the creative process for narrative artists in all media. It may arise in the daydreaming imagining that precedes invention or recurs during the composition process. It may be a component of flow. An author's empathy with her subject is neither automatic, nor is it the only rhetorical stance available to creators. Although work by psychologist Marjorie Taylor suggests that successful creators of fictional worlds and imaginary characters may be endowed with higher empathy than the general population (Taylor et al. 361), and although Freud associated authors' evocation of readers' sympathy with their daydreaming and creativity ("Creative" 425–7), there is still much to be learned about authors' empathy as a component of imaginative labor.

Authors' intentions in their worldmaking, though frequently contested by critics and often elusive, matter a great deal to our everyday procedures of judgment of the legitimacy of "readings," or interpretations of narrative texts. While critical inquiry shies away from certainty about authorial intentions, warned off by more than half a century of training in avoiding that fallacy, it is still the case that interpreters rely on a sense, often attributed to the implied author, of what *must have been* meant. This generally agreed-upon zone of possibility is not immutable. It changes over time, and it can certainly be altered by the composition of a reading community, as many teachers who have ventured behind bars to discuss fiction with incarcerated students can attest. Resistant reading practices and wave after wave of perspectives dignified as "new approaches" have inculcated a degree of openness to shifts with respect to authors' likely intentions. Yet we readers of literature still agree that we can recognize a wrong interpretation, of the kinds that hinge on misunderstood vocabulary, lack of familiarity with context, missing key plot details, application of inappropriate generic frames, or over-hasty reading with unjustified jumps to conclusions.

Take for example a mistaken reading of Ian McEwan's *Atonement* (2001), one that misses the startling revelation that the author inside the novel, Briony Tallis, has been *inventing* a story about the past that readers have been invited to understand as *true* in the storyworld. For most readers the metafictional reveal evokes surprise if not dismay, but not if you miss the twist! Remarking on this kind of error, often in a classroom setting, ordinarily takes the form not of an argument about interpretation but of an attribution of intentions: "McEwan wants us to be shocked when we learn that Robbie and Cecilia's deaths have been suppressed in Briony's narration." The shock involved in a "right" reading of *Atonement* is empathic in the sense that it provokes two overlapping emotions (in addition to the surprise that inheres in McEwan's metafictional gambit, an affect of narrativity attributable to the impacts of form and techniques). Accurate narrative empathy could include fresh grief for the loss of Robbie and Cecilia, renewed anger at the deceptive Briony, and a desire presumably shared by Briony to "undo" or "unlearn" the facts of the case, which we can infer from her effort to rewrite it in atonement. We can go on to argue about whether Briony's narration in *Atonement* succeeds as expiation or demonstrates egoistic self-regard to the end, but a guide to the proper reading of the novel will insist that Robbie and Cecilia die separately during the war, that Briony invents a future for them, and that McEwan requires that we notice the twist at the end of his novel where this has been revealed. To the reader who missed it, one can only counsel going back and re-reading, always a useful exercise (and rewarding in this instance, as McEwan embeds the origins of the author Tallis's created imagery in its mundane sources from his character's experiences). McEwan invites empathic inaccuracy in order to correct it later.

Similarly, empathic inaccuracy can be baked into a fictional world and overtly referenced internally to the fiction. In Margaret Atwood's *Oryx and Crake* (2003) the central character and focalizer (Jimmy/Snowman) has earlier misunderstood the genocidal motives of his boyhood friend, the genius genetic engineer Crake. Atwood's fictions frequently employ layered time-schemes that demand that a reader set the feelings and knowledge of earlier and later selves in juxtaposition with one another. Atwood invites the reader to share in Jimmy's uncomprehending response to Crake—here the reader may respond with accurate empathy, duped with Jimmy into admiring or feeling jealous of Crake. Yet Atwood also reveals the apocalyptic consequences of Crake's schemes for the surviving Snowman, and here again, the reader may empathize with Snowman's bitterness towards Crake. Jimmy's empathic inaccuracy with respect to Crake can be shared for a time by the reader, but few readers will end up sympathizing with Crake all the way through the novel, and virtually all comprehending readers will stop trusting Crake long before Jimmy does. In these experimental fictions, empathic inaccuracy becomes part of a metaknowledge exercise, where an author deliberately solicits readers' empathy only to reveal it as mistaken, just ahead of the characters in the story's belated realization. The strategy can have many effects, ranging from the frisson of metafictional twists, as in *Atonement*, to the unsettling of human sympathy (especially connecting with others through art) orchestrated by the linked stories of Edwidge Danticat's *The Dew Breaker* (2004) (see below 223–28).

Beyond explicit thematizing, empathic inaccuracy as a phenomenon of reading remains elusive. First and most fundamentally, there is no way to cross-check actual readers' feelings with verifiable realities, because the target worlds and their inhabitants are nonexistent. One could interrogate a living author about intentions, but as Wimsatt and Beardsley long ago cautioned, "critical inquiries are not settled by consulting the oracle" ("Affective Fallacy" 487). When a reader really gets the wrong end of the stick, attributing feelings or perspectives in the absence of textual cues, teachers and critics often feel justified in correcting the underlying attitude revealed by the misreading, or at the least arguing with the interpretation as a bad one. The stance of correction does not assist understanding the phenomenon, however. While it is certainly the case that a literary education involves the development, over time, of critical tact that guides the educated reader away from making interpretations so idiosyncratic that they isolate, threading the needle of a prized originality means that trained readers routinely offer unexpected readings. We call them fresh readings, and we admire critics who can produce interpretations that alter our perspectives on texts, especially of canonical works that have accrued a long history of set interpretations. A hypothesis: *Interpretive distinctiveness may originate with empathic inaccuracy that prompts the critic to regard texts anomalously*. For example, I am fairly certain that Jane Austen does not mean her readers to worry about the sources of the Bertrams' wealth in West Indian sugar plantations, but Edward Said's empathically inaccurate feeling with the distant and scarcely inscribed Caribbean slaves of *Mansfield Park* (1814) has permanently altered the critical response to Austen's novel (*Culture and Imperialism* 84–97).

Narrative empathy for fictions requires the active imaginative extension of readers towards nonexistent beings (usually, characters) and possible worlds crafted by authors who also exercise empathy in their fictional worldmaking. The co-creative compact involved in experiencing fiction can render some of its most significant results when readers share intensities of character identification, extend themselves through role-taking or perspective-taking with alien others, or lose themselves (albeit temporarily) in the immersive reading experience, sometimes called transportation. Indeed, immersive reading's reputation as the lowly opposite to trained critical reading practice may stem from its capacity to generate inaccuracy: transportation relates to a fantasizing tendency in which readers get "lost in a book" and may indeed disregard details of the text that disrupt their immersive pleasures. With respect to literary theory, empathic inaccuracy is distinct from *misreading* in its ordinary, commonsense form and its deconstructive (DeManian) or creatively Oedipal (Bloomian) forms .... Empathic inaccuracy can be situated within a constellation of related but distinct literary-theoretical concepts, each of which could be considered as offering opportunities for empirical study. For example, in relation to narrative techniques, one might query whether incidences of empathic inaccuracy correlate with external or internal representations of characters' mental lives. Narrative unreliability, a prized effect of modern fiction, certainly evokes empathic inaccuracy from naïve readers. All ironic techniques run the routine risk of being taken "straight," without readers' perceiving the necessity of reversing the effects, and this opens up opportunities for empathic inaccuracy.

No one text reliably invites narrative empathy from all its readers; *empathic inaccuracy* explains a part of that variance. Empathic inaccuracy contributes to the grounds for two prominent critiques of narrative empathy, false empathy and failed empathy, for it is a form of misdirected narrative empathy, not empathy that is missing altogether. The *absence* of an empathetic response to a novel inviting empathy I have previously described under the term "failed empathy" (Keen, *Empathy* 159–60), which deserves separate comment. Readers' temperaments and empathetic dispositions vary, so narrative empathy faces constraints arising from differences in individual readers' identities and experiences. Fully functional healthy humans exhibit a range of empathic dispositions. The empathy scales used to study both real-life and fantasy empathy register unresponsiveness through self-reporting queries that allow subjects to pick "does not describe me well at all" for questions about emotional fusion, pity, or compassion in reaction to witnessing others' conditions (Davis, "Multidimensional"). Among people who score in the normal to high range on self-reporting empathy scales such as Davis's Interpersonal Reactivity Index (IRI), most possess a fairly high degree of confidence in the rightness of their identification of others' feelings and point of view. Because there are so many component versions of empathy (Batson, "These Things"), one must take care with definitions and the scope of the phenomenon measured.

Possessing the ability accurately to assess another's minds or feelings can lead to empathetic resonance but it need not do so; indeed, in some circumstances, such as performance in one of the helping professions such as surgeon or emergency responder, a cool and efficacious response may be more desirable than empathy, which always runs the risk of tipping over into aversive personal distress. Failed empathy includes a range of behaviors from total unresponsiveness, to weak unmemorable, non-persistent responses, to apathy and inaction (inefficacy if we regard narrative empathy as a strategic element of the rhetorical choices of writers). It stems from many factors outside readers' and authors' control. In the psychological literature about human empathy, overt and implicit biases (such as the *here-and-now* bias, the *familiarity* bias, and the *similarity* bias) operate to effect or block empathy for others. Reading novels that invite readers to transcend barriers of difference and distance has often been recommended as an antidote to the biases that cause empathy to fail. Thus, in the moral sentimental story-line about the civic and moral benefits to be garnered by empathetic reading practices, failed empathy certainly has the appearance of inadequate reading. Yet failed empathy is very common, as readers who have abandoned novels that haven't compelled interest can attest. Teachers and theorists putting stock in facilitating the various forms of emotional fusion and cognitive sharing that contribute to narrative empathy should take care not to judge its absence too harshly. Not everybody empathizes readily; no novel, story, or film evokes empathy from every reader. Failed empathy is an ordinary and everyday occurrence among even devoted novel readers. Indeed, in the practice of literary study that many college and university professors train students to emulate, the deliberate cultivation of a coolly analytical mode of critical reading may disable empathic responses, a result not necessarily to be deplored.

False empathy, by way of contrast, can seem more blameworthy than failed empathy, and may be subject to a degree more self-suppression as a result. We can really only be sure that false empathy has occurred in certain non-fiction narrative situations, as for example when the first-person voices and real experiencing creators of autobiographical works or *testimonio* directly contradict a reader's misidentification of "what they must have been feeling." Though textual purists are on solid ground defending a reader's response to a fictional work's ambiguities of emotional invitation, typically we defer to the authority of the experiencing writer about her own emotions. The nonfiction circumstance informs at least the social dynamic of discussion when disclosing narrative empathy felt in response to a fictional work might be judged by the others in the group as condescending, over-reaching, or as a symptom of one's white-savior complex. A morally neutral variant of false empathy would describe its likely causes and effects, including empathic inaccuracy. Instances of false empathy occur frequently enough that literature teachers need only a prompt to proffer examples, such as this astonishing report (on Facebook) from Anne Fernald: "A significant minority of one class thought Clarissa Dalloway's main conflict was regret over deciding not to marry Hugh Whitbread." The patronizing false empathy criticized by postcolonial, feminist, and critical race theorists has only the most tenuous relation to the false empathy that arises from immaturity. Normative judgments about right reading should have no part in theorizing, because (as every classroom teacher of literature who allows discussion of fiction knows) different readers, not only inexperienced students, respond with different degrees and targets of emotional engagement when they read the same words in the same order in the same fictional texts. Though the discourse may provide a stable prompt, the storyworlds co-created by the imaginative work of readers differ infinitely. Each engaged reader makes his or her unreal version of the story and its characters, thus empathic inaccuracy is a built-in liability of fictional worldmaking and readerly co-creation.

4

FROM NARRATIVE AND THE EMBODIED READER

Embodied Readers' Emotional Responses

Though machines can follow instructions and artificial intelligence can produce something like a human response to a prompt, narrative requires an embodied reader to complete its communication. Our visual, auditory, and in the case of Braille readers, tactile perception contribute to the cognitive micro-processes of reading (Barrett; Zwaan, "Embodiment"). Because we become expert in the processing of phonemes, morphemes, words, and phrases, literate people often forget that their bodies are very much involved when we apprehend stories. Yet we are certainly aware of our physical preferences: for example, we may prefer to read a book held in the hands rather than the same words displayed on a screen; to listen to a human actor read rather than a computer; to view a film in a digital format that allows us to manipulate the size of the image or the pace of the screening; or to watch the narrative as part of a shared com munal event in a movie theatre. [Literary scholars tend to pay little attention to these aspects of reading. As Andrew Elfenbein observes, the mechanics of reading comprehension have been studied in greater depth by cognitive psychologists than by literary scholars, acknowledging that "many aspects of this process are indeed routine, automatic, and quasi-mechanical" (Elfenbein 485), thus they have a bearing on critics' responses to literature, as he demonstrates.] We are reminded of our reading bodies when fatigue or discomfort disrupts the illusion of being transported and we are no longer "lost in a book," or—the polar opposite—when immersion in a story evokes an emotional response that suggests how deeply we have invested our imagination in co-creating a storyworld. Narrative activates neural representations of imagined visual and motor experiences in our brains, which along with neurons, are part of our body. Narrative's readers bring not

DOI: 10.4324/9781003264071-6

just their senses and cognitive capacities, but also their bodies and emotions to the task of imagining and responding. Much remains to be learned, as Anne Mangen and Adriaan van der Weel point out, about the "psychological, ergonomic, technological, social, cultural, and evolutionary aspects" of embodied reading ("Evolution" 116). My investigation begins at the point where a narrative evokes an intense bodily reaction from a reader.

In recent years, psychological and neuroscientific research into human cognition, affect, and embodied consciousness has influenced narrative theory, and in a fine example of the two-way traffic of ideas, narratologists' work on the impact of genres, literary techniques, and fictionality has stimulated scientific examinations of real readers' responses to narrative. [Victor Nell's *Lost in a Book* offers … a description of the phenomenon called both immersion and transportation by psychologists (Green et al., "Emotion").] As a result of these conversations and collaborations, in my own area of research—narrative empathy—we know a great deal more in 2017 about the relationship between experiences of emotional fusion with fictional characters and storyworlds and readers' subsequent attitudes (and even prosocial behavior) than was known in 2007 when *Empathy and the Novel* was first published. [For prominent examples, see the work of David Kidd and Emanuele Castano on the impact of literary reading on theory of mind (ToM); Angus Fletcher and John Monterosso on the effects of free indirect discourse (FID); Dan R. Johnson on consequences of transportation into a fictional story; Natalie Phillips's literary and neuroscientific studies of readers' attention when reading passages from Jane Austen; and Mangen and van der Weel's fascinating studies of reading on paper and on e-reading devices …. [B]oth Keith Oatley and Raymond Mar's labs have been especially productive. See also the work of Alice Hall and Cheryl Bracken; Dolf Zillman; Maral Tajerian; and Tamir et al.] Yet there is much remaining to be investigated about the empathic responses of real readers to narrative, especially when we take into consideration the intersectional identities of readers, including their gender and ethnicity, and their underlying dispositions or temperaments. In addition to multiple competing axes of identity, readers' differing personal qualities, distinct cultural contexts, and individual experiences of the world all shape readers' co-creation of the narratives that they read. [On intersectionality, see Crenshaw; for literary applications, see Lanser, "Are We There Yet?"; Warhol, "Feminist"; and Keen "Intersectional."] … [R]eaders' (and listeners' and viewers') co-creation of and responses to narrative delivered in film, in games, through oral storytelling, or through print forms take place in brains and bodies. Embodied reading—as opposed to machine reading—is the only kind of reading that human beings can perform, and notwithstanding disciplinary training in analytical habits of mind, all embodied readers have feelings. Imagination involves a blend of cognitive and affective capacities, linked to bodily responses that reinforce reactions to, feelings about, and appetite for narrative fiction. How, why, to what degree, and to what ends narrative engages those feelings remains a fascinating puzzle.

Though there are good reasons to take an interest in the potentially positive impacts of narrative, some reading experiences clearly have negative emotional valences. Narratives can make you feel sick to your stomach. They can disrupt your sleep and give you nightmares. They can make you cry. [The salutary effects of purgation, alleviation of emotion, or restored balance associated with the Aristotelian term *catharsis* put a positive interpretation on the result of experiencing pity and fear as a result of watching a tragedy.] Not all narrative aims to induce pleasure, as narrative theorists since Aristotle have understood. Philosophers and literary theorists have approached the topic of unpleasant, dysphoric responses to narratives from a number of angles, exploring the bittersweet sensation of enjoying the release of weeping about a fictional character's situation, as in Robyn Warhol's *Having a Good Cry: Effeminate Feelings and Pop-Culture Forms* (2003), or querying the paradox of fictional emotions, when we are transported into imaginary worlds, as in E. M. Dadlez's *What's Hecuba to Him? Fictional Events and Actual Emotions* (1997). [On the status of fictional emotions, see Yanal; Jenefer Robinson; cf. Walton.] Sianne Ngai's *Ugly Feelings* (2005) investigates what she labels the "unprestigious negative affects" of irritation, envy, and disgust. Psychological science helps provide a context for understanding the depth of imaginative engagement (as evidenced by immersion or transportation), the strength of emotional responses (including empathy), and the short- and longer-term effects of their reading.

Narrative Personal Distress

In this chapter I seek to redress the neglect of one intense form of reaction to narrative: personal distress. The time is ripe for a reconsideration of the particular forms of readers' narrative empathy that invite intense, aversive bodily responses to fictional representations of others. In the psychological literature, personal distress is regarded as an empathic reaction, but a form of empathy oriented primarily towards the self (though it is stimulated by reaction to another). It causes aversion from the source: people experiencing personal distress seek to avoid or discontinue contact with the cause of their feelings. [The source of personal distress does not have to be another sensate being. *Einfühlung* can involve 'feeling with' inanimate objects, especially for unpleasant states such as freezing, burning, being separated, fragmented, or crushed. Art objects can evoke *Einfühlung*. When a reader shudders, shivers, gasps, quails, or flinches with intense *Einfühlung*, this can be a form of aesthetic or narrative personal distress registered in the body]. Unlike other-oriented empathy, which could lead to mature sympathy or even prosocial action on behalf of others, personal distress shows when the people feeling it push away, tune out, or refuse to engage. In an important article enumerating and describing different phenomena that go by the name empathy, psychologist C. Daniel Batson describes personal distress as "Feeling Distress at Witnessing Another Person's Suffering" ("These Things" 7). As Batson elaborates, personal distress expresses not feelings for (sympathy) or feelings like the other's feelings (empathy as traditionally understood), but "feeling distressed *by* the state of the other" (8; italics in original). Perhaps not surprisingly, personal distress has been linked to compassion fatigue and burnout (Thomas 375–6). Developmental psychologist Nancy Eisenberg defines personal distress as "a self-focused, aversive, affective reaction to the apprehension of another's emotion' that is 'believed to result in egotistically motivated behavior," unlike the other-directed moral emotion, sympathy ("Emotion Regulation" 672). In contrast to empathy, personal distress does not lead to prosocial behavior, and may even contribute to anti-social responses (673). Personal distress is associated with increased levels of physiological arousal, lower levels of coping skills, and executive (decision-making) dysfunction (Eisenberg and Eggum 76). For some people whose dispositions involve high-intensity negative emotionality and a low ability to regulate their emotions, personal distress can overwhelm them with vicarious negative feelings (Eisenberg, "Emotion Regulation," 677–8). Escaping the source of the feeling motivates people experiencing personal distress to avoid engagement (Eisenberg and Eggum 72).

Influenced by these and other definitions, in my earlier work on narrative empathy, I declined fully to address a literary corollary to personal distress, reasoning that a reaction that causes the reader to abandon the book or walk out of the movie theatre could not and should not be considered an important form of narrative empathy. I asserted:

> An over-aroused empathic response that creates personal distress (self-oriented and aversive) causes a turning-away from the provocative condition of the other. I hazard that personal distress caused by novel reading leads people to stop reading, to put the book down, or to disengage full attention by skipping and skimming.
>
> (*Empathy* 4–5)

Though I further observed that "None of the philosophers who put stock in the morally improving experience of narrative empathy include personal distress in their theories" (5), … [I recognized] that personal distress contributes to aesthetic emotions such as disgust. [Negative emotions such as disgust certainly contribute to aesthetic responses, and not only through catharsis. See Ngai 332–54, and the earlier influential discussion of disgust as a mechanism by which bourgeois subjects differentiated themselves from low domains, in Stallybrass and White's *The Politics and Poetics of Transgression* (1986).] I concluded that "personal distress has no place in a literary theory of empathy" (Keen, *Empathy* 5). Yet each of the reactions that exhibits personal distress, from shutting the eyes, to covering the ears, to turning away, to putting down the book, all the way to walking out of the movie theatre, qualifies as a behavior of the body, expressing aversion with voluntary and involuntary responses (such as changes in heart rate, blood pressure, palm sweat, and clenching in the gut). These responses of embodied readers deserve attention.

In this chapter I re-evaluate and revise my earlier judgment. Specifically, I report on the feelings of readers who remember experiencing empathic personal distress in response to narratives. My approach is not empirical, but it is open-ended, so it has the virtue of broadening our sense of the range of narratives that can be considered distressing, rather than zeroing in on singular, notorious examples. I discuss what my correspondents actually did in response to their personal distress, in particular whether they continued with the narrative that had caused the aversive reaction. I draw from their reports ideas about narrative personal distress that could inform narrative theorists and psychologists of narrative impact.[12] In conclusion, I compare this account of personal distress (grounded in psychology) with educational theories that assert the value of emotionally challenging literary reading, asking whether narrative personal distress (NPD) does harm or benefits students. Because there is a relative dearth of research on personal distress in the psychology of narrative impact or in investigations of readers' empathy, I draw on findings from mass media studies about evocation and regulation of emotions. Emotion regulation is 'essential to keep high levels of vicarious emotional arousal from turning into personal distress' (Eisenberg and Eggum 73), but people with different dispositions vary in their ability effortfully to manage their response to arousing stimuli (74–5). While this means that narrative personal distress may be avoidable for better regulated readers, it may also suggest that reading extremely emotionally arousing narrative, the kind that causes gasps, tears, racing heart, and even nausea, could help acclimatize students to regulation of their emotions. Readers' responses to narratives are often mixed, with feelings that ebb and flow, or emotional intensities that overlap with cooler reactions to style or form. A common trajectory is to move from character identification to narrative empathy to personal distress on behalf of that character. Can a blend of narrative empathy with narrative personal distress hold off, delay, or diminish the rejection and avoidance of the emotion-provoking Other? Or is NPD actually harmful?

I draw in this and subsequent paragraphs on the reports of the life-long readers that I reached through the VICTORIA listserv discussion in a query posted on 26 January 2016 under the header 'empathy so intense you stopped reading' (Keen 2016). Because I was corresponding with volunteers from among the Victorianists subscribed to this academic discussion, it is not surprising that Thomas Hardy's name came up as especially provoking of distressing empathy. He was the most-mentioned Victorian-era author, though Louisa May Alcott, Charlotte Brontë, Wilkie Collins, Charles Dickens, Fyodor Dostoevsky, George Eliot, Elizabeth Gaskell, George Gissing, Leo Tolstoy, Anthony Trollope, and H. G. Wells also received nominations. Authors who trap their characters (such as Tess Durbeyfield, Jude Fawley, and Maggie Tulliver) in unbearable situations evoked dismay that led to discontinuation of reading. Cruelty to orphans and animals came up frequently, as did scenes of injustice. For example, a research assistant at the University of Glasgow reported:

> The other moment of significant distress came during my Masters when first read Collins's *The Woman in White*. The scene in which Fosco writes a note in Marian's private diary, signifying that he's read the entire thing, left me sick and shaking with unexpected rage. I had to step away from the novel for an hour or two, but ultimately stayed up the entire night to finish the book to ensure that Fosco got his comeuppance.
>
> (Boucher)

This sample highlights two important points about narrative personal distress (qualifying as NPD because it was so intense that it interrupted reading). First, it caused two strong physical reactions, nausea ("sick") and fury "'shaking with unexpected rage") that caused the reader to put the book away. Second, it illustrates the emotional elements of narrativity with which narrative empathy and narrative personal distress may intersect. Narrativity is the set of qualities (such as having a narrator, evoking temporality, relating events, and characterizing active agents) that help readers or viewers perceive a text as narrative (Keen, *Narrative Form* 120); the core affective drivers of narrativity are curiosity, surprise, and suspense (Sternberg, "Narrativity" 37). The report suggests that NPD can begin with surprise (if we take shock to be an extreme form of that affect) and can then stimulate curiosity and suspense. Returning to the novel and staying up all night reading to find out how the malefactor will be punished suggests that not all NPD causes a dead end to reading. Indeed, it may turn into a strong driver of emotional investment in a narrative.

Like narrative empathy, narrative personal distress seems to hit some readers with a powerful reaction and others not at all. This correspondent explained her reasons for reacting so strongly to a scene in Collins's novel that others may find innocuous (compared with some of the excessively violent representations that are often cited as most shocking in discussions of distressing or disgusting narratives). She writes:

> What sparked this particular response in me was the fact that I grew up in a house where I was allowed very little privacy. For an awkward, aspiring writer insecure in her own skill, it was extremely frustrating and embarrassing to know that anything I attempted to write down (be it a diary or a work of fiction) would be secretly read by my mother. I developed a very elaborate system of code and shorthand just so I could write in peace. My reaction to Fosco stems very much from my own personal feelings about violations of privacy.
>
> (Boucher)

Any further theorizing of NPD should, in my opinion, acknowledge from the out-set the remarkable variability in responses that most likely stems from the variety of personal experiences that readers bring to their co-creation of the storyworld and its characters. It should also acknowledge that the effects of NPD, like those of narrative empathy, may be only temporary. This reader, who after all returned to the novel and read all the way to its satisfying conclusion, may have been spurred by her NPD to a stronger investment in the novel.

Some accounts of narrative personal distress did validate my original intuition that NPD permanently stops reading. If narrative personal distress interrupts transportation (or immersion) in a narrative storyworld, enjoyment, narrative empathy, and the benefits of full engagement with a text may also suffer. [Transportation (immersion) has been positively linked to empathy, enjoyments, and even increased pro-social helping behavior (Hall and Bracken; Dan Johnson).] Tender readers report weeping, gasping, sobbing, and needing time to recover from such a reading or viewing experience. Correspondents from the VICTORIA discussion described throwing a distressing book in the trash (Moody), tossing a book down (Hill), throwing it across the room (Goldfarb), turning a radio off (Hoyle), and walking out of a movie theatre or classroom film screening (Williams). I can attest personally to the impulse to walk out in the middle of a narrative, having left screenings of both *My Life as a Dog* (1985) and *Saving Private Ryan* (1998). In both cases, violent representations were the trigger. I know to avoid films that depict violence against women, especially rape, but I confess that violence against male bodies only truly began to trouble me after I became the mother of a son. The development of reading and viewing habits over time may be conditioned by early experiences of NPD, leading to avoidance of certain authors, genres, or texts. Yet those preferences can also be altered or augmented over the course of a lifetime. [The lack of longitudinal studies of real readers and viewers of narrative cries out for redress.] Several correspondents remarked specifically on never going back to a particular author after an especially distressing reading experience.

The novels, stories, films, radio serials, and nonfiction narratives that evoked narrative personal distress exhibited great variety … and the unpredictability of the elicited list should give educators pause as they contemplate the difficulty of anticipating how students may respond to works on a syllabus. Still, certain hot-button stimuli do crop up. Many of my informants spontaneously focused on cruelty to animals, reporting personal distress as a response to reading, for example, Anna Sewall's *Black Beauty* (1877), "Raspberry Jam" by Angus Wilson (1949), and *The Story about Ping* by Marjorie Flack (1933). Some remembered responses were to representations of cruelty directed against children and women, with rape and abuse standing out, but it must be acknowledged that, mirroring the gender proportions in the reading public, the vast majority of my correspondents were women (Bowker 2010). Racism, violence, and psychologically intense evocation of danger, as in horror films and thrillers, bothered some readers. Altogether, VICTORIA correspondents reported a wide range of recalled sensations, including claustrophobia (Richardson), breathlessness, wincing (Nevins), shuddering (Karpenko), and unbearable fellow-feeling that resulted in crying uncontrollably (Struve, Pederson, Klimaszewski), dry heaving (Holzer), having nightmares (Becker), and yelling aloud (Pennington). While extreme sadness was the most frequently reported experience, some reported horror (Galvan, Heather), rage (Moody), or anxiety (Lewis). Several respondents used the term "traumatic" to describe the impact of distressing reading (Schintgen, Sutton-Ramspeck). About Toni Morrison's *Beloved* (1987) one correspondent reported, "there are parts of that book that make me feel as if my insides are tearing and bleeding" (Klimaszewski).

Many of the people who wrote to me about their experiences of narrative personal distress are scholars, either graduate students or established faculty. As a result, some of them recalled NPD experiences in the classroom, and some related learning the hard way to avoid reading aloud passages guaranteed to cause choking up or actual tears while teaching. Most teachers believe that it is important to remain articulate, as the performance of expertise and the necessary focus on others' understanding discourage episodes of weeping or even speechlessness. Recollections of narrative personal distress from their student days remind us that strong aversive emotion reactions to narrative can come at a cost. One faculty member recalled being "thoroughly traumatized by the horrific rape in the book" [Kosinski's *The Painted Bird*] as she had "never been by anything in a book before or since." In this case, the NPD silenced her. She writes, "as a rather shy freshman, I didn't even feel I was in a position to articulate my horror" (Sutton-Ramspeck). Regarding Cormac McCarthy's *Blood Meridian* (1985), another correspondent recalled an episode from her undergraduate days:

> A number of the students found the graphic violence so gratuitous and sickening that they could not finish the text; one student in particular stands out in my memory, as she had to drop the class very late in the semester because the book sparked a nervous breakdown.
>
> (Boucher)

Struggling through the novel and the course, this correspondent challenged her professor "on every aspect" of the novel, a behavior she describes as "extremely out of character" (Boucher). In this case the NPD brought on not silencing but unruly engagement, which might be regarded as a positive impact.

The Pedagogy of Discomfort

This possibility that narrative personal distress provoked strong participation should make us wonder whether NPD has other salutary effects, despite the fact that personal distress is expressly dissociated from altruistic, other-oriented pro-social response in the psychological literature. Possibly a group experience of a distressing narrative can be harnessed to the social drivers of communal feeling for positive purposes. So, for example, the beneficial consequences of NPD felt as a result of reading *Black Beauty* can be seen, within a guiding context, in commitment to a cause and action in the world. In a course entitled "Victorian Animal Dreams," a professor reports:

> somehow the experience of all of us feeling the pain communally and trying to do both communally and individually what we can for the alleviation of animal suffering makes it bearable—or more bearable. One student in the class has rescued three horses, the oldest of which is just out to graze in a meadow in his old age, like *Black Beauty* at the end of the novel. Many of the students rescue animals and/or are involved with Students for Animals on campus.
>
> (Morse)

The creation of a purposeful communal response to shared distress not only results in specific positive actions on behalf of animals, but gives students who may feel overwhelmed by emotion from the narrative an alleviating focus for their feelings. Given the presence of a teacher or informed guide, does narrative personal distress have pedagogical uses that outweigh its negative consequences?

Clearly, an educational context makes a difference, both in terms of providing a purposeful context and in impelling readers to finish the narratives. The most common consequence of narrative personal distress is discontinuance of exposure to the distressing narrative, a strategy that works for ordinary reading but not when the text is required, or even highly regarded. When the narrative is a canonical classic, informants usually report persevering with the reading eventually, but doubts remain. Having been deeply disturbed by *The Mill on the Floss*, another professor reports:

> I didn't revisit the novel for many years, didn't read it, didn't teach it, so I guess that counts as aversive. After twenty-five years, though, I thought I'd give it another go. I've taught it six semesters running—and I think I've made my peace with it, at least aesthetically. Every semester, though, I see a student or two reliving my trauma!
>
> (Melnyk)

Teachers of literature routinely impel students to continue reading texts that discomfit them, and indeed many faculty regard inducing discomfort as one of the prime uses of literature and purposes of education. [For a nuanced discussion of the uses of potentially offensive art, see Aldama and Lindenberger.] At the university level, moving students out of their comfort zones to confront alternative perspectives, world views, and experiences is a routine goal of education in the arts, humanities, and social sciences. As Irina Popescu [argues] in *The Chronicle of Higher Education* (2016), "history is unsettling. The present is unsettling. It unsettles with its crimes against humanity, its wars, its sex trafficking, even its presidential debates. There should be more being said about the power of discomfort." A major source of commentary on discomforting subjects, what Philip Fisher calls "hard facts." lies in literary texts. Most teachers of literature strongly agree with what Popescu asks: "Shouldn't reading Harriet Jacobs's slave narrative be uncomfortable?" Many professors of literature go further, embracing forms of discomfort that may not be dignified with the automatic moral prestige of witnessing to the experience of slavery. They introduce students to works intending to horrify, disgust, shock, or test boundaries of propriety, to the degree that any such limitations still survive in a largely permissive reading and viewing culture.

When shock art is taught, whether in visual or textual media, it is nearly inevitably presented as purposeful representation … with core assumptions that makers use techniques to invite or provoke reactions from an audience or readership that has the capacity to respond or even change as a result of the encounter with the artwork. These ideas carry over to narrative literature. Arguably, Cormac McCarthy and those who teach his works both mean to harness readers' shock for ethical purposes. Quentin Tarantino and Bret Easton Ellis employ violence aesthetically; students in discussions debate the morality of their choices. In the logic of many curricular expectations, teaching Toni Morrison, Keri Hulme, Margaret Atwood, and countless other novelists who take on tough subjects such as child abuse, rape, torture, and violence against women and enslaved people provokes discussion and learning through perspective taking. Many faculty accustomed to assuming that the end result of catharsis justifies the pity and fear evoked by classic texts feel some qualms when considering the risks of teaching modern and contemporary narratives such as Toni Morrison's *Beloved*, Chinua Achebe's *Things Fall Apart* (1958), and Virginia Woolf's modernist novel *Mrs Dalloway* (1925). Though many of the arguments in favor of unfettered reading lists come from civil libertarians, defending extreme representations as part of the exercise of free speech, others come from the pedagogical field, where teachers introducing global, multicultural, or disadvantaged perspectives have included non-canonical readings that deliberately challenge students' complacency and to complicate their thinking about the world they inhabit.

What happens when that discomfort tips over into traumatic pain? The teachers reporting students disabled by reading may be witnessing NPD. The most extreme cases of personal distress as a consequence of assigned reading have led to a national discussion of trigger warnings for students in courses, referring to "explicit alerts that the material they are about to read or see in a classroom might upset them or, as some students assert, cause symptoms of post-traumatic stress disorder in victims of rape or in war veterans" (Medina). Regarded by some as necessary, compassionate signals to help trauma victims avoid painful flashbacks or withdrawal into numbness, trigger warnings have also been castigated as politically correct "vindictive protectiveness" that fails to prepare students for professional life and, worse, teaches them to "think pathologically" (Lukianoff and

Haidt). Though it is not my purpose to discuss the efficacy or inadvisability of trigger warnings here, I hypothesize that the student complaints that have led in some cases to calls for trigger warnings arose from experiences of narrative empathy in the form of NPD, felt as a result of exposure to evocative course materials. But we should ask, which narratives, in what circumstances, and for what proportion of readers? Is the triggering level of NPD something that can be consistently anticipated, and if so, what subjects or techniques evoke it? I suspect that there are as many and as diverse cues in narrative that invite personal distress as there are pathways to less aversive forms of narrative empathy, sympathy, and pleasurable emotional fusion.

If reading narrative sometimes provokes reactions that go beyond disquietude to suffering or even life-threatening anguish, however, there are still merits to weight the other side of the scale. The cognitive and affective dissonance believed to stimulate greater learning, compassion, and understanding, starting when students encounter unfamiliar or unpleasant subjects in the classroom, and extending to experiences that may occur during service learning activities in the community or wider world, is a phenomenon embraced by the pedagogy of liberal learning, not only in literary studies. The experience of personal distress may indeed be a foundational element of the learning encouraged by the AAC&U's LEAP initiative, and may contribute to students' cultivation of "Personal and Social Responsibility, Including Civic knowledge and engagement—local and global; Intercultural knowledge and competence, and Ethical reasoning and action" (AAC&U). Liberal arts pedagogy encourages students to overcome both latent familiarity and here-and-now biases to extend the empathetic circle to people different from them selves. For some tender readers, this may require getting past a personal distress reaction and taking the risk of exposure to unfamiliar storyworlds. For if, as novelist Tim Parks observes, "when we open a novel, as with any encounter, we move into an area of risk" (ix), we ought to understand the full range of possible responses, including flinching, shuddering, weeping, gasping, feeling nauseated, perseverating, and experiencing sleeplessness, that can ensue as a result of intense personal distress provoked by narrative. Confronted with the self-focused states of subjects experiencing personal distress, psychologists show that personal distress does not lead to altruism in the same way that other-oriented empathy does (in the real world). [For the difference between narrative empathy and real-world empathy in provoking altruism, see Keen, *Empathy and the Novel*; see also Carrera et al.] Yet many literature teachers place stock in the ability of narrative to change attitudes, reduce bias, and stimulate prosocial behavior in the real world. We should add to our queries about narrative personal distress a hard look at the assumptions underlying the desired, and presumably productive, cognitive dissonance that teachers seek from challenging reading. We need to develop a robust set of pedagogical practices not only to mitigate potential damage to vulnerable readers, but also to channel both narrative empathy and narrative personal distress in a way that promotes positive intellectual growth.

Hypotheses about Narrative Personal Distress (NPD)

- NPD may cause strong physical reactions that cause the reader to put the book away and permanently interrupt the reading.
- A great variety of narratives have evoked NPD.
- NPD affects some readers with a powerful reaction and others not at all.
- The variability in responses stems from the variety of personal experiences that readers bring to their co-creation of the storyworld and its characters.
- If NPD interrupts transportation (or immersion) in a narrative storyworld, enjoyment, narrative empathy, and the benefits of full engagement with a text may also suffer.
- Reading extremely emotionally arousing narrative could help acclimatize students to regulation of their emotions.
- A blend of narrative empathy with narrative personal distress could hold off, delay, or diminish the rejection and avoidance of the emotion-provoking Other.
- NPD can engage with narrativity and drive reading, beginning with shock (surprise) and stimulating curiosity and suspense.
- The effects of NPD, like those of narrative empathy, may be only temporary.
- The development of reading and viewing habits over time may be conditioned by early experiences of NPD, leading to avoidance of certain authors, genres, or texts.
- NPD may have pedagogical uses that outweigh its negative consequences.
- A group experience of a distressing narrative could be harnessed to the social drivers of communal feeling for positive purposes.
- The student complaints that have led to calls for trigger warnings relate to NPD felt as a result of exposure to evocative course materials.
- Diverse cues in narrative invite NPD, just as there are multiple pathways to less aversive forms of narrative empathy, sympathy, and pleasurable emotional fusion.

5

FROM LIFE WRITING AND THE EMPATHETIC CIRCLE

In this essay I consider the potential of nonfiction narrative, especially life-writing and *testimonio*, to expand the empathetic circle of readers through varieties of authorial strategic empathy, revisiting my claim in *Empathy and the Novel* (2007) that writing perceived as *fictional* is especially effective in evoking readers' empathy (88–9). In a very fine essay in the journal *Narrative*, Leah Anderst calls attention to my exclusion of "all variety of narratives that announce themselves as referencing the real world rather than an imagined world of fiction" (273). This is a fair criticism, though my work on the novel necessarily focused on theorizing the role of fiction in invoking narrative empathy. Especially in her readings of Alison Bechdel's *Fun Home* (2006) and Doris Lessing's *Under My Skin* (1994), Anderst goes on effectively to redress the gap she identifies, attending "to the ways that affective responses, and empathetic responses in particular, are also operative in autobiographical narratives" (273). While the empirical research on fictional narratives, especially literary ones, has endorsed my earlier proposal that fiction has a special capacity to evoke empathy, in this essay I consider the proposition that we should also see nonfiction life writing as sharing with fictional narrative the capacity to invite feeling responses and to evoke readers' empathy. I do acknowledge that *nonfictional narrative* has been given short shrift in existent empirical research programs, and the distinctiveness of life writing as a mode of nonfiction has not so often entered into empirical comparisons of the impact of fiction and nonfiction.

There are two reasons for this, I believe. First, the category of nonfiction is often caricatured as a unitary, nonliterary, dry, factual mode in studies that employ textbooks or factual reportage as the exemplary items to be compared to fiction—and the interests of readers of nonfiction thus seem to be very different from those of readers of fiction. Second, the formal similarities between literary biography,

DOI: 10.4324/9781003264071-7

autobiography, memoir, and *testimonio* on the one hand and fictional narrative genres on the other have typically been either over-looked or glossed over. Out of these oversights, categorical problems at the levels of genre, readership and/or audience emerge. Some studies starkly juxtapose fiction and nonfiction readers as if they were two mutually exclusive groups, but experience and conversations with many booklovers tell me that a single reader can enjoy and appreciate both fiction and nonfiction, that many novel readers also enjoy forms of life writing and creative nonfiction, and that many nonfiction readers read both dry, factual informational texts and more affectively-charged narrative forms such as history, biography, and memoirs. Some of these readers surely respond with empathy to both fiction and nonfiction life writing. This is just a matter of the common-sense observation of readers' behavior and personal testimony, and is thus a start in the right direction. Yet there is a lot of work still to do in theorizing and in studying empirically how readers respond emphatically to nonfiction narratives of actual people's lives—especially if we want to understand how that experience is similar to or different from their experience of reading fiction.

A brief review of the most-cited empirical study, by Raymond Mar and Keith Oatley, comparing the narrative impact of fiction and nonfiction, sets the stage for this work. There are huge gaps in our knowledge. In order to consider the pathways to narrative empathy that life writing invites by means of affective strategies and cognitive perspective-taking, I will go on to reprise my theory of narrative empathy, defining key terms in my discussion of narrative empathy and fiction and suggesting how my approach might be adopted to help us think about that special kind of nonfiction narrative that we call life writing.

Nonfiction readers have gotten a bad rap in some of the existing empirical studies. This often-cited study by Mar and Oatley, "Bookworms versus Nerds: Exposure to Fiction versus Non-Fiction, Divergent Associations with Social Ability, and the Simulation of Fictional Social Worlds," suggests that

> [w]hile frequent readers are often stereotyped as [being] socially awkward, this may only be true of non-fiction readers and not readers of fiction. Comprehending characters in a narrative fiction appears to parallel the comprehension of peers in the actual world, while the comprehension of *expository non-fiction* shares no such parallels. Frequent fiction readers may thus bolster or maintain their social abilities unlike frequent readers of non-fiction.
> (694; *emphasis added*)

Controlling for age, English fluency and intelligence, Mar and Oatley looked at how "[l]ifetime exposure to fiction and non-fiction texts" revealed differences in "performance on empathy/social-acumen measures" (694). In general, fiction print- exposure positively predicted social ability, while non-fiction print-exposure was a negative predictor. The degree of one's "tendency to become absorbed in a story also predicted empathy scores" (694). The assumptions about non-fiction immediately evident here are its lack of an immersive quality, its expository nature, and the absence of characters that readers may strive to understand. Yet clearly life writing in all its modes shares these specific qualities with narrative fiction, and helps to differentiate from nonfiction. This leads to the possibility that life writing may engage the narrative emotions of more socially adept "bookworms" as readily as does fiction.

As I have recently written in *Narrative Form: Revised and Expanded Second Edition* (2015), "[n]arrative emotions, considered as an aspect of narrative form, differ from the feelings attributed to fictional characters. Those attributions may be made directly by a narrator employing [a] thought report or psycho-narration about a character's emotions" (152). [This essay builds on and extends my previously published treatment of nonfiction narrative] … to include, beyond characters, the represented persons who are the subjects of life writing, as for example when Richard Ellmann writes of James Joyce: "He is by turns gay, morose, trusting, suspicious, uxorious, and misogynous" (2). Like fictional characters, the represented persons of life writing possess feelings that may be revealed through the narrated or quoted monologue attributed to them; biographical subjects also invite inferences from readers responding to external cues delivered through actions or characterization. So if "Stephen Dedalus dresses in black because he is in mourning, and his speech and thoughts reveal that he still grieves for his mother" (Keen, *Narrative Form* 152), James Joyce's feelings may also be inferred from Ellmann's assertion that after his mother's death, "[h]e dressed in black, a Hamlet without a wicked uncle" (Ellmann 143). Representations of emotions certainly pertain to both fictional and non fictional narratives when the latter center on human agents.

Narrative emotions, however, differ from representations of emotional responses. Again, from *Narrative Form*: "They are forms of affect and they inhere in devices of storytelling" (152). I would assert that narrative emotions are involved in readers' experience of both fiction and life writing—but almost certainly not in that of the expository prose that represents nonfiction in Mar et al.'s oft-cited study. Narrative emotions go beyond the character identification that makes a story 'relatable' in the parlance of today's students. If it is the case that "[n]arrative emotions are tied up with fictional characters because those actants normally play the role of active agency in plots" (152), as I have argued, then historical persons represented as the active agents in life writing also may evoke them. In both the fictional and nonfictional context, narrative emotions also

> belong to the readers who respond to the techniques of storytelling with curiosity, suspense, and surprise. They are shared across the narrative transaction by authors who seek to evoke feelings in readers employing the powers of narrativity…. [T]he kinds of feelings that drive reading or viewing [are] the core affects of narrativity.
>
> (152)

In my view a common sort of narrativity is shared by fictional and nonfictional narrative texts, especially memoir, biography and autobiography, and *testimonio*, as well as narrative history. This statement represents an extension of my own theorizing about narrative emotions, but also fits in with understandings of narrativity that do not concern themselves with fictionality.

Definitions of two fundamental concepts must precede any discussion of narrative emotions: *narrativity* and *affect*. An important definition of affect for literary studies arises from the field of ethics, and indeed the term is used differently across disciplines. Among scholars of ethics, Brian Massumi's influential distinction is widely respected. Massumi suggests that emotion should not be synonymous with affect (as in much social scientific usage, where the two terms are often used interchangeably). In his translation of Gilles Deleuze and Félix Guattari's *A Thousand Plateaus* (1987), Massumi draws on Spinoza to define affect as "a state of mind and body marking the transition from one state to another with either increase or diminishment in the body's ability to act" (xvi). I have argued in *Narrative Form* that, for narrative theorists, this distinction also applies to narrative: "One connection occurs in the drive to keep reading or viewing. The core bodily affects of desire, pleasure, and pain may be translated into the realm of narrative form by means of *narrativity*" (153). To elaborate:

> plots consist of related events and their beginnings allude to states of affairs that are undergoing change. Change and disruption are thus the natural states of narrative, which cannot exist for long in stasis. Something has to happen in order to stimulate the unspooling of related events that constitute plot, and those changes of state invite readers to experience versions of affect. Although a dictionary definition of affect (as a noun) makes it synonymous with feelings or emotions, its Latin root (and its meaning when it is a verb) emphasizes affect's role in *influencing action*. This is one reason why the core narrative affects, curiosity, surprise, and suspense, relate to narrativity.
>
> (153; *emphasis added*)

As for narrativity, it consists of the qualities that establish a text as narrative: having the events that constitute a plot; possessing a narrator whose discourse makes up the text; arrangement of narrated events in a fashion that suggests temporality, normal or abnormal in its order; characterizing active agents, whether human or otherwise (153).

We note that fictionality is not a distinguishing feature of narrativity, but the experiences and attitudes of readers may establish make-believe as a *preference* in reading. As for the formal techniques of narrative that can be identified by their qualities, named, and distinguished from one another, these only take on any power as narrative techniques when they are activated by reading or viewing—and so readers' predispositions are important. The ingredients of narrative-ness remain inert until a reader or viewer enters the scene.

Once the scenario for a narrative communication or transaction exists, then the collection of techniques and contents arranged by a maker into a narrative can be activated. They combine to produce curiosity, surprise and suspense, the three core affects of narrativity as Meir Sternberg argues ("Narrativity" 637). Each of these affects is experienced by a perceiving reader or viewer: they are stimulated by a text but do not exist independently of a reading or viewing experience. (See the discussion in *Narrative Form*, 153–4) … Represented emotions need real, embodied audiences in order to exist. As I have earlier argued, "intrinsic formal qualities of narrative evoke the affects of narrativity in actual readers or viewers. How individual techniques of narrative form actually work in real readers is a matter for both theorizing and testing through empirical study of narrative impact" (154). These studies ought to tackle not only *how* we read but also *what* we read. This principle brings us back to the challenge of nonfiction, or factual narrative, as it has been studied by narratologists. I agree with Monika Fludernik that a "division between factual and fictional narratology does not make much sense" (134). Fludernik and I concur that the formal distinctiveness of fiction, theorized by Dorrit Cohn, is difficult to pin down—beyond the implicit existence of real-world referents. Yet real readers strongly feel that there is a difference between fictions about imaginary beings and narratives that offer factual accounts of real persons.

So, for example, it has been observed that the immersion reading of fiction invites higher levels of narrative empathy than such a reading of other kinds of texts, or even than our experience of people in real life. I believe that some readers find it easier to share feelings with *fictional* characters than with *real life* individuals, in part because our fiction reading doesn't demand anything of us. We can let our caution and skepticism relax when we read fiction: it doesn't matter if we are fooled by it because we go into the experience knowing that it is unreal (Keen, *Empathy* 168). The controversies around successful books such as *Three Cups of Tea* or other memoirs that have later been revealed as fictionalized suggest that the label under which readers experience a story conditions their responses and their expectations. If you have believed in the real man in the story, maybe even going so far as to donate to his charity, and then you have found out that his memoir was exaggerated or even invented from whole cloth, you may feel defrauded. Yet if you are not a very young child, you are far less likely to feel tricked or taken advantage of when you recognize that a first person narrator in a fictional autobiography never really lived—although there are some interesting cases involving fictional works that were misunderstood as autobiographies.

I have hypothesized that the "no strings attached" expectation invoked by the paratextual label, "fiction" releases the readers to make empathetic connections without fear that they will be required to reciprocate, make commitments, or act in the real world. Here I add a hypothesis about the paratextual labels of certain subsets of "nonfiction," those subsets of life writing that exist right on the borders of their sister genres of fiction: with near-fictional autobiographies (related in the first person) we have the life writing genres of memoir, autobiography, and *testimonio*; with the near-third-person *bildungsroman* we have biography. These generic words matter because they often appear physically on books themselves (beneath the title or in the back-cover identifiers), determining where they will sit in bookstores or how metadata identifies them in search engines. The empirical research on the impact of paratexts is indeed fascinating and well worth our attention.

Appel and Malečkar hypothesize that the conditions set by paratexts *trigger different needs*, a need for cognition in reading nonfiction and a need for affect when reading fiction (459). Before we even start reading, they think, we are guided by paratexts *to expect* to be transported more fully into, more thoroughly immersed in fictional worlds. Story labels affect the mode and degree of our transportation (474). This is a different question than the one asked by studies comparing the underlying dispositions of fiction and nonfiction readers (are they bookworms or nerds?). It is no surprise that we find voluntary novel readers tend to have greater empathy while nonfiction (factual) readers tend to have lower empathy, but this contrast in itself does not argue for a causal relationship arising from the genre. However, if the paratext alone sets us up to engage more cognitively with nonfiction and more emotionally with fiction, then the modest generic label does condition very different kinds of reading experience. I would hypothesize that subgenres of nonfiction focused on the perspectives of human agents, including memoir, *testimonio*, and biography may attract (or form) higher-empathy readers than dryer, more factual and overtly argumentative or analytical forms of nonfiction. But that comparative work, providing an opportunity for future collaborative scholarship, has yet to be done.

Research on the impact of reading has been remarkably enriched by such collaborations. Ulrike Altmann and her collaborators performed a neuroimaging study, which revealed readers' activation patterns as they read factual narratives, patterns which suggested that an action-based reconstruction was elicited; the brain areas involved in fiction reading, on the other hand, suggested the operation of constructive simulation, which is closely tied to the way our brain imagines future events. This work supports the suggestion of Mar et al. that factual and fictional works orient readers toward real-world interactions and imaginative simulations, respectively (173). Anne Mangen and Don Kuiken's very suggestive study "Lost in an iPad: Narrative Engagement on Paper and Tablet" also has some interesting implications for the connection between immersion and *nonfiction*, for they did find that *nonfiction read on an iPad* disrupted transportation, indirectly impeding empathy (154).

One of the most powerful emotional effects of reading or viewing narratives occurs when the qualities of narrativity mesh with representations that evoke sensations of narrative empathy.

Narrative empathy is a special case that we may get with narrative transactions moving from maker to audience. I acknowledge the legitimate narrative emotions that occur when the actual reader *differs* dramatically from the implied or ideal reader of a text: indeed, I think experiencing the potential of an expanded perspective to some degree piggybacks on our ability to be a successful reader of a text that does not seem to script us into its narrative audience. As a matter of narrative form, narrative empathy depends for an accurate definition on multiple stages in the narrative transaction .... (See above 8).... Narrative empathy's shared feeling enables a reader or viewer to contagiously experience the emotions and sensations of a representation. It is intensified by the core affects of narrativity, so that readers or viewers may feel, for example, that the curiosity experienced by a detective in a mystery novel mirrors their own drive to figure out "whodunit?" Suspenseful narratives may make readers feel breathless, and we may even experience the "bodily matching" of our racing heart as a response to heightened suspense. Yet an important principle in the study of narrative form and its various impacts holds that we should not blend the effects of form and theme as if they were causally linked. A reader does not *have to* empathize with the detective's curiosity in order to experience the narrative affect of curiosity about "what's next." Indeed, the core affects of narrativity often operate along sympathetic lines: a character feels scared, while a reader shares in the suspense without becoming actively fearful. Perhaps most obviously of all, the reader may be surprised by a narrator's revelation of something about a character or plot that wouldn't be surprising at all to the fictive individuals within the story world.

...

Authors' empathy appears to be involved in the creative process for writers, dramatists, film-makers and other narrative artists, including life-writers. This comes into play during the daydreaming imagining that may precede or accompany composition. One way in which it may be exhibited is through autobiographical representations, that is, when a writer self-narrates. I am not a life-writer myself, but I am a sometime poet, and I think that as a writer one can sometimes engage in acts of memory of a past self that empathize with that earlier person, but that our memories of our past selves may just as readily feel estranged, embarrassed for, or even alienated from that younger person. I employ Dorrit Cohn's terminology of dissonant or consonant narration to suggest the distance (or closeness) between the narrating self and experiencing self that is the object of the narration. Even in life writing (or in my writerly experience the poetry of personal memory) an author's empathy with her subject is not automatic. It is not the only rhetorical stance that a writer may wish to deploy. There is some evidence that successful creators of *fictional* worlds and their imaginary inhabitants may simply be more highly empathetic individuals, when measured against the general population. Whether lifewriters (historians, biographers, memoirists, and journalists involved in creating *testimonio*) are also more highly empathic than the general population is an open question. This would be a promising research question to be taken up by scholars seeking a project. Consulting the letters, writing journals, and interviews of writers can reveal traces of evidence about authors' empathy, although a researcher must always remain attentive to the context, especially in the case of interviews. It would be no surprise to discover Oprah Winfrey eliciting confessions of empathy from authors, since this influential tastemaker places a high value on empathy and coaches her wide viewership to read empathetically. Narrative empathy has a reputation for enhancing a work's sales, in part as a result of Winfrey's advocacy. Narrative empathy can also accomplish a great deal more in its readers than just stimulating an appetite for more reading if a writer chooses to unleash its power. Authors can employ narrative empathy *strategically* in order to reach different audiences with specific hoped-for results in mind. On reflection, and in response to Leah Anderst's challenge, I concur that a lot of life writing vividly illustrates the use of "strategic narrative empathy," a concept I have previously theorized and summarize here in order to consider how it might function in nonfiction.

Authors' efforts to use strategic narrative empathy show their ambition to reach target audiences with representations that sway the feelings of their readers (Keen, "Strategic" 478–80; see Chapter 2 above) .... Sometimes motivated by the desire to effect social change or raise awareness, narrative artists employ representational techniques aimed at moving their readers ... quite vividly ... in works of life writing, and especially in *testimonio*. This is especially the case in nonfiction narratives that link up with the advancement of human rights ....

...

Let me just broach one example by referring to a powerful work of *testimonio*, Dave Eggers' *What Is the What* (2006), which relates the story of Valentino Achack Deng, one of the Sudanese Lost Boys. Will its evident ambassadorial empathy, which includes on its last page a direct address to its contemporary reader, still work in another generation when the Lost Boys are gone? Does nonfiction that employs ambassadorial empathy for a contemporary purpose gain power in the historical moment of its publication?—do its readers actually act, taking steps to support the charitable organization promoted in the novel? Then, what happens as time passes? Does ambassadorial empathy expire and cease to evoke an emotional response after the immediate context no longer pertains? Do we read old life writing the same way that we read fiction—*more empathetically* because we can't be asked to act? Or does the real-world referentiality of new or recent life writing reinforce our empathetic and altruistic response?

As I explain in *Narrative Form*, the term altruism was coined by Auguste Comte to describe other-directed reflective emotions that lead to our working on behalf of others, with ethical consequences. [see Keen, "'Altruism'."] Today it is considered the costliest form of pro-social behavior, as the altruist acts on behalf of another at some personal cost or risk. Because real-life empathy has been linked to altruism, many people believe that narrative empathy works the same way (see Keen, "Altruism Makes a Space for Empathy"). This belief motivates many arguments about the potential impact of emotionally engaging narratives (*Narrative Form* 160–1), arguments that may have a special legitimacy when referring to life writing that comes out of contemporary circumstances which can be directly addressed, whether personally or politically.

For example, Kay Schaffer and Sidonie Smith argue that as personal narratives about human rights abuses raise the consciousness of an expanding world readership, these texts can "prompt acts of engagement with persons having experienced rights abuses" (226). However, I have previously observed, for the writer or maker, deploying narrative emotions can be a high-stakes gamble, asking if the tactic of evoking readers' or viewers' emotions works reliably? Furthermore, does it work as a driver of desirable social change? (Keen, *Narrative Form* 161). In Rachel Ablow's account, "Much of the work that has been published since the 1970s has been rather more skeptical regarding the progressive potential of literary emotion" (301); Lauren Berlant criticizes authors who make emotional appeals to compassion as a spur for political action or social change (2–4). I have also expressed skepticism about the idea that narrative empathy is strongly linked to real-life altruism. The purported impact of narrative empathy on readers' or viewers' subsequent selfless behavior on behalf of others is in fact a good subject for future research into narrative impact. It would be especially interesting to know whether the responses set off by such paratextual labels as "fiction" or "nonfiction" result in different levels of helping behavior, or impulses towards altruism, in readers who experience empathy. I am also very curious as to whether the nonfictional frame of life writing alters the duration of the emotional impact that a text can have over the years. For surely at least one kind of strategic narrative empathizing should survive the passing of time.

. . .

PART II
Empathetic Readers

Empathetic Readers

All the essays reproduced in this section reflect my continuing interest in real readers, whom I theorize as active co-creators of the texts that they read, following Louise Rosenblatt. Very often, when literary critics refer to "the reader," they mean either the implied reader projected by the text under discussion, or they mean an entity quite like themselves, to whom they attribute their own responses and interpretations. Readers' empathy can't be experienced by textual projections, so my discussion of implied readers focuses on what a text appears to invite when empathy-evoking techniques appear in it. Furthermore, a singular empathetic response, even one felt by a smart and sensitive critic, shouldn't be regarded as a universal, predictable, or even a common result of reading a text that invites empathy. In the essays collected here I advance arguments intended to develop improved understanding of the impact of narrative fiction on diverse actual readers.

The opening essay excerpted in this section, "Intersectional Narratology," offers an argument about the multiple competing identities of real readers, which requires a method that can accommodate the different directions and locations of a rich set of texts, contexts, and identities while framing global hypotheses about the workings of narrative in the world. This approach emphasizes the complex overlays of narrative form, contexts of creation and reception, and identity that work together to provoke diverse responses to narrative. The influence that readers' differing identities have on their responses to fiction, especially the fictional characters with whom they empathize, is my subject in two essays, "Empathy in Reading: Considerations of Gender and Ethnicity," and "Readers' Temperaments and Fictional Character."

DOI: 10.4324/9781003264071-8

A core part of my argument in *Empathy and the Novel* cast doubt on the moral philosophical contention that empathy felt in response to fiction reading leads reliably to altruistic action in the real world. "Novel Reading and the Empathetic Angel of our Nature" extends that argument in a response to Steven Pinker's ideas about the improvement, over millennia, of human beings' treatment of one another. In his book *The Better Angels of Our Nature: Why Violence has Declined* (2011), Pinker describes a cultural shift, especially since the Enlightenment, towards greater empathy and improved human rights practices. To be clear, Pinker does not place much weight on the rise of the novel as a contributing cause. My essay reopens the matter of the psychology's empathy-altruism hypothesis, applied by analogy to narrative empathy felt in response to novel reading. Reviewing the available evidence for narrative impact that might contribute in the long run to the cultivation of good world citizens and the development of nonviolent societies, I inject a note of caution into the hopeful argument that novel reading helps form a more altruistic and peaceable citizenry.

As all of the essays excerpted in this section emphasize that the study of real readers' behavior, especially the long-term impact of reading on people's beliefs and behavior, will require further research, careful experimental design, and rigorous theorizing.

6

FROM INTERSECTIONAL NARRATOLOGY IN THE STUDY OF NARRATIVE EMPATHY

This essay seeks to explore why further understanding narrative empathy requires adoption of an *intersectional narratology*, a method that can accommodate the different directions and locations of a rich set of texts, contexts, and identities while framing global observations about the workings of narrative in the world. Since exploration of narrative empathy takes place at an interdisciplinary crossing point (of literary studies and psychology), a communication challenge deriving from competing definitions of the term "empathy" often arises. The legitimacy of the kind of intersectional research I propose in this essay depends upon baseline terminological clarity, a clarity that rarely exists when scholars from different disciplinary contexts discuss empathy. To reach that end of greater clarity about the disparate phenomena discussed under the label of empathy, I discuss here psychologist C. Daniel Batson's authoritative description of different concepts called empathy. Because Batson, a preeminent figure in the field of empathy research, does not comment on empathy for nonexistent beings, I further extend each concept to gloss its application to the study of narrative empathy. Further communication across disciplinary lines can be improved if parties know which version of "empathy" we mean when we write and speak about it.

Two other terms demand immediate attention: *intersectional* and *narratology*. Robyn Warhol has urged feminist critics to "take what Kimberlé Crenshaw named an 'intersectional' approach because white privilege, class privilege, heteronormativity, and other positions of relative power complicate hierarchies of gender" ("Feminist" 9). Though Warhol makes a strong case that feminist narratology has already branched out to "include race, sexuality, nationality, class, and ethnicity as well as gender, the components of intersectional analyses" ("Feminist Approach" 9), she prefers the term "narrative theories" to narratology because it "still connotes for many a theoretical approach cut off from questions of history

DOI: 10.4324/9781003264071-9

and context" (9). I pitch my tent on the ground of postclassical narratology, which opens "the fairly focused and restricted realm of narratology to methodological, thematic, and contextual influences" (Alber and Fludernik 9). Postclassical narratology has been profoundly shaped by feminist narrative theory. Its transdisciplinary embrace of cognitive and affective theories of narrative also makes it accommodating to a developing theory of narrative empathy.... (See above 8). In this essay I suggest how an intersectional narratology necessarily complicates research questions about narrative empathy, in the end strengthening conclusions we may draw about its formal techniques, its impact on readers, and its effect on real-world changes in attitudes and behavior.

... Intersectionality, a feminist concept examining "the relationships among multiple dimensions and modalities of social relations and subject formations" (McCall 1771), meshes well with a narrative poetics that is open to diverse effects of narrative techniques in various texts, contexts, and modes, following Meir Sternberg ("Proteus"). Like intersectional analyses of discrimination (Crenshaw), for which the concept was first formulated, my version of intersectional narratology seeks to understand why certain positions and concepts are privileged while others suffer from inattention or disparagement. In her foundational rendering of feminist intersectionality for narrative theory, Susan S. Lanser emphasizes the discernment of the way "systemic, structural, and institutional 'traffic.' ... operates to the advantage or disadvantage of individuals and groups according to their social positioning" ("Are We There Yet" 34) .... [I]ntersectional narratology need not aim primarily at uncovering discriminatory representations, but may also focus on the status of the representational vehicles carrying meanings. It thus extends the feminist project of scrutinizing non-mainstream texts to complicate observations based on a limited canon.

In its application to narrative empathy, intersectional narratology enables discussion of the complex overlays of narrative form, contexts of creation and reception, and identity that work together to provoke diverse responses to narrative, among divergent readers of a wide variety of texts. It complicates rather than schematizing, and it risks proliferation of axes rather than insisting on neat taxonomies. It still remains narratology as long as it seeks evidence of impact of narrative techniques, manifestations of theme in form, and as long as it discerns dominant, residual, and emergent forms in historical contexts. As Lanser writes, intersectional feminism "can now map and be mapped by narrative patterns across time and space, accounting for vectors of difference to create a narratology that is deeply locational and therefore cross-cultural and historical" (32). An intersectional narratology would skeptically examine claims for universal impacts of narrative techniques, but it would welcome evidence that shows the narrative arts contributing to an expanded empathetic circle, especially if that extension benefited vulnerable members of disparaged outgroups. For when narrative empathy reaches across boundaries of difference, geographical and temporal distance, to evoke shared feeling, what—if anything—happens as a result? Propositions, derived from the science of real-life empathy, include changed attitudes, greater tolerance, reduced fear of the other, and increased helping behavior or altruism.

An intersectional narratology brought to bear on narrative empathy extends rhetorical narratology's interest in transactions between authors and readers, makers and audiences, emphasizing the challenges to theorizing of substantial differences among real human beings. Yet it also accommodates a sense of shared human experiences derived from the behavioral sciences, where much of the empirical work on empathy has been carried out. The psychology of narrative impact examines ranges of possibilities, discovers clusters of frequent experiences, and records outliers among readers' responses to emotionally evocative texts. These empirical techniques support intersectional narratology's project of discerning differences stemming from multiple competing axes of identity and experience in subjects. I concur with Lanser that "the *articulation* of women—and men—into distinct pluralities opens multiple new avenues for historical, cross-cultural, and intra-cultural inquiry" (33; emphasis in original). Intersectional narratology enables the theorist to employ markers of identity, technique, or impact derived from contextual, feminist, and queer narrative theories, rather than sticking to a single binary contrast. The emergent queer narratology has already usefully complicated the binary starting point of much early feminist narrative theory. Further openness to the multiple intersecting axes of readers' subject positions and the protean possibilities of narrative techniques (Sternberg) characterizes intersectional narratology. This makes it especially adaptable to the study of narrative empathy. Just as empathy involves both affective and cognitive responses, the study of narrative empathy inquires how the blend of affective *feeling with* and cognitive accuracy in mind-reading relates to multiple aspects of readers,' characters' and authors' identities.

Empathy: What It Is and What It Does

In contemporary discourse, empathy has many definitions, components, and roles to play in accounts of human emotional responsiveness, communication, social behavior, and altruism. It is one of the factors, for instance, attributed to the decline of violence against women (Pinker, *Better Angels* 409–15) and gays (447–54) in the latter part of the twentieth century and in the early decades of the twenty-first century. C. Daniel Batson, one of the most influential authorities on empathy in psychology, has recently highlighted eight of the possible phenomena known as empathy, as the term is currently used in psychology and to a lesser degree in philosophy (see Wispé). His essay represents an important disentangling of competing meanings that imply different research methodologies and assumptions about empathy's real-world impact. Here as in subsequent paragraphs, I extrapolate from Batson's real-world empathy between human subjects to narrative empathy, where some of the agents involved are made out of words. Discussions of narrative empathy ought to establish firmly to which version of empathy they correlate, and this discussion should make that definitional task easier for intersectional narrative theorists to accomplish. Although only some of the phenomena listed by Batson are obviously involved in narrative empathy, where the eliciting prompt of empathetic feeling is a construct or effect of narrative (including fictions) rather than another actual person in the real world, a review of the phenomena using Batson's categories freshens our sense of their links to literary response as well as their inherent complexity. This complexity encourages the development of an intersectional narratology, especially as it pertains to narrative's impact on vulnerable populations. An intersectional narratology would skeptically examine claims for universal impacts of narrative techniques, but it would welcome evidence that shows the narrative arts contributing to an expanded empathetic circle.

Batson's overview of the eight psychological states that correspond to different versions of empathy begins with a cognitive definition, "Concept 1: Knowing Another Person's Internal State, Including His or Her Thoughts and Feelings" (4). Sometimes called cognitive empathy, this phenomenon has been studied by William Ickes for its degree of successful mind-reading, or "empathic accuracy" ("Empathic Accuracy" 57), since most humans estimate with relative ease what a person close to them is thinking or feeling, in everyday mind-reading. For narratologists, knowledge of internal states correlates with matters of narrative situation and narratorial reliability or unreliability. An intersectional narratologist might investigate whether the age, gender, ethnicity, and literary experience of a reader makes a difference in the response to a first-person narrator such as Katniss Everdeen in Suzanne Collins's *Hunger Games* trilogy (2008–10). In a recent discussion, an 11-year-old girl resonated with the emotions of narrativity, especially curiosity and suspense. She took Katniss's narration at her word. An 18-year-old young woman in the same conversation felt no sympathy, distrusted Katniss's self-reports, and reported a cooler response to the narration. The 18-year-old was alert to the gaps in Katniss's (a consonant narrator's) own self-knowledge, which had a distancing effect for her. Would an olive-skinned reader, or one who had lost a parent in an industrial accident, recognize Katniss's internal states more readily? A larger and more diverse sample of readers could help an intersectional narratologist test some of the many existing suppositions about conditions that increase the likeliness of cognitive empathy.

For narratologists concerned with form, questions about cognitive empathy and narrative technique often suppose differing impact of first- and third-person narration. In narrative empathy for fictional constructs, I have argued, empathic accuracy for characters can be vouchsafed by third-person narrators' representation of characters' consciousness (*Empathy and the Novel* 136). When a narrator generalizes in a reliable fashion about a character's thoughts and feelings, using psycho-narration, readers have little reason to doubt it. Similarly, in fiction employing either quoted (interior) monologue or narrated monologue (free indirect discourse), in which the words of the characters' thoughts appear, narrative empathic accuracy will be high. However, the potential that Batson acknowledges, that "you could be wrong, at least about some nuances and details" (4), increases radically in less reliable first-person-narrative situations (Keen, *Empathy and the Novel* 137), or when readers bring their individual preferences, memories, experiences, predictions, fantasies, and feelings to the task of co-creating fictional characters by filling in the gaps (Keen, "Readers'" 295–6). Thus experiences of narrative empathy, which cannot be verified by cross-checking with real people about their actual feelings, involve greater likelihood of what I have named *narrative empathic inaccuracy*, the strong conviction in reader's empathy that divergently attributes emotion or state of mind to a fictional persona, at cross purposes with an author's apparent intentions (*Empathy and the Novel* 137).

Batson's second concept, "Adopting the Posture or Matching the Neural Responses of an Observed Other," refers to the rapid, automatic, and unconscious mimicry of others' bodily or facial positions ("These Things" 4). Some psychologists believe that the neural substrates of this widespread animal behavior underpin other more cognitive, conscious forms of empathy in humans, though not necessarily to higher-order concern, sympathy, or altruism (Blair and Blair 139). Motor mimicry in an audience certainly occurs during dramatic productions, in film viewing (such as facial close-ups or action sequences of acrobatic parkour), and probably in response to graphic narrative representations of nonhuman characters (Keen, "Fast Tracks" 135, 137). As Batson comments, "the problem of anthropomorphism arises precisely because we humans have the ability—and inclination—to make such inferences" about what others think and feel, "even about other species" ("These Things" 5). It is possible that descriptions of characters' disposition in space in imagined locations of prose or verse fictional storyworlds call upon readers' motor mimicry. Reports of painful bodily experiences or descriptions of dysphoric facial expressions, even of fictional characters, can elicit physical responses in the reader's own body (Warhol, *Having* 62–63). Though often regarded as a behavior of sentimental women responding to affecting stories (Radway, *Reading the Romance*), such experiences are also reported by male readers. When my husband read John Muir's account of Mr. Young hanging from a cliff in Alaska with dislocated arms (40–1), he grunted aloud and adjusted his own shoulders to make sure they were still in their sockets. Does a gender difference between reader and protagonist alter the degree of motor mimicry experienced when reading a novel such as *The Hunger Games*? When Collins manipulates the pace of her narration, employing expansion as Katniss stands immobilized on the metal circle at the start of the games for 60 seconds (148–9), do readers' differing axes of identity, including experiences of timed athletic contests, alter their degree of motor mimicry? Pace of reading, heart rate, sweating, and visible signs of bodily posture alteration could all be studied with the assistance of a psychologist.

Concept 3 of Batson's survey addresses the more affective element of emotion-matching and emotion-catching: "Coming to Feel as Another Person Feels" ("These Things" 5). Identifying this well-documented aspect of human behavior as *emotional contagion* suggests that the same feeling spreads from person to person, whereas the older terminology of sympathy, dating back to David Hume and Adam Smith's influential eighteenth-century accounts, does not demand an exact match in feelings. (Hume and Smith do also describe instances of motor mimicry under discussion of sympathy, compassion, and fellow feeling). Since empathy in some contexts appears as a virtual synonym of sympathy, this concept clearly has a literary history (Keen, *Empathy and the Novel* 39–55). The version of emotion-catching and matching that Batson describes comes closer to empathy as theorized by the neuroscience of mirror neurons, comprising a shared manifold for intersubjectivity (Gallese, "Roots" 171). Mirror neurons work quickly, giving an onlooker a fast physiological version of the observed subject's action, expression, or feeling. That is, if humans have a mirror neuron system like other primates, then witnessing or even hearing about another's feelings may prompt fast emotion-matching and catching without an extensive educational process. This kind of empathy and its narrative correlate could be studied by adepts in neural imaging. To what degree biological differences among subjects, let alone social and cultural aspects of identity, alter this affective emotion-matching is an open question. Intersectional narratology could focus on contentions that appear in essentialist binary formulations, such as the argument that female readers are more empathetic than men. (The culturally promulgated assumption that women are more empathetic than men [Baron-Cohen 1–2] is not borne out when physiological measures of empathy are employed [Lennon and Eisenberg 197, 203]. Cognitive science on gender difference in empathy affirms that men and women have equal empathic capacities, and acknowledges that sufficient motivation to accurately read others' thoughts and feelings alters performance, which accounts for perceptions of gender differences in empathy if females are more motivated by gender-role expectations than most males [Ickes et al. 107–8].)

The remaining concepts enumerated by Batson more obviously correlate with aspects of narrative empathy. Batson's concept 4 draws on the original meaning of empathy as a translation of *Einfühlung*, as theorized by late nineteenth- and early twentieth-century aesthetics: "Intuiting or Projecting Oneself into Another's Situation," as Batson describes aesthetic empathy (6). Batson pushes the definition towards human perspective-taking, lightly glossing the target of *Einfühlung* as "some inanimate object, such as a gnarled, dead tree on a windswept hillside" (5). Aesthetic empathy remains an important effect of fictional storyworlds. Fiction readers and writers know that setting can evoke narrative empathy, both through its connection with a human perspective and through a feeling for the landscape, buildings, rocks, and trees. Suzanne Collins opens the last novel of trilogy, *Mockingjay* (2010), with a prompt to *Einfühlung*:

> I stare down at my shoes, watching as a fine layer of ash settles on the worn leather. This is where the bed I shared with my sister, Prim, stood. Over there was the kitchen table. The bricks of the chimney, which collapses in

> a charred heap, provide a point of reference for the rest of the house. How else could I orient myself in this sea of gray?
>
> Almost nothing remains of District 12.
>
> (3)

The disorienting ruins of the firebombed house and its surrounding mining town employ the association of a human-built environment with human culture (hearth and home), as well as with the missing people. Though the passage alludes to family, Collins directs the reader's attention to the fate of destroyed objects. Although a reader who has gone through a house fire or aerial bombardment would possess empathetic reference points for this scene, the gray ash alludes to the televised scenes of the aftermath of the Towers' collapse in the 9/11 attack. (In 2001, Collins's original readers were between five and ten years old.) Do readers who remember 9/11 more readily make this poetic connection? As Rae Greiner has recently argued, the "the formal protocols of empathy align with those of poetry" (420), actively relating the *unalike* human perceiver and inanimate object of perception, analogously with metaphor: "With its fusion of subject and object, empathy accomplished the work of metaphor, while sympathy, with its emphasis on context—one's adjacency to or distance from others with whom one does not merge—calls the attributes of metonymy to mind" (421). It will take a serious effort to resuscitate psychologists' interest in the early twentieth-century version of aesthetic empathy. Batson dismisses it: "Such projection is rarely what is meant by empathy in contemporary psychology" (6). However, for literary studies, *Einfuhlung* has a specific literary history, from Vernon Lee's early theorizing to the mid-twentieth-century work of romanticist Richard Harter Fogle to recent work by Greiner. (Greiner persuasively argues that the realist novel's representational aims accord more with *sympathy* than with empathy). Congruently, in contemporary neuroscience, the study of brain response to verbal directional prompts may provide a basis for understanding how empathy for things and others rests on a foundation of physical orientation (Zwaan and Taylor). This has a bearing on some of the most vivid effects of fictional storyworlds on aesthetic empathy in immersion reading. For example, studies of the effects of video games suggest that moving in the three-dimensional space of the game may activate spatial orientation mirror neurons (Tajerian).

Deliberate perspective taking, or in Batson's terms for concept 5, "Imagining How Another Is Thinking and Feeling" (7), involves sensitivity to another's point of view. Related to the aesthetic projection of *Einfühlung* (concept 4), but moving away from inanimate targets, the "imagine other" condition of empathy involves one person's "feeling into" another's thoughts and feelings. This definition of empathy focuses on the other person, with an awareness of the separate being of that individual. Rather than experiencing emotional fusion with the other, the empath who engages in perspective taking employs observation of the other and knowledge of that person. Empathy in this sense is a more obviously cognitive operation that depends on having a theory of (another's) mind (ToM). For narrative theorists exploring the phenomenon of character identification, this mode of empathy transposes quite neatly to the kind of narrative empathy that follows on effortful attention to a fictional character's actions, circumstances, speech, represented thoughts, and reported or inferred motives. Much (but not all) of the philosophy of empathy refers to perspective taking (see Coplan and Goldie).

The closely related concept 6, "Imagining How One Would Think and Feel in the Other's Place" (Batson 7), also receives emphasis in philosophical accounts of empathy, in part because of its appearance in Adam Smith's *A Theory of Moral Sentiments* (1759) under the older term sympathy. This version of empathy is also cognitive (since it involves active imagining), but it is rooted in role-taking (putting oneself in the shoes of another) rather than taking the perspective of that person. It answers the question *How would* I *feel?* rather than *How does* s/he *feel?* Batson notes that the "imagine-self perspective is in some ways similar to the act of projecting oneself into another's situation" (concepts 4 and 5), but asserts that the two stances should not be confused, as "the self remains more focal here than in aesthetic projection" (7). Like perspective-taking empathy, role-taking empathy is likely to be involved in readers' experiences of narrative empathy. Indeed, many readers reporting strong sensations of character identification phrase their experiences in terms of how they would feel themselves in the position of the character. Some theorists of narrative empathy regard this form of empathy as more "categorical," more dependent on matches with the self and group identity, and therefore less other-directed and less likely to lead to the ethical expression of compassion than "situational" empathy (Hogan, "Epilogue" 134–36), which is closer to perspective taking (Batson 7, concept 5). An intersectional approach to experimental design might well be able to examine these possibilities, which have been theorized but not subjected to empirical testing.

If role taking is more egotistical than perspective taking, personal distress is more self-focused than either. Personal distress is an empathic reaction that focuses on one's own sensations to the point of diverting attention from the suffering other's experience. As concept 7, Batson describes it as "Feeling Distress at Witnessing Another Person's Suffering" (7). As Batson explains it, personal distress expresses not feelings *for* (sympathy) or feelings *like* the other's feelings (empathy as defined by concepts 1–6), but "feeling distressed *by* the state of the other" (Batson 8; emphasis in original). Personal distress as described by developmental psychologist Nancy Eisenberg is an aversive emotional response that leads to avoidance. It can have little to tell students of narrative empathy, since true aversion leads to cessation of the reading or viewing that evokes the response (Keen, *Empathy and the Novel* 4–5). Many younger readers of Suzanne Collins's *Hunger Games* abandoned *Mockingjay*, the third novel of the trilogy, in which representations of violence escape the game arena and take over the primary fictional world. Collins's interrogation of just-war theory and her unsparing account of the costs of violent resistance to an unjust regime drive many of her young readers away. If the ability to be transported by fiction is one of the key precursors to narrative empathy, then proneness to personal distress rather than other-oriented empathy may become an obstacle to immersion reading. The effects of personal distress continue when the reading is not abandoned. Educational circumstances that compel reading of an upsetting fiction or viewing of a distressing film to continue in the face of an aversive response can block the impulse to get away from the stimulus, but they cannot dictate a spirit of receptiveness or openness in readers and viewers (see chapter 4 above).

Batson's eighth and final concept will be familiar to literary scholars, for it is best known as sympathy, with an emphasis on the feeling component rather than the cognitive knowing another's perspective described in concept 6. "Feeling for Another Person Who Is Suffering" (Batson 8), or for the fictive equivalents of persons in narrative, has been discussed under the older terms pity, compassion, fellow feeling, and sympathy. Related to empathy in some social psychology as the concerned outcome of an other-oriented feeling *for* another, empathic concern expresses an appropriately "congruent" emotion that needs to match the other's feeling exactly: feeling sorry for a frightened person or gratified for a joyful person would exhibit sympathy. Many philosophers regard sympathy as an ethical expression of what begins as empathy, a more mature and other-directed concern than the motor mimicry, emotional contagion, or feeling-matching that Batson describes in concepts 1 through 3. As a goal of fictive representation, sympathy has had a prominent role to play in literature, with important statements in its favor by Henry Home, Lord Kames, Percy Bysshe Shelley, and George Eliot (Keen, *Empathy and the Novel* 44–55) and historic exhibits in the narratives of George Eliot, James Joyce, Harper Lee, Doris Lessing, Maya Angelou, Toni Morrison, and hundreds if not thousands of other novelists. Some influential commentators on the social impact of the realist novel persistently refer to its *empathy*-inducing qualities (Hunt 27–34; Nussbaum, *Cultivating* 90; Pinker, *Better* 177). It must be acknowledged, however, that to the perpetual bedevilment of those who would distinguish empathy from sympathy, the terms have often been conflated or reversed. As Keith Oatley, an expert guide to the emotions involved in fiction reading, remarks, in his *Such Stuff as Dreams: The Psychology of Fiction*, "In modern usage, sympathy is generally taken as separate from empathy (feeling with), and usually means feeling for someone in their predicament" (118). Oatley associates literary experiences of character identification with empathy, and readers' recollection of emotional memories with sympathy (126), and I concur with that difference, although I think that character identification does not inevitably lead to empathy (or vice versa).

Strangely, Batson does not address fantasy empathy. One of the most widely used empathy scales is Mark Davis's Interpersonal Reactivity Index, or IRI (Davis, "Multidimensional" 85). Davis's multidimensional scale includes subscales measuring personal distress, empathic concern, perspective-taking, and fantasy empathy.

The fantasy empathy subscale measures subjects' "tendency to imaginatively transpose" themselves "into fictional situations" (Davis, *Empathy* 57). David acknowledges that fantasy empathy exhibits congruence with perspective taking (58) but rightly insists that the questions elicit experiences of "imagining oneself in the place of *fictitious* characters appearing in books, movies, and plays" (58; emphasis mine), a key difference often glossed over in discussions of narrative empathy's relation to altruism or prosocial behavior. (While Martha Nussbaum asserts that experiences of narrative empathy [with the right kind of novels] will produce good world citizens [90], other theorists find examples of the prosocial impact of empathy in fiction itself. For example, see Hoffman (225), where he uses the actions of fictional characters engaged in altruistic acts to demonstrate the efficacy of empathy).

. . .

Theoretical Intersections in Narrative Empathy

Batson's disentangling of empathy-related concepts reveals the complexities of empathy research. Even under the big umbrella of "psychology," the study of empathy can involve expertise in both affect and cognition. The neural substrate and chemical bases of empathic responses have been studied by neuroscientists, while social and developmental psychologists have charted much of empathy's roles in social behavior and moral development. Philosophers in a variety of traditions (ethics, moral sentimentalism, utilitarianism, aesthetics) have theorized empathy, sometimes in collaboration with cognitive scientists or developmental and social psychologists. The study of empathy is automatically interdisciplinary, even if not all empathy researchers undertake the task of answering questions and posing problems that navigate disciplinary boundaries. As relative latecomers (or belated returners) to the scientific and scholarly conversation about empathy, literary theorists find some assumptions congenial and some alien, some conclusions predictable and some startling, some running counter to our own disciplinary commitments, some affirming our beliefs, and some challenging our deepest convictions. Developing an intersectional narratology will assist researchers in the discovering and disseminating findings about narrative empathy in an interdisciplinary field.

For instance, while studying narrative empathy as a feature of immersion fiction reading, junctions of narratology, feminism, affective studies, and cognitive science could help us answer how, under which circumstances, and in response to which techniques, individuals as distinct from one another as we are can experience the emotional fusion and intense recognition of shared feeling. Introspective testimony from readers and viewers who have experienced narrative empathy (or not!) in response to an emotionally evocative text should receive our respectful attention, but we should not make the error of mistaking our own intense reading experiences for universal or predictive phenomena. They are instead starting points for an intersectional narratology of narrative impact. Thus variable cultural contexts, individual differences among people, readers' temperamental dispositions, as well as their gender and sexual orientation, would emerge from the brackets into which classical narratology placed all evidence about actual audiences. Though this procedure would render the convenient construct "the reader" irreducibly complex, fluid, and extremely resistant to simplification and schematization, it would encourage confidence in future discoveries about narrative empathy.

Intersectional narratology participates in the extension of feminist narratology's project, responding to Ruth Page's challenge: "To make a more convincing discussion of the ways in which gender might intersect with the characteristics of narrative form, considerably more empirical data are needed, about the tellers and receivers as well as the tales themselves" ("Feminist narratology?" 52–3). This data originates from many sources, including the work of David S. Miall, Melanie Green, Raymond Mar, and their collaborators. Literary scholars have begun and should continue the project of communicating their empirical findings, as well as collaborating with researchers in other disciplines. So, for instance, empathetic effects of narrative have been evaluated by means of experiments in discourse processing, in the psychology of narrative impact, and through philosophical introspection, but the conflicting data on gender and empathy have not yet been systematically investigated with respect to either literary responses of female and male audiences or gendered narrative forms (more common in psychology is the opposite effort, to control for gender rather than contrasting male and female responses).

Among other questions, the relation of narrative empathy to altered attitudes and prosocial action in the real world, often theorized by philosophers such as Martha Nussbaum, deserves the respect of experimental scrutiny. Research in neuroscience, cognitive science, developmental psychology, and discourse processing has advanced our knowledge of both empathy and narrative empathy, but much remains to be discovered. Regarding narrative, Fong and Mar remark, "empirical research investigating the social outcomes of reading is in its infancy" (61). Regarding empathy, two of the neuroscientists who have extended our understanding of its neural substrate enumerate the gaps: "A second big issue is the link between empathic brain responses and sympathy or compassion, that is, feeling *as* and feeling *for* the other. Thirdly, it is an open question how empathic brain responses relate to prosocial motivation and behavior and finally, almost nothing is known about the plasticity of the empathic brain, that is, about the trainability of empathy and compassionate motivation, all issues that should have considerable practical impacts on society" (Hein and Singer, "I feel" 157). Note that these scientists point out what is *not known* about the chain of responses reputed to exist between empathy and sympathy and empathy and altruism, let alone how those relations change when empathy, in psychology's empathy-altruism relation, is replaced by *narrative* empathy. Literary scholars and reception theorists can add nuance to the discussion of empathy-inducing texts, which have often been hedged about with canonical barriers that suggest only the most high literary narratives can have ethical effects. What if escapist reading also benefits readers by shifting perspectives, opening up attitudes, and prompting more generous feelings and actions toward others? The answers to these research questions about narrative empathy will be of immediate interest to many, including feminist and queer theorists, who hope to show how narrative literature, broadly defined, can expand the empathetic circle in the real world.

A conjunction of cognitive narratology, feminism, and affective studies occurs when studying narrative empathy: whenever we ask how, under which circumstances, and in response to which techniques, beings so different from one another as we are can experience the emotional fusion and intense recognition of shared feeling mediated by fiction .... [N]arrative empathy felt and exercised by makers (novelists, graphic narrative artists, filmmakers, the amateur videographers of the "It Gets Better" project) motivates fictional and nonfictional utterances aimed at specific target audiences ....

Matters of identity, experience, and context combine with the possibilities enabled by readers' and viewers' embodied minds to condition potential responses to the invitations of narrative technique (Keen, "Readers' Temperaments"). In novels, stories, and film fictions, narrative empathy overarches narratological categories: a range of techniques might be operating at once to produce the likelihood of empathy. It can involve fictional characters; point of view and narrative situation; handling of pace, duration, and seriality; and storyworld features such as settings. An intersectional narratology begins with some contextual premises: the willingness to combine inquiry about a narrative technique—for instance use of a second-person "you" narration—with data from outside the text. Does familiarity with the conventions of 1930s documentary films, which commonly address the viewer, train a reader to accept a "you" role as an addressee? Does a habit of playing Xbox Live with friends make a reader of fiction more flexible about the overlap in addressee and avatar in "you" narratives? In co-creating a "you" narration, does a queer reader feel more or less likely than a straight reader to naturalize it representationally into a "he" or "she," or do other experiences and aspects of identity complicate a queer/straight binary? Does a female and feminist reader accustomed to cross-reading books for boys more easily sustain the sense of "you" as narratee? Do any of these differences correlate with—or cause—heightened or diminished sensations of narrative empathy?

While classical narratology typically focused its attention on forms, techniques, taxonomies, and communication models, feminist narratology re-evaluates these theories in light of gender. This matters to a theory of narrative empathy not because empathy is an exclusively or especially female trait: it is not tied to biological sex. Males and females show similar ranges of empathic responsiveness on physiological measures (Lennon and Eisenberg 197, 203). Cultural contexts, however, can motivate the expression of empathic concern by females more than by males. The gendering of genre plays a role in reaching readers that have been acculturated to regard experiences of emotional fusion as desirable or as a response to be suppressed. This in turn has a bearing on the marketing and reception of emotionally evocative fiction. Gendered conventions that appeal to the ostensibly female, feeling reader or a male excitement-seeking reader thus make up a culture-bound component of narrative empathy. To return to my example of second-person narration, if gender is one of the axes of identity that orients readers' co-creation of fictional worlds, do female (or feminist) readers make feeling readers prone to identify with characters who look like, feel like, dress like, speak like "you"? Or is the word "you" enough all by itself to erase barriers of difference? A feminist narratologist, in cooperation with an analyst of discourse processing, or a psychologist of narrative impact, could design a study to find out. To my mind, devising those studies is preferable to simply believing that we already know the answers.

...

Seeing what isn't working the way we expect can lead to alternative explanations. So, for instance, the cultivation of the sympathetic imagination through rendered perspectives of fictional characters is a linchpin of narrative ethics. Yet cognitive scientific efforts to verify this theory by studying the empathetic impact of role-taking instructions during fiction reading have not yielded robust results. Cognitive science surprises us by showing instead that exercises in *visualizing mental imagery* more reliably produce empathetic effects and (short-term) helping behavior. In other words, a more vivid and absorbing storyworld, visualized in the mind's eye, may intensify the ethical effects of reading where the injunction to "walk in the shoes" of a character may not (Johnson, "Transportation" 150–5). Joining a fictional world as a temporary visitor may involve effects as robust as those often attributed to character identification.

One possible yield of experimental scrutiny could be the challenge to re-evaluate previously disparaged aspects of reading (such as escapism and fantasizing) as an aspect of narrative empathy. We could ask whether an experience of narrative empathy facilitates cross-reading over generic categories that usually imply a gendered readership, or other barriers to imaginative access to fictional worlds. We could discover whether narrative empathy felt for a minor character opens a path for critical resistant reading. We could extend the fascinating work begun by psychologist Shira Gabriel, in which she and her graduate student Ariana Young demonstrate that immersive reading of fantasies such as Stephenie Meyer's *Twilight* (2005) and J. K. Rowling's *Harry Potter* books (1997–2007) gives children the experience of belonging and thereby enhances empathy: "The current research suggests that books give readers more than an opportunity to tune out and submerge themselves in fantasy worlds. Books provide the opportunity for social connection and the blissful calm that comes from becoming a part of something larger than oneself for a precious, fleeting moment" (Gabriel and Young 993). [Not widely known outside of the psychology of emotion, the term *amae* describes the comforting feeling of attachment and belonging that receives more emphasis in collective cultures than in individualistic societies (Doi).] While *amae* and empathy are linked in some psychological studies of Japanese subjects, Gabriel and Young are the first to suggest the link as an effect of fiction reading. Their finding challenges hierarchies of literary quality and taste that would regard *Twilight* and *Harry Potter* as unlikely sources of socially beneficial reading experiences. An intersectional narratology could ask if the temporary shedding of identity that occurs when readers intermingle with fictive beings in fantasy worlds opens readers to empathy across social difference by way of *amae*. Freed from the strictures of representational identity aesthetics, we could admit that fans of *Twilight* include middle-aged moms and adult gay men as well as 13-year-old girls, and that they seek not images of themselves but to get out of this world (Blackford).

...

Reports from diverse readers make any discoveries about shared experiences or predictions about impact more persuasive. One critic's introspection about narrative impact on herself may begin the process of analysis, but one reader's impressions should not inevitably be construed as *the* reader. Thus, in applying intersectional narratology to narrative empathy, reports from more readers than one should be analyzed. This would obligate narrative theorists to attend to readings that may strike professional literary critics as erroneous. When the movie of *The Hunger Games* (2012) came out, a subset of young viewers objected in tweets to the film Rue, played by a young black actress ("Hunger Games Cast Subjected to Racist Attacks"). They had read Rue as white, having misread, skipped, or forgotten the clear descriptions in the novel that render Rue as having "bright, dark eyes and satiny brown skin" (*Hunger* 98). Their sympathy for the character, to whose death Katniss responds humanely and subversively, was disrupted by the accurate representation of her race. Intersectional study of this failure in strategic narrative empathy could address readers' and viewers' age, gender, race, reading level, skimming and skipping, and disposition to fantasy empathy. The condemnation of the evident racism of the young viewers' tweets does not help us understand how the novel permitted an empathetic response while the film blocked it.

Formalist analysis can and ought to intersect with accounts of the experiences of actual and various readers. Gender and sexual identity are among the conditioning factors that contribute to readers' collaboration in fictional worldmaking, but so are underlying temperaments and individual life experiences (Keen, "Readers'" 296). I recall here Eve Sedgwick's first axiom, "*People are different from each other*" (22, emphasis in original). Sedgwick saw women and queer and effeminate men as especially adept at "the refinement of necessary skills for making, testing, and using unrationalized and provisional hypotheses about what kinds of people there are to be found in one's world" (23). This observation suggests that feminist and queer readers (as well as women writers and gay and lesbian authors) cultivate skills of interpretation that can contribute to an intersectional narratology. Individual male straight readers, too, should be recognized as possessing differences that escape what Sedgwick castigated as "inconceivably coarse axes of categorization that have been painstakingly inscribed in current political and critical thought" (22). We *are* all different from one another, but in our embodied humanity we also share the narrative habit: stories are part of the natural habitat that we spin out of ourselves as we respond with emotion and calculation, moodily and rationally, to a world populated with other beings. Narratives are extraordinarily effective devices for opening the channel of fellow feeling and breaking through barriers of difference thrown up by distance, time, culture, experience.

7

FROM EMPATHY IN READING

Considerations of Gender and Ethnicity

Reader-response criticism meets intersectional narratology

Considerations of gender and, to a lesser degree ethnicity, have been associated with emotional reading habits for more than a century. The emotional reader, as opposed to the coolly rational evaluator of literary texts, has often been characterized as weepy, immersive, escapist, undiscriminating, voracious, and female (Warhol, *Having* 29, 48; Walsh "Why we Wept"). The ethnic reader—contrasted with an implicit white Western educated reader—appears either as an aspirational figure of the colonial world, modeling his reading on an imperial standard and yearning for escape from the margins (Naipaul, *A House for Mr. Biswas* [1961]) or as an injured party, shocked to find those like herself invisible, or dehumanized if represented at all in the pages of literature. [For instance, Jamaica Kincaid depicts and redresses such readerly experiences of erasure in many of her fictional and autobiographical works, such as *Mr. Potter* (2002).] These representational and critical phenomena have contributed to the disrepute of emotional reading habits in the twentieth and twenty-first centuries. The educated reader learns early to focus on theme, form, and theory, training that puts distance between naïve, emotional reading practices and approved literary critical discourse, especially when practiced at the university level. Meanwhile, because emotional reading habits are attributed to female and non-white readers—Oprah's readers—women critics and non-white academics may also shy away from reporting on the feeling of reading, to avoid being branded as middlebrow. Feminist critics, cultural theorists, and postcolonialists have been eager to dismantle the hierarchy of values implicit in denigration of feeling reading, but relatively few have been willing to risk endorsing the emotive, affective path. Hard-won equality in modes of reading and interpretation associated with New Critical close reading, formalism, Marxism,

DOI: 10.4324/9781003264071-10

structuralism, deconstruction, and high theoretical forms of post-structuralism has come at the cost (for female and non-white critics, as well as for working class white male critics) of disavowing emotionality.

The Affective Fallacy labeled and deprecated by Wimsatt and Beardsley in 1949 has had a very long run as an often repeated (less often examined) fundamental of literary-critical practice, warning students from confusing the poem with the results of reading the poem (21). Impressionism, relativism, and psychologizing the text seemed to mid-twentieth-century critics a risk of considering readers' responses. Even among reception theorists, we find defensiveness about a focus on the results of reading. Wolfgang Iser writes, "the reproach of the 'Affective Fallacy' cannot be applied to a theory of aesthetic response because such a theory is concerned with the structure of the 'performance', which precedes the effect" (Iser, *Act* 26–7). The emotionality of aesthetics as experienced by a subject encountering an artwork, theorized by Vernon Lee in the early twentieth century and rendered moribund by the formalisms of mid-century, was not resuscitated by an 'affective stylistics' which placed greater emphasis on textual cues than on unruly feelings of readers (Fish 123ff). As Steven Mailloux observes of Iserian reception theory and Fishian affective stylistics, "What becomes invisible in many such readings is the sociopolitical context constituting the reception of a text at particular historical moments. This form of reader criticism often assumed an ideal reader unencumbered by particular characteristics of class, occupation, race, nationality, gender, and age" (48). The informed reader's most important characteristic thus becomes a literary competence expressed by objectivity.

However, as Rita Felski has brilliantly demonstrated, even the most arid discourses of high-theoretical debate reveal emotional drives: to label an ardent feminist critique as symptomatic of the "hermeneutics of suspicion" is not to escape rhetoric driven by passion, nor pleasurable sensations (Felski, "Suspicious" 215–6). Furthermore, an affective turn can now be observed in many disciplines (Keen, "Introduction" 18–30). Philosophers (Dadlez; Feagin; Robinson, *Deeper*), neuroscientists (Damasio, *Descartes'*, Lane and Nadel), and even cognitive scientists (Mark Turner) have rehabilitated emotion as an aspect of rationality. The research programs that have opened up questions of affect allow a return to an area of reader-based theorizing that never entirely eschewed the feeling of reading: David Bleich's subjective criticism, which at least acknowledged gender as an aspect of reading, and Louise Rosenblatt's transactional theory of reading, which strongly emphasizes emotional responses of readers to literary texts. This chapter carries forward the project of analyzing readers' empathy (Keen, *Empathy and the Novel* 65–99) by means of an *intersectional narratology*, an analytic method that can accommodate a rich set of multiple, competing aspects of identity that provoke divergent responses to texts intended to evoke empathy (Keen, "Intersectional"; see chapter 6, above). The elevation of empathy as a desirable human quality causing improved concern for and action on behalf of others has encouraged claims that *narrative empathy* for fictional characters—including experiences of intense identification and emotion-sharing with bodily effects—leads to altruism. As I have earlier argued, narrative empathy evoked by fictional texts does not present a standard or predictable pattern (Keen, *Empathy and the Novel* 65–84). Many factors, from the underlying dispositions of readers, to personal histories, to aspects of culturally formed identity (including gender and ethnicity) alter the intensities of this aspect of reader response. Employing an intersectional narratology complicates research questions about narrative empathy, in the end strengthening conclusions about formal techniques eliciting narrative empathy, about its variable impact on readers, and its effect on real-world changes in attitudes and behavior. For narrative fiction evokes a great diversity of responses, from a wide range of personalities: actual readers include the trained academic readers who may bring dispassionate analytical habits that take emotional responses offline; immersive readers who seek the transportation often expressed as being "lost in a book"; attentive readers; skimmers and skippers (Price 5); and low-empathy individuals who respond in an emotionally disengaged fashion to works that many others find intensely moving (Keen, *Empathy and the Novel* 72–3). This variation can be accounted for in part by differences among readers, differences in experience, identity, and temperament or disposition (Keen, "Readers' Temperaments" 302–10).

The revived reader-response practices of this decade contribute to an intersectional narratology by embracing the different directions and locations of a rich set of texts, contexts and identities while framing global observations about the workings of narrative in the world. The old-school Iserian formulation in which the responses of a singular idealized "reader" (*Implied Reader*) represent univocal illustrations of reception has already been qualified by more than three decades of work on specific differentiated reading communities (Gilligan; Radway, *Reading*; Long; Colclough; and William Johnson) and by more recent empirical studies of readers' self-reports and bodily responses to narrative (Andringa, "Interface"; Miall "Feeling"; Zyngier, et al, *Directions*; and Lázló, *Science*). Rhetorical narratology by Peter Rabinowitz earlier opened up consideration of the different stances or positions with regards to the text an individual reader may occupy in his description of authorial and narrative audiences (Rabinowitz, *Before* 96–100), and Brian Richardson has theorized the multiple implied readers a single text may invoke (Richardson, "Singular"). Following the lead of Robyn Warhol, who has urged feminist critics to "take what Kimberlé Crenshaw named an 'intersectional' approach because white privilege, class privilege, hetero-normativity, and other positions of relative power complicate hierarchies of gender" (Warhol, "Feminist" 9), I seek further to open theorizing about "the reader" in reader-response theory to considerations of gender and ethnicity, at least, with other axes of identity complicating any blanket assertions about what "the reader" feels, perceives, remembers, and contributes to the task of co-creating narratives through reading. I review the available research and suggest that attention to intersectional identity in representations and in readers enriches both narrative ethics and an updated transactional account of reader response. The intersubjectivity involved in rhetorical narratological models of narrative empathy such as my own points towards a diversity of responses to emotionally evocative fiction, responses that can be better understood if the identity of a monolithic "reader" can be opened up to the complications of diverse readers' intersectional identities. This in turn should assist future theorizers of reception in integrating results from empirical studies of narrative impact, especially if those experiments attend to the interactions of identity and readers' responses, interactions that have been expected to produce divergent interpretations. However, our commonalities may turn out to be more substantial than our cherished distinctive individuality. An intersectional narratology ought also to be able to identify significant crossroads where narrative calls upon shared humanity, if they exist.

Some practitioners of reader response criticism take recognition of readers' individuality further than I do, admitting an infinitely variable and divergent set of responses, where understandings of and responses to texts are as unique and numerous as the actual readers. Perhaps because of my commitments to rhetorical narratology and communications models for narrative dynamics, I discern evidence of patterns in responses, patterns that demonstrate how fictional texts elicit recognizably related understandings from cohorts of readers. Textual content and narrative technique do put some limits on the possible interpretations of a text. A common-sense test of a reading's legitimacy is to discover whether another reader of the same text at least recognizes the interpretation, though different, as arising from the same textual starting point. The destablilization of hierarchy implicit in an intersectional approach discourages a published, canonical, or otherwise institutionally sanctioned interpretation from becoming the litmus test of a right reading, but it need not devolve into a multitude of mutually incomprehensible interpretations. For at the same time, rhetorical narratology's commitment to discovering how authors employ textual strategies to invite readers' imagining of a storyworld invests significance in the communication vehicle, the fictional text, which places some limits on the possibilities. The basis for this theoretical stance I locate in the transactional theory of Louise M. Rosenblatt.

Transactional Theory and Narrative Empathy

Of Louise M. Rosenblatt, Wayne C. Booth writes in a foreword to the 5th edition of her textbook *Literature as Exploration* (1995), "I doubt that any other literary critic of this century has enjoyed and suffered as sharp a contrast of powerful influence and absurd neglect" (vii). One purpose of this essay is to revisit Rosenblatt's transactional theory of the literary work, articulated in her 1978 book, *The Reader, the Text, and the Poem*, and emerging from work begun in her influential textbook *Literature as Exploration* (1938), especially in the 1968 second edition. (Rosenblatt altered her textbook modestly between its original edition in 1938 to its last edition in 1995, but an early revision for the second edition added her terminology of transaction, developed *The Reader, The Text, and the Poem* (1978) and other articles.) Rosenblatt's theorizing is an often-unacknowledged point of origin for modes of interpretation that recognize the role of the reader as co-creator. As Rosenblatt writes, "a text, once it leaves its author's hands, is simply paper and ink until a reader evokes from it a literary work" (*Reader* ix). Text and reader are dynamically interfused (viii), and while texts offer both openness and constraint (x), readers possess particular attributes that make their contributions unique (15). In Booth's words, Rosenblatt "saw the folly of ignoring diversity of response" (Booth, "Foreword" ix) that emerges when literary reading is construed as an individuated experience, yet she also defended critical judgments about better and worse readings, writing

> There is, in fact, nothing in the recognition of the personal nature of literature that requires an acceptance of the notion that every evocation of a text is as good as every other. We need only think of our successive readings of the same text, at fifteen or thirty or fifty, to know that we can differentiate. Undisciplined, irrelevant, or distorted emotional responses and the lack of relevant experience or knowledge will, of course, lead to inadequate interpretations of the text. The aim is to help the student towards a more and more controlled, more and more valid or defensible response to the text.
> (Rosenblatt, *Exploration* 267)

As I acknowledged in *Empathy and the Novel*, my theorizing of narrative empathy is indebted both to Rosenblatt's transactional theory (65) and to one of her major influences, John Dewey (93). Rosenblatt advances a case for readers' unique contributions to both meaning-making and aesthetic experience, without displacing the text or the teacher who guides readers towards more valid interpretations. Her theory underscores both the perspective-taking that imaginative responses to literature (often labeled "the poem" in Rosenblatt's work) requires; she insists that the practice of reader-focused pedagogy contributes to inductive study of literature (*Exploration* 272) and the formation of citizens suited to participate in democratic societies. She writes, in words that have inspired generations of literature teachers, especially those laboring in secondary school classrooms.

> When there is active participation in literature—the reader living through, reflecting on, and criticizing his own responses to the text—there will be many kinds of benefits. We can call this growth in ability to share discriminatingly in the possibilities of language as it is used in literature. But this means also the development of the imagination: the ability to escape from the limitations of time and place and environment, the capacity to envisage alternatives in ways of life and in moral and social choices, the sensitivity to thought and feeling and needs of other personalities. The youth will need to grow into the emotional and intellectual and aesthetic maturity necessary for appreciating the great works of literature in our own and other languages. As he does this, he grows also into partnership in the wisdom of the past and the aspirations for the future, of our culture and our society.

> The great abstractions—love, honor, integrity, compassion, individuality, democracy—will take on for him human meaning.
>
> (Rosenblatt, *Exploration* 276)

The "transaction" of transactional theory has a purposeful direction. The individual reader contributes to the enlivening of the text and its co-creation, but the practice of encouraging sensitivity to the textual cues of intersubjectivity points, for Rosenblatt, in an improving direction. Rosenblatt has not travelled far from George Eliot's cultivation of the reader's sympathetic imagination; the Deweyan pedagogical theory that inspires Rosenblatt's work directly infuses the themes of moral sentimentalism with early twentieth-century convictions about democracy and education. In recent years, narrative empathy has often been identified as the driver of the transactional reading that turns the naïve youth into the good world citizen, in Martha Nussbaum's phrase (Nussbaum, *Cultivating* 90).

Narrative empathy, glossed as the sharing of feeling and perspective-taking induced by reading, viewing, hearing, or imagining narratives of another's situation and condition (Keen, "A Theory" 207), involves readers, texts, and authors, and it is well-suited to interpretation through a transactional theory, in which readers "interanimate" the words put together by authors (Rosenblatt, *Reader* 53). The reader's behavior is less firmly governed by the text or the writer than purely formalist descriptions of narrative technique or biographical accounts of authorial intention suggest, and this may be especially true of the range of responses that we relegate to the affective or emotional side of narrative impact. Yet response in a transactional account does bear serious relation to textual parameters: reading may lead to offline daydreaming, to be sure, but engaged fiction reading itself involves co-creation of a storyworld and its denizens from the tacit cues of the text. These include techniques deployed by authors in an attempt to evoke readers' empathy. Intersectional axes of identity play a role in narrative empathy's core experiences: mental simulation during reading, the aesthetics of reception (the feeling of reading), and divergent responses to formal narrative strategies. That the temperaments and dispositions of actual readers in all their variety have a profound impact on the co-creative work of reading narrative fiction I take as axiomatic, in an extension of Rosenblatt's transactional theory of reading (Sedgwick 22; Keen, "Readers'" 302–10). This insight has recently received empirical validation. For example, gender difference in readers' responses has been verified by cognitive scientists and analysts of discourse processing, but not always in the ways we might predict. Özen Odag, for example, reports on studies of emotional involvement of readers which show,

> contrary to expectation, and as opposed to both feminist theory and widespread survey results, male participants score higher than females on questionnaire scales assessing emotional involvement. At the same time, the personal remindings of readers disclose no differences in how closely men and women approach characters. Likewise surprisingly, the *category of a literary work* [fiction and non-fiction] seems of negligible importance for the

> two sexes, while the *thematic focus* of a text appears to have an impact on female reading in particular.
>
> (Odag, "Of Men" 308, original emphases; see also Odag "Emotional Engagement" 1)

Odag's counterintuitive results showed male readers are more emotionally involved than women, especially with the driver of narrativity, suspense (317), though they did confirm women's greater involvement with narratives of inner worlds than externally-narrated stories (while men had moderate to high emotional participation across those distinctions of technique) (319). Though Odag's work disconfirms many expectations about gender and reading, it does suggest male readers' predisposition to enjoy plot and the emotions of narrativity, and female readers' interest in characters result in similar intensities of affective engagement, with differentiated experiences of plot-driven narratives focusing on externalities (325). Odag concludes, "it became clear that (certain) men can in fact be more engaged during reading than (certain) women. And it became evident that men and women are not always different from each other but astonishingly similar in how closely they approach characters in narrative" (325).

Study of narrative empathy should be ready to parse both similiarities and differences in responses that a given text may evoke in readers who themselves vary in ethnicity, gender, and other aspects of identity. For Rosenblatt, there is no such thing as a generic reader, for "each reader is unique, bringing to the transaction an individual ethnic, social, and psychological history" (*Exploration* xix). Her distinction between efferent and aesthetic reading differentiates between purposeful reading that carries away meaning (efferent) and affective, associative experiences of texts (aesthetic) that unfold in individual and individuated readers. Following Rosenblatt, I hold that aesthetic readings thus differ from one another as much as readers do. Balancing the diversity of aesthetic responses, including the effects of narrative empathy, with the inevitable narrowing of efferent readings founded in a more limited range of meanings remains a challenge for applications of Rosenblatt's transactional theory.

"The Reader... He"

Can readers who experience divergent aesthetic readings arrive at mutually comprehensible efferent readings, or interpretations of meaning? How much do individual differences, including differences of gender and ethnicity, alter empathetic responsiveness? Do the responses of readers marked by differences of identity command attention and respect? Dissent and reading against the grain certainly persist, and teachers committed to balancing individuality with democracy in classroom probably do not vote down minority views. The process of discussion need not elevate the opinions of one gender or the responses of a privileged ethnic group. Yet the possibility of the tyranny of the majority persists in discussion and interpretation of literary works. Whose views prevail? A typical literature classroom at the university level almost certainly has more women than men in it, and it is more likely than ever to be led by a female professor. Do the aesthetic and efferent readings of female and nonwhite audiences register as equally legitimate in the cacophony of responses, or do white male voices still, in the second decade of the twenty-first century, still dominate? There are reasons for concern. In the professional area of book reviewing, works by male authors are still more frequently reviewed, and male reviewers are more frequently published, in *The London Review of Books*, *The Nation*, *The New York Review of Books*, *The New York Times Book Review*, the *Times Literary Supplement*, *The Atlantic*, *The New Republic*, and *Harpers* (VIDA, "The Count 2012"). This list cites some of the journals studied by VIDA, Women in Literary Arts, a group founded in August 2009 "to address the need for female writers of literature to engage in conversations regarding the critical reception of women's creative writing in our current culture" (VIDA, "Mission & History"). More than a century of feminism and at least a half century of women in the professions and the academy have not yet brought equality of opportunity to published opinion about books. That this circumstance should persist even though census polls of readers discover higher rates of reading among women than men (a pattern verified by the market surveys of the publishing industry and studies of library usage) gives us pause, or ought to. [The National Endowment for the Arts' *Reading on the Rise* (2009) reported that "male reading of literature grew at an 11% rate between 2002 and 2008, after declining from 1982 to 2002" (when there was a low of only 37.6% of male readers, compared to 55.1% of female readers). In 2008 the gender gap had narrowed but was still evident: 41.9% of men had read at least a single work of literature, whereas 58% of women were self-reported literary readers. Market research for the US publishing market in 2011 found (from a sample of 80,000 unique consumers) that women bought 59% of all books, 62% of all fiction, 70% of mysteries, 89% of romances, 54% of biographies. Only in the category of graphic novels do male consumers account for a majority of sales (67%) (Bowker Market Research, "The Magic and Mystery"). A 26 January 2011 Harris Interactive Poll reported that 72% of US circulating library visitors were women, in contrast to 58% of men. Women are also the majority of library-card holders. See American Library Association, "Public Library Use".] If empirical data on rates of reading analyzed by gender were our guide, we would consistently assume that "the reader" is a woman or a girl. Instead, referential practices aimed at avoiding sexist language usually gloss over differences among readers by referring to them in the plural. What might we lose sight of by omitting gender difference from studies of emotional responses to reading?

Rosenblatt herself consistently refers to a singular male reader, even as she imagines the protean potentiality of *his* transactional role in co-creating the meaning of the literary text: "We cannot simply look at the text and predict the poem," she writes, "for this, a reader or readers with particular attributes must be postulated: for example, the author-as-reader as he is creating the text; the author as he reads it years later; contemporaries with different backgrounds; other individuals living in specific places, times, and milieus" (*Reader* 15). The plurals admit women and men, but the direct references to readers always revert to the male pronoun: "The transaction is basically between the reader and what he senses the words as pointing to" (21); "As he engages with the text, the reader, as we have seen, sets up hypothetical frameworks, entertains expectations as to what will follow, and uses these as guidelines for selecting out from alternative responses" (137); "The reader, it can be said, provides at that point in his life or in that social situation, a particularly receptive context, a kind of amplifier, for what he derives from the text" (157). While the insights as to the role of the reader's activity and the impact of the reader's identity remain persuasive, the limitation to a universal male as representative human actively works against Rosenblatt's insistence on readers' diversity. This rhetorical choice (or capitulation to 1970s house style) in *The Reader, The Text, and the Poem* renders the singular human being as male by default. It has in my opinion contributed to the relative neglect of Rosenblatt's theorizing in literary studies, perhaps especially by the first wave of feminist reader-response critics. [For example, Jane Tompkins' (ed.) *Reader-Response Criticism* barely acknowledges Rosenblatt beyond the bibliography. Her work receives serious consideration only in David Bleich's contribution; Tompkins mentions her to brush her aside (x). Steven Mailloux observes that first wave reader response critics kept debating the reader-text binary opposition as if Rosenblatt had not already offered a pragmatic antifoundational epistemology in her transactional model. (Mailloux 40–2).] Her belated plea, in her 1995 preface to the 5th edition of *Literature as Exploration*, indicates Rosenblatt's awareness that assumptions about the universal applicability of terms in the male gender had changed over the years. She writes, "A reminder of when the book first appeared is the generic *he*, then taken for granted, no matter how feminist, as in this case, the writer might be. To remedy this would have required a total rewriting. I must simply assume that my readers are sufficiently free of old patriarchal attitudes to keep in mind my statement" that each reader is unique (*Exploration* xix). In retrospect that total rewriting might have been worth the effort, for she is often passed over in silence by feminist critics who almost certainly owe something to Rosenblatt. [Rosenblatt's home base in a school of education may have also contributed to her diminished reputation, despite the manifest impact of her theorizing on secondary school literature pedagogy. On the impact of Rosenblatt's Deweyan transactional theory through *Literature as Exploration*, a textbook widely adopted by educators for over a half century, see Connell 27.] Drawing attention to Rosenblatt's anticipation of the concerns of early reader-response criticism, as Wayne C. Booth does, leads to the recognition that *Literature as Exploration* "having incorporated and transformed close reading, respect for the canon, and multiculturalism" also boasts radical interdisciplinarity and "the deep cultural embeddedness of every writing and reading act" ("Foreword" xi–xii). It is well worth explicitly updating Rosenblatt's transactional theory in order to keep her contribution relevant.

Rosenblatt's gender neutrality under the guise of a universal male reader thus should be revisited and revised. When actual readers' responses to reading narrative fiction are studied, gender differences are sometimes revealed .... While I doubt that the underlying cause of gender differentiation in literary response is biologically based, except insofar as our biological sex interacts with our environment in the form of our social world (including aspects of culture embedded in narratives), it is certainly the case that cultural expectations predispose females towards expression of emotions, but not necessarily on the potential for affective response.

This cultural context has an impact on empathy and by extension on narrative empathy (a variant of empathy sometimes described as fantasy empathy [Davis, "Multidimensional'], as narrative empathy involves sharing feeling with unreal beings in imagined worlds). Janet Strayer and Nancy Eisenberg's literature review of empathy research suggests that cultural factors associated with gender expectations rather than physiological differences between female and male brains explain apparent differences between degrees of empathy felt and reported by males and females (Eisenberg et al., "Physiological" 380–5). They found that pen-and-paper surveys or those with live interviewers interacting with subjects showed the greatest divergence between male and female empathy, while studies relying on physiological measures (such as skin conductance and heart rate) showed insignificant differences between the biological sexes. The impact of cultural expectations about the performance of gender shows when data is elicited through self-report or interviewer questioning. Notwithstanding influential claims about male and female brains (Baron-Cohen 1–2), individual men (and women) are distributed over a wider spectrum of low to high empathy measures than men in contrast to women .... An intersectional narratology encourages the addition of gender difference to the axes of unique identity that a reader brings to the interpretive and affective transaction in reading. In its application to narrative empathy, intersectional narratology enables discussion of the complex overlays of narrative form, contexts of creation and reception, and identity that work together to provoke diverse responses to narrative, among divergent readers of a wide variety of texts. Complicating rather than schematizing, intersectional narratology hazards proliferation of axes rather than insisting on neat taxonomies. As Lanser writes, intersectional feminism "can now map and be mapped by narrative patterns across time and space, accounting for vectors of difference to create a narratology that is deeply locational and therefore cross-cultural and historical" ("Are We There Yet?" 32). This practice, while complicated, opens possibilities for fresh discoveries about the correlates of narrative empathy.

Raymond Mar, Keith Oatley and Jordan Peterson, controlling for gender and tendency to become immersed in a story, discovered that fiction readers of both genders, not women, have higher empathy (Mar et al., "Exploring" 424). This finding supports my hypothesis that the perception of fictionality by a reader enhances the likelihood of narrative empathy (Keen, *Empathy and the Novel* 88–9), but it confutes the notion that female readers of fiction are more empathetic than male readers. While others have found in thematic preferences of male and female readers (Odag, "Of Men" 208) support for the idea that prototypical female and male responses to core emotions of narrativity (curiosity, suspense, and surprise) reveal sex-based differences, we should take care not to generalize beyond the verifiable point that a tendency towards fantasy empathy predisposes subjects of both sexes to experience narrative empathy (Mar et al., "Exploring" 417). Hierarchical linear regressions performed by the Mar group demonstrate that "fiction print-exposure predicts performance on an empathy task, even after gender, age, English fluency, trait Openness, and trait Fantasy are statistically controlled" (420). The Mar lab has found that readers who immerse more deeply in fictional worlds had higher degrees of print fiction exposure and greater ability to infer another's mental state, an expression of cognitive empathy. This finding gains support from the research of Dan R. Johnson, who has discovered that subjects who were more transported into a story exhibited higher affective empathy and were more likely to engage in pro-social behavior (Johnson, "Transportation" 150). That is, Johnson shows "a direct link between reading narrative fiction, affective empathy, and helping behavior" (154). A habit of fiction reading correlated in both studies with empathy, and in one case with helping behavior, on behalf of both male and female readers. To discover what readers of both biological sexes have in common as they respond to fiction, or to pin down how they differ, a researcher ought to augment Rosenblatt's respect for the reader's role in the transaction with attention to gender identity and other axes of identity, disposition, and circumstance. In time we may be able to establish whether the apparent gender differences reflected in reading habits, preferences for certain genres, and reported emotional responses are artifacts of our assumptions about the sexes or verifiable differences predictive of specific effects.

Readers in Color

The role of race and ethnicity in reader response and transactional theory is more difficult to discover than that of gender, though aspirations about the ethical impact of reading literature pervades Louise M. Roseblatt's work. For example, in *Literature as Exploration*, Rosenblatt writes,

> Literature offers a release from the provincialism of time and space. In this way it may exert a powerful influence on the youth's future behavior. In a heterogenous, democratic society, more and more explicitly seeking to create new social and economic patterns, literature can perform an increasingly important function.... More than ever before it is essential that the individual be liberated from the provincialism of his particular family, community, or even national background.
>
> (Rosenblatt, *Exploration* 184)

Rosenblatt holds up awareness of diversity, discovery of the different goals that individuals may pursue, discovery of temperament, trial-and-error vicarious imagining of alternative outcomes, and occasionally, a transformative reading experience of a singular book as the potentialities of literary reading (212–3). Cultivation of the role-taking imagination is, for Rosenblatt, one of the core affordances of the experience of literature, developing sensitivities to the temperaments and circumstances of "different kinds of people" (176). The Deweyan project of cultivating human sympathy in order to forge a democratic nation, capable of resisting the sadistic appeals of totalitarianism, is at the heart of Rosenblatt's thinking:

> Lack of such imaginative sympathy is probably back of many of our present-day difficulties. No matter whether the problem is just distribution of taxation or universal civil rights or federal-state relations, the basis of any ultimate decision should be its meaning for actual human lives. It is easy enough to understand the possible effect of a point of view on ourselves and on the human beings with whom we feel the kinship of family, class, nation, or race. We must also develop the capacity to feel intensely the needs and sufferings and aspirations of people whose personal interests are distinct from our own, people with whom we have no bond other than our common humanity.
>
> (177–8)

Where Rosenblatt differs from Martha Nussbaum, who shares this moral sentimental agenda and believes in the efficacy of a certain kind of literary reading in creating good world citizens, or from Lynn Hunt, who sees in eighteenth-century novel reading the birth of human rights discourse, is in Rosenblatt's modesty. While she asks, "is not humanitarianism ultimately the result of this sense of the prime importance of the human being, based on the ability to transcend selfish interests and to feel the needs of others?" (178), she also recognizes of the limitations of literature: "It would be absurd to suggest that literature was the cause of this" increase in humane practices (178) .... Rosenblatt sees the human influence, not books alone, as the "most powerful and lasting" (*Exploration* 179) influences on readers' ability vicariously to enter into the experience of others (178). Throughout Rosenblatt's work, a universalizing impulse avoids defining the "youth" as possessing a racial or ethnic identity, though as I have discussed above, he is male and by implication American. We could attribute a tacit whiteness to Rosenblatt's reader without controversy. Yet recently Rosenblatt's work has been seen as anticipating (without directly contributing to) the ethical turn in literary theory, drawing on an unusually interdisciplinary base for its time: "She attempted to break through the provinciality and disciplinarity of literary studies by demonstrating what reading might mean if it were recognized as a social process, as a transaction between and among human beings," according to her most ardent contemporary advocate (Flynn 68).

This makes it worth asking, does race or ethnicity enter into the transactional experience of reading? Because of the demonstrable racial bias of arguments about the contrasting abilities of members of different racial groups (Jacoby and Glauberman), researchers in reader-response may have shied away from asking questions based on readers' race and ethnicity. There is a dearth of research in the area. If gender has the appearance of influencing reader response, an appearance not consistently verified by empirical investigations, the race and ethnicity of readers also contributes to their intersectional identities. I have mentioned above several influential *literary* accounts of what it is like to be a nonwhite reader encountering canonical western texts. Given this influential testimony, I believe it is worth asking whether readers from an in-group respond differently than readers from an out-group, concerning the same text? I have argued that authorial strategic empathizing allows individual texts to appeal to different audiences, near and far (Keen, "Strategic"). When those audiences differ in race or ethnicity, can—or should—distinctive reading responses be correlated to such markers of identity? Are readers identified with a particular in-group necessarily biased readers about an out-group, or can experiences of narrative empathy overcome bias in the face of difference? Literary study has often vouched for the salutary ethical effects of reading about characters that differ from the reader in race, ethnicity, and nationality, but the studies in social psychology and social neuroscience find that intergroup bias can be difficult to overcome (Avenanti et al.).

What effects of narrative empathy might be diminished or enhanced by depictions of otherness marked by race or ethnic difference? That racial bias in a subject reduces empathetic responsiveness to the pain of other races is a well-validated observation in social psychology, cognitive science, and social neuroscience (J. Feagin et al.; Cosmides et al. 173–9; Avenanti et al. 1018). The susceptibility of empathy to in-group bias may extend to narrative empathy, though I have argued that authors of fiction employ techniques of ambassadorial and broadcast strategic narrative empathy to evoke sympathy from readers beyond the in-group (the audience for bounded empathy) (Keen, "Strategic" 480–90). Many of the studies showing racial or ethnic bias in empathic responses rely on images (e.g., Xu et al.), but how implicit or overtly described racial/ethnic identity in *prose* narrative effects readers' empathy is less well understood. Yet recent fMRI studies of failures in intergroup empathy do employ short narratives about, for example, Arabs and Isarelis (Bruneau and Saxe; Bruneau et al.), that would be recognized by narrative theorists as very short fictions. The responses in the brain areas of members of ingroups and outgroups reading very short narratives about representative characters can be understood as a new form of reader-response study. A few labs focus specifically on the impact of narrative fiction, seeking to validate the belief that empathetic engagement with representations of outgroups reduces bias, changes attitudes, and leads to prosocial behavior. For example, encouraging recent news comes from Dan R. Johnson and his students, who report that reading narratives that employ counter-stereotypical characters is effective in reducing Americans' implicit prejudice against Arab-Muslims. Johnson found that reading short fiction was "particularly effective at reducing implicit prejudice in low dispositional perspective takers" and he hypothesizes that reading fictional narrative "appeared to provide a safe haven from intergroup anxiety" for low empathy individuals (Johnson et al., "Reading"). This result is important because it shifts the focus from high empathy individuals with a tendency to immerse readily in narrative fiction and engage in character identification to those less prone to perspective taking when reading fiction. Within every ingroup and outgroup, people whose dispositions (and experiences) make them less ready empathizers exist. It may be that their responses to reading fiction differ sufficiently from high empathizers to deserve separate study. Indeed, differences in dispositional empathy may cut across more obvious markers of identity such as ethnicity. An intersectional narratology can address dispositional differences and could reveal commonalities not immediately apparent to view when cruder binaries of sex or race divide subjects.

Intersectionality, which accounts for "the relationships among multiple dimensions and modalities of social relations and subject formations" (McCall 1771), meshes well with a narrative poetics that is open to diverse effects of narrative techniques in various texts, contexts, and modes. In an insight that Meir Sternberg developed in discussion of insets and quotations altered by their local context, he develops a principle that is widely applicable to narrative form, the "many-to-many correspondence between linguistic form and representational function" (Sternberg, "Proteus" 112). Like intersectional analyses of discrimination, for which the concept was first formulated in legal studies (Crenshaw), my version of intersectional narratology seeks to understand why certain positions and concepts are privileged while others suffer from inattention or disparagement. Is it really the case that women make more feeling readers, or those steeped in the great tradition make the best world citizens? In her foundational rendering of feminist intersectionality for narrative theory, Susan S. Lanser emphasizes the discernment of the way "systemic, structural, and institutional 'traffic' .... operates to the advantage or disadvantage of individuals and groups according to their social positioning" ("Are We There Yet?" 34). This means, in my extension, that intersectional narratology need not aim primarily at verifying folk wisdom or received theories about how men and women read, or how representations contribute to the perpetuation or eradication of biases. Drawing on the psychology of narrative impact and studies of fantasy empathy in diverse audiences, further research might explore how the intersectional identities of readers (including their gender, ethnicity, and dispositional empathy) puts them in the position to respond feelingly to writers' bounded, ambassadorial, or broadcast strategic narrative empathy (Keen, "Strategic"). An intersectional narratology can take seriously the actual responses of a wide array of different readers, without predispositions about how their identities predict their reading experiences. A reader-response criticism attentive to the complex crossings of identity can revivify transactional theory and its commitments to democracy.

8

FROM READERS' TEMPERAMENTS AND FICTIONAL CHARACTER

Narrative theory has long been at odds with ordinary fiction reading when it comes to character. Characters, says the formalist or poststructuralist theorist, are nonhuman word-masses (Forster, *Aspects* 44), existents (Chatman 19–21), actants (Greimas 5–6), narrative-men (Todorov 66–70), Nobodies (Gallagher xiii–xix), or the products of semes traversing proper names (Barthes, *S-Z* 67). Yet readers persist in regarding characters as more human than "substantial hypothetical beings" (Hochman 26), more like friends or neighbors than Forster's species *Homo Fictus* allows (*Aspects* 55). This tendency shows every time regular readers talk about fictional characters, and there's really nothing that narrative theory can do to stop it. Instead we ignore it. Narrative theorists have chosen functional, thematic, and linguistic approaches to character over the analysis of readers' reports of self-recognition in fictional characters, or what might be described as naïve engagement with readily identifiable character types. [Early Norman Holland is an exception to these generalizations (see *Dynamics*; *Five Readers*).] This work rarely reckons with the behavior and beliefs of ordinary readers of fiction, though it implies effects on ideal audiences (Rabinowitz, *Before*; Phelan, *Narrative as Rhetoric*; Richardson, "Other Reader's"). For instance, in cognitive narratology, recent work on modes for representation of fictional consciousness contributes to models of narrative communication and accounts of human mind-reading ability (Herman, ed., *Emergence*; Palmer, *Fictional* and *Social*; Young, *Imagining*), though the experiences of actual readers remain in the black box. [Psychonarratology has begun to bring work in social cognition into conversation with studies of narrative form: this work has the praiseworthy element of empirical study of real readers (Herman, *Story;* László, *Science*).] Common readerly practices such as liking and hating characters, connecting with or distrusting characters, have been relegated to the book group or the blog, if they are discussed at all. These ubiquitous means

DOI: 10.4324/9781003264071-11

of engaging with narrative fiction deserve attention. This essay calls for a revival of reader-response studies, informed by evidence of the high degree of variability in reactions to fictional characters.

In an historical moment where reading overall and fiction reading in particular suffers precipitous declines, attention to what the remaining ordinary readers do with and to fictional characters could then change the direction of theoretical engagement with "character." [For statistical analyses prepared with the assistance of the United States Census Bureau, see the National Endowment for the Arts reports, *Reading at Risk* (2004); *To Read or Not to Read* (2007), and an optimistic update, *Reading on the Rise* (2009).] Rather than increasing the distance between theorizing about fiction reading and the experiences of actual readers, we acknowledge the shaping influence of readers on character. This influence includes aspects of identity such as gender and class. Feminist standpoint theory suggests that personal identity influences all aspects of scholarly work (D. Smith), including reading practices, which need not acquiesce to the apparent textual demands for a compliant reading style (Fetterly). This is not simply a matter of gender, however. The pressures exerted by readers on the imaging and judging of fictional characters derive from the multiple intersecting axes of their subject positions (Crenshaw). As I will argue here, the way we co-create fictional characters in reading also depends on inner qualities of temperament, defined as "constitutionally based individual differences in reactivity and self-regulation, in the domains of affect, activity, and attention" (Rothbart and Bates 99–100). Constitutional differences involve a combination of heredity, individual development, and experience. These contribute, in the form of temperament, an affective, attentional, and activational core to personality, which itself includes "much more than temperament, particularly the content of thought, skills, habits, values, defenses, morals, beliefs, and social cognition" (100). Far from rooting responses in a biological substrate alone, developmental and social psychology complicate the picture by admitting multiple variables contributing to consistent personality traits. These temperamental differences express themselves not only in the ways people respond to other people (cautiously, shyly, warmly, defensively, openly, etc.), but also in the way they construct imaginary human-like persons in fictions.

What would happen to narrative theories of fictional character if they admitted the full temperamental range of actual readers, and the evidence of divergent ways that readers respond to the imaginary beings in storyworlds? Privileged reading modes (the analytical or symbol-seeking) would yield to the more numerous skimmers, skippers, and escapist immersion practices (Price). Taxonomies of character types would verge on chaos, for how could narratology account for all the non-textual detail added by readers? The relative tidiness of models based on description of textual strategies would give way to messier schemas admitting readers' variant responses to representational techniques. As a starting point, narrative theories of fictional character should accommodate evidence of readers' empathy (and other emotional responses to fiction reading).

Narrative empathy means feeling with fiction (Dadlez; Feagin). [Robinson's *Deeper than Reason* updates the philosophy of aesthetic emotions through a sustained engagement with current psychology of the emotions.] A common experience of immersion readers, a frequently, though not universally, cultivated effect of fictions, and a desired outcome of many novelists, filmmakers, and storytellers, narrative empathy features in accounts both of emotional triggers in imaginative experiences of reading (Hogan, *Cognitive* 186–90) and of empirical studies of shifts in readers' feelings while encountering literary texts (Miall, *Literary* 69–88). Several of my conclusions in *Empathy and the Novel* bear on readers' experiences with fictional characters. There I discuss the puzzle that many readers experience intense emotional fusion with narrative texts, but that no one narrative text evokes empathy from all its readers (Keen, *Empathy* 169). It is widely understood that readers' cultural contexts and individual experiences influence the degree of their responsiveness to the emotional appeal of texts (170). This has not restrained theorists from extrapolating the profound impact of character identification and emotional fusion on readers' subsequent behavior as citizens of the world. Paying heed to readers' divergent experiences of fictional characters discourages such generalizations....

My convictions about narrative empathy thus shape my temperamental theory of character, about which I offer four propositions that map onto the subsequent sections of this essay. First, I discuss the relative roles of readers' own temperaments and experiences and authors' constructions in shaping readers' responses to character. By temperament I mean the interior qualities of a person's mind and affective style (or feeling tone), not necessarily their performative or public personality. This topic admits with some leniency a wide range of potential responses to characters and questions the notion that fictional character is entirely controlled by writers and texts. Second, I assert the likelihood, based on studies in developmental psychology, that human temperaments shape reading more than reading shapes people's temperaments. This places the popular notion of fictional character as a means of character-shaping for readers under skeptical pressure. Third, I nominate Baruch Hochman's early cognitive theory of fictional character, *Character in Literature* (1985) as a bridge between formalist theories of character and practices that acknowledge the range of responses predicted by temperamental character theory. Fourth and finally, I sketch the lineaments of a practical theory of temperamental character, with a discussion of its classroom applications and implications for literary criticism.

Fictional Character and Narrative Empathy

Fictional character is a nearly unanimous nominee of fiction readers for the title role in their stories of feeling with fiction. Narrative empathy may precede character identification or work against the grain, as when readers experience narrative empathy with figures otherwise evoking dislike or discomfort (Keen,

Empathy 74–5, 170). In my earlier studies, a focus on narrative technique has sometimes zeroed in on empathetic aspects of characterization (as, for instance, in the rendering of facial expressions and bodily postures in comic books and graphic narratives). Fictional character, however, is not a narrative technique, but a product of it. Fictional character resides somewhere between the discourse and the storyworld, a projection of fictional worldmaking and the site of readerly creative collaboration. Axiomatically, readers are different from one another (Sedgwick 22). The resultant divergences in how we flesh out the text's words into the illusion of persons usually fall into the great bracketed area of reading phenomena experienced but not studied, acknowledged but not sanctioned by theory. Temperamental character theory ventures into that chaotic zone.

Character causes trouble for narrative theory. It is the mobius strip that disrupts formal taxonomies of level and function. Character is difficult to separate from plot, as Henry James announced back in 1884: "What is character but the determination of incident? What is incident but the illustration of character?" (*Art of Fiction* 13). It is hard to place tidily when one works within narratology's story/discourse convention, for characters seem to belong to one realm (the storyworld), while characterization belongs to the other (discourse or narration). Character is frequently renamed according to the role it plays (narrator, narratee, focalizer or reflector, narrative agent—each of which may contribute to characterization). Under narrative situation's various roles, character gains narratological status: we can more readily discuss narrator and narratee as characters, and characters in their roles as focalizers or reflectors, than character as the word-wrought projection of something very like a human being.

Yet if character is hard to disentangle from plot, the narrated domain, and the intricacies of narrative situation, it is equally hard to confine to the textual realm, for character notoriously escapes the boundaries of the text itself, and not only through sequels and other transfictional reanimations. Ordinary readers do things to and with character that evade description by narrative theory when they respond to characters as persons. Who has not wondered what it is like for Charlotte Lucas to submit to sexual intercourse with the odious Mr. Collins? (On this subject Austen is silent: We know only that Charlotte has chosen the coldest room in the house for her parlour.) Cognitive theories of character suggest that the mental models of storyworld participants (Herman, *Story*) depend in part on readers' general knowledge of schemas and stereotypes, including modes of social person (Fowler), brought to the reading experience. Recent theories of virtual narrative emphasize the degree to which the reading of plot depends upon readers' active imagining of potential storylines that do not come to pass (Ryan, *Narrative*). These theories authorize the active reader's content-rich projection and invention of counterfactual events and consequences—the alternative possibilities that a plot brings alive in the mind, driving reading forward. It is impossible to imagine how such virtual narratives cluster around live plot possibilities, if not through readers' imagining of the behavior of characters unbound from textual limitations.

The value of these cognitive theories inheres in their description of a dynamic process that restores a position for readers in narrative theorizing about character. Their limitation lies in their inability to account for different results of reading, especially in different kinds of readers or audiences (Rabinowitz, *Before*; Phelan, *Narrative*; Richardson, "Other Reader's"). We can label a reader as actual, implied, resisting, belonging to the narrative audience or not, but in critical practice most of our knowledge about what actual readers do with fictional characters comes from introspection and our observations from teaching. This has an impact on our theorizing of character. Uri Margolin observes, "While the model reader and professional literati will give the literary [models] precedence, ordinary readers tend to give precedence to entrenched actual-world models" (54). Ordinary readers often subscribe to a mimetic or representational theory of character that defaults to human and folk-psychological settings, even when the characters reside in fantasy lands (Bortolussi and Dixon 153). This does not mean that ordinary readers are honor-bound to treat characters as realistic representations of persons, though they may. James Phelan has explained how mimetic, thematic, and synthetic functions of character coexist: readers may exert considerable influence in activating or ignoring those functions, even while adhering to the instructions of the text (Phelan, *Reading*). The mix may depend more on the temperament of the reader than is usually acknowledged. And there's the unpredictable afterwards, when fictional characters called up by a finite word set persist in the reader's imagination, inviting reassessment, creative revision, speculation, further adventures.

The mimetic or representational theories of character offered by cognitive, semantic, and communicative approaches (Margolin 52–7) can only go so far in describing what readers contribute to character and even reader-response theories dedicated to describing the dynamics of co-creation leave a lot out of the description. Bodily responses, immediate feelings and long-term moods, memories that distort dimensions and traits of narratives, gap-filling imagining that goes further than the textual evidence supports, and out-right supplemental fantasizing: these effects of texts on readers are rarely discussed, though they may be signal qualities of what Victor Nell calls ludic reading. I am in agreement with the observation of psychonarratologists Marisa Bortolussi and Peter Dixon: "It is entirely conceivable that some readers impose on the text character constructions that are discordant with the text" (153). They go on: "There is no objective and reliable method for measuring the degree of consonance between the textual configuration and the construction, other than common sense and communal consensus," concluding that "Understanding character constructions should therefore not be confused with hermeneutic, evaluative activities regarding the validity of any construction" (153).

While literary theories of character and characterization have tended in the twentieth century to de-emphasize feeling connections between readers and person-like constructs of narrative, in the same period philosophers, educational psychologists, and various defenders of the humanities have not hesitated to offer a different view. They have embraced the readiest connections between readerly selves and fictive beings, assuming that character identification invites rehearsal of moral dilemmas (Booth, *Company We Keep*; Paul Armstrong) and out-and-out imitation (there are fearful versions of this thesis, mainly directed against video games, as well as a more hopeful didacticism. [See for instance McGinn, who argues that the novel ought not to be ignored by moral philosophy, in *Ethics, Evil, and Fiction*, and Gregory's nuanced account of how stories generate moral effects in readers, in "Ethical Criticism" 37–61]). They have optimistically argued that narrative empathy with fictional characters results in the formation of good world citizens (Nussbaum, *Cultivating* 90). Because "character" in the English language is something that narrative fictions and real human beings both possess, there has been a great deal of what Meir Sternberg calls "package-dealing" ("Universals" [II]) in contemporary discourse about the uses of character, the formation of character, the correction of bad character, and aspirations for reformed character. This ought to attract narratology's attention, for narrative theorists can contribute both a precision of terminology and a disentangling of confounded concepts to this conversation. It is remarkable how rarely this happens. Even as contemporary theories of identity have emphasized its constructedness, its fluidity, and performative nature (Goffman; Butler), character education programs have advocated narratives' didactic potential. Character education is often taught in American primary and middle schools by means of stories illustrating core values, with the aim of shaping children's values and behavior, as well as supporting academic success. Between underlying human temperaments and predictable outcomes in the form of response to narrative lies a great gulf, often bridged in educational psychology by hopeful constructions of the impact of didactic tales on children (Character Counts) and convicted criminals (Trounstine and Waxler).

Advocates of virtue ethics (Slote, *Ethics*), ethicists of care (Noddings), and defenders of the humanities (Steiner) argue that reading about characters forms (or reforms) character. The widespread dissemination of character education curricula, using illustrative fictions, suggests that in K-8 classrooms, fictional characters are expected to have a positive impact of children's moral development—on their characters. Developmental psychologists (Narvaez) and experts in outcomes assessment have begun to take on the task of evaluating these claims, with mixed results. Evidence-based assessment of character-education programs has revealed gains in academic performance but not the desired improvements in behavior, attitudes, and values (Institute of Education Science [IES]). For instance, the story-based character-formation curriculum "Lessons in Character" was found "to have potentially positive effects on academic achievement. It had no discernible effect on behavior or on knowledge, attitudes, and values" (IES, *What Works*). Younger readers may not be so malleable, or they may be deriving different lessons from their reading than the intended inculcation of virtues. Developmental psychologist Darcia Narvaez has demonstrated that young children arrive at entirely different morals or lessons than adults when invited to interpret didactic narratives on their own (43–54). We should beware conflated definitions: In English a person's moral and ethical quality, the aggregate of an individual's traits, and a fictional person inhabiting a story world all go by the name of character. An accident of vocabulary does not guarantee that fictional characters exert shaping influence on readers' characters.

Readers' Temperaments and Experiences Versus Authors' Constructions

Readers' temperament plays a larger role than has usually been acknowledged in their responses to fictional characters. This in turn has a bearing on theories of character.... The empirical literature is nearly silent on the subject of those fiction readers in whom character identification and emotional engagement fail to occur. ... I contend not only that temperament should play a role in future theorizing about character, but also that it already inflects theorizing about character that does not acknowledge its influence. This happens when critics and theorists generalize from their own experiences without acknowledging the roles played by their own personalities and inward bearings in their reading habits.

Psychology normally treats human character under the umbrella term *personality*, one basis of which, temperament, especially concerns me here. [A major journal of the American Psychological Association is *The Journal of Personality and Social Psychology*. It publishes empirically based articles on attitudes and social cognition, interpersonal relations and group processes, and personality processes and individual differences. The *Journal of Personality* publishes scientific research on personality and behavior dynamics, personality development, and individual differences in the cognitive, affective, and interpersonal domains.] Aspects of temperament can be assessed using a wide variety of scales, many of which focus on the so-called Big Five categories of traits: extraversion, agreeableness, conscientiousness, neuroticism, and openness (McCrae). According to developmental psychologist Jerome Kagan, "A personality type is a pattern of traits, each determined by a combination of temperament, personal experience, and the contexts of daily life. Temperament makes a more substantial contribution to feeling tone than to the public personality ... The developmental journey that leads to a relaxed or tense feeling tone requires a more substantial contribution from temperament than does a sociable or shy posture with others" (Kagan and Snidman 218). Temperament begins in infancy with an inherited neurochemical make-up that affects the excitability of the amygdala (22–3). It renders some human beings low-reactive (bold) and some high-reactive (shy), and although experience has a modest impact on it, studies in developmental psychology have shown that fewer than 5% of infants from low-reactive or high-reactive temperamental groups grow up to develop the behavioral and biological characteristics of the other type (23). While not absolutely fixed, temperament prevents the development of a contrasting profile most of the time (23). Three points must be underscored before tackling the application of personality psychology to narrative theory. First, the existing research on underlying temperament casts doubt on the likelihood of change from one temperamental style to another. An introverted infant is unlikely to grow up into an extroverted adult. Second, although this school of thought is premised on the notion that all human beings possess temperaments, it is dedicated to task of understanding individual differences. It does not seek to model a singular, general human mind. Third, most of the research in developmental psychology concerns the responses (of the infant and the older child) to the strange and unfamiliar.

If we take narrative as comprising a set of devices for activating curiosity, suspense, and surprise (Sternberg, *Poetics* 264–320), we can hypothesize that readers' temperament will likely play a role in their engagement with fictional events and characters, and in their responsiveness to degrees of strangeness and unfamiliarity (or their opposites). We usually handle these differences, if we acknowledge them, under the heading of tastes, which is to say, not at all neutrally. An implicit hierarchy of literary merit rests upon assumptions about the ostensible complexity of character, with sketchy and stereotyped characters engaged in predictable actions typifying despised low-brow genres and complicated, changeable and category-resistant characters populating serious literary fiction. This categorizing has been matched, at least until the recent past, by a tacit stereotyping of readers by their tastes: the sophisticated, trained reader who engages with narrative enigmas and appreciates the character who surprises in a convincing way, versus the ordinary reader who prefers that characters and plots live up to their generic contracts without disturbing deviations from the norm. We have been in the habit of thinking of these differences as a matter of education, but what if they actually reflect readers' temperaments?

All of this leads me to the intersection of two vexatious problems for narrative theory: First, the often-contested nature and status of fictional character; and second, the question of how much credit, responsibility (or blame) individual readers have for co-creating fictional worlds. If readers cannot help making people in their minds out of the limited textual cues inscribed by authors who encode characters in words, why does literary critical practice circumscribe their imaginative license? We learn early in our educations that we are not to ask how many children had Lady Macbeth. We know what we gain by this rigorous convention—quotable evidence over vague impressions, analysis of passages over reactions and opinions. But what do we lose by insisting on the textual nature of fictional character? When we suppress the experience of having characters come to life in our minds, what questions do we omit to ask about them, and about ourselves? Parallel questions about narrative empathy suggest the pressure exerted by textual conventions. Can we locate empathetic narrative techniques and demonstrate predictable responses to their deployment? Does narrative empathy work because fiction invites emotional engagement, or because readers possess certain temperaments that they impose on authorial constructs? I argue that readers' individual temperaments, in addition to their historical and cultural context, their experiences, and chance distinctions of their identities, have a little-acknowledged but profound impact on their responses to fictional characters. Like narrative empathy, temperamental character begins and ends within individual and unique human beings.

Temperament Shapes Reading More Than Reading Shapes Temperament

It is reasonable to wonder what we can know about individual temperament, beyond the low-reactive and high-reactive types discussed by Kagan and Snidman. One area in which human beings have temperamental variation lies in the relative intensity of their empathy. In this area, individual's personalities are subject to analysis using instruments called empathy scales. The most widely used of these is Mark Davis's Interpersonal Reactivity Index (IRI), a multidimensional measure that can be used to evaluate subjects' perspective-taking, empathic concern, personal distress, and fantasy empathy (*Empathy* 55–8; see also the recently devised Toronto Empathy Questionnaire, Spreng et al.). While perspective-taking, empathic concern (sympathy) and fantasy empathy ("the tendency to imaginatively transpose oneself into fictional situations" [57]) most likely contribute to a reader's receptivity to character identification, other aspects of empathy have been demonstrated to correlate with attitudes towards fiction. Low empathy subjects tend to be less gifted at person-to-person mind-reading and less fond of fiction-reading as an activity (Baron-Cohen 144–7; his scale, 209, 219). High-empathy individuals are better at perceiving causal relations between narrated events (Bourg). High empathy subjects enjoy fiction while low-empathizers prefer non-fiction (Mar and Oatley et al., "Bookworms"). [See also the follow-up research, controlled for personality types and gender difference (Mar, Oatley et al., "Exploring" In this work the Mar lab demonstrates that "fiction exposure still predicted performance on an empathy task . . . exposure to fiction was positively correlated with social support" whereas "Exposure to nonfiction, in contrast, was associated with loneliness, and negatively related to social support" (407).] Other matters of emotional temperament enter into the reading experience, not always in the way we might predict. For instance, Raymond Mar, the leading North American investigator of cognitive, social, and emotional outcomes of exposure to narrative fiction, has discovered that frequent fiction readers are no lonelier than non-readers, a finding that confutes commonsense stereotypes about book worms (Mar, "Stories"). Many more questions remain to be investigated. Does a reader's disposition alter reading choices, for mood maintenance or manipulation? If fiction reading (or exposure to fiction) has an effect on an individual's behavior (an enduring idea), is that effect strong enough to last more than an hour or a few days? A high empathy reader is demonstrably more likely to engage in character identification: does it therefore follow that an experience of character identification on the part of a *low* empathy reader will profoundly alter his role-taking imagination? Or does the high-empathizer have to be drawn to fiction in the first place to enjoy potentially beneficial outcomes of reading fictional characters? These are all open questions.

The potential outcomes of reading fictional character extend beyond character identification and imitation. They convey warnings about hazards represented by deceptive, manipulative, or malign characters. They invite safe role-playing imagining of actions that would be hazardous in real life. They permit rehearsal of potential future emotional states and experiences, and so forth. Each one of these outcomes could refract differently through the lens of temperament, with bold and shy readers making different use of the opportunities to travel with characters. Though the governing principle of character education by way of fiction takes a simple view of fiction reading as formative of character and behavior, real world responses to fictional character may be more shaped by disposition than a shaper of them.

Hochman's *Character in Literature* as an armature for temperamental character

...

The cognitive character theory of Baruch Hochman, outlined in his book *Character in Literature*, provides an armature for discussion of responses to fictional character that allows space for readers' temperamental differences and varied opinions but still affords a teacher the opportunity to ask for textual evidence to support students' judgments about fictional characters. Hochman offers as a sequence of juxtapositions the following pairings, representing scales of greater and lesser degree, and inviting judgments on the parts of readers about the characters they encounter in fictional worlds:

stylization	Naturalism
coherence	Incoherence
wholeness	Fragmentariness
literalness	Symbolism
complexity	Simplicity
transparency	Opacity
dynamism	staticism (inertness)

(89)

Each pairing opens possibilities for readers to make judgments about characters, supported by textual evidence, without occluding personal responses that may arise from readers' temperaments and experiences. Experience in the classroom suggests that students will make a variety of judgments about the same fictional character: some will find a character more whole, while others will see a fragmented figure; some will make a case for a stylized, symbolic reading, while others recognize a natural, literal rendering of the very same character. The point is not to adjudicate right and wrong readings, but to invite discussion of evidence that does not preclude personal feelings about characters. In a recent MLA volume, *Options for Teaching Narrative Theory*, I describe an exercise for classroom application of these alternatives to help my students think about characters as constructions made out of words, since I am inviting them to supply textual evidence to support their judgments about characters' qualities (Keen, "Undergraduate" 19–32).

Hochman's multiple scales for evaluating character leave space open for actual readers' temperamental response to fictional character. The alternatives do not embed implicit value judgments about better or worse kinds of character or better or worse responses to them. In practice, while students sometimes agree about how to categorize a character, very often they come up with persuasive cases for alternative placements of a character on one of Hochman's scales. This has obvious benefits for teaching argumentation, but it also helps me square my commitment to an analytical approach to character with my conviction that readers' responses to narrative fiction vary a great deal more than most narrative theories can accommodate.

Aspects of Temperamental Character in Theory and Practice

What would happen if fictional character were reexamined through the lens of temperament? Temperamental character theory would not allocate fictional characters to categories (in a manner analogous to the medieval humors: choleric, melancholy, sanguine, and phlegmatic), for that would simply replace one typology with another. [Typologies by fictional character type were once a popular mode of literary analysis. Occasional this intersected with an early form of reader-response criticism. For instance, early in the twentieth century, Arthur Jerrold Tieje theorized seven varieties of romance, four kinds of realism, and four unclassifiable genres by means of "shallow or deep" sentiment evoked by characterization ("Theory" 74).] Instead it would ask how the personality, disposition, and experience of *readers* filter narrative fiction for evocative cues about fictional persons. This call differs from the critical practice of reading characters through trait attribution, or humanizing characters (Knights, "How Many?"; Ross, Cámara Arenas). In his influential critique, L. C. Knights focuses especially on what he regards as the psychologizing errors of critic A. C. Bradley. As a consequence of this critique, generations of students have been counseled to attend to the words out of which characters are wrought rather than making assumptions about the personalities and lives of fictional beings. Yet the social psychology of attribution suggests that people habitually employ commonsense theories of others' behavior, often overestimating the extent to which a person's behavior is due to internal factors of disposition.

Such a theory would acknowledge the scripts about social persons that all readers bring to the apprehension of character (Fowler), and it would seek ways to discern the points of contact between models of social person and textual representations. It would ask how readers choose *with* or *against* the grain of narrative technique and authorial intentions to construct impressions of fictional beings that sometimes obey but also sometimes escape the constraints of characterization. It would rely on the cognitive and affective psychology of intersubjectivity to account for the abundant assumptions brought to the understanding of character by readers of markedly different temperaments and tastes. It would avoid assessing readings of character as right or wrong. It would also seek to discover points of contention arising from the common deployment of narrative fiction for purposes of character education (by advocates of moral education and virtue ethics). It would consider the evidence from developmental psychological studies that show the minimal impact of environmental influences on underlying temperament and how rarely the use of exemplary characters in illustrative narratives results in demonstrably changed attitudes and behaviors. It would attempt to disentangle what fictional character ought to be from what it actually is for readers of various temperaments.

This includes our own temperaments, and they may be the hardest of all to reckon with. Our attitudes towards fictional character may indeed be vexed by contrary impulses in our own pleasure reading and analytical practices: this is worth examining, but we should also take care not to elevate our own temperaments— or our training— as exemplary. We might ask whether theories of character have been skewed by the population of high-empathizers gravitating towards novel-reading and narrative theorizing. Has the experience of empathetic character identification, familiar to virtually all immersion novel-readers, shaped theories of character? Overall, I think we have to say that they have not: rather the converse. Narrative fiction, broadly construed, remains committed to the project of representing human beings moving through social worlds. Most narrative theories of character operate in an arid zone that admits few readerly feelings and underplays the gap-filling fantasizing by which most readers flesh out fictional characters from scant verbal cues. Since few of us, in our teaching, are ready to go all the way with a Bleichian subjective criticism (Bleich), this presents a pedagogical challenge for the uses of a temperamental character theory. It is certainly not meant to be diagnostic: that is, temperamental character theory should not become a process for discovering readers' temperaments through their responses to characters—at least not in the literature classroom. How, then, can discussion of fictional character allow a broader and unrulier range of responses from readers without devolving into a purely subjective report on feelings about fiction? How can a measure of disciplined, evidence-based analysis be recaptured for the sake of shared discussion, without reinstating the purist regime of textualism announced by L. C. Knights? Acknowledging these challenges takes a step in the direction of developing a methodology to admit temperamental character theory to the practice of literary criticism in our writing and classrooms.

Certainly, temperamental character reading can be trained away. If we adopt non-mimetic approaches to narrative in our classrooms, we may succeed in directing our students to the textual instantiation of character, to the words and phrases about paper-people (Chatman 122–38). We can slow the immersion readers down, drag them up to the narrative surface, force them to analyze the language, and din the conventions of literary discourse into their heads. However, the emotional powers of narrativity, operating through suspense, curiosity, and surprise (Sternberg, *Biblical* 264–320), will be working against this project the whole time, hooked onto the intuitive recognition of fictional characters as persons. The drive of narrativity can be contained, but not suppressed. Perhaps the time has come to wonder whether real readers' practices deserve a place in narrative theorizing.

...

(On the paradox of fiction, see below 161)

Even though readers know perfectly well that fictional characters are make-believe, they go on caring about them, lending them the bodies that they do not possess, feeling with them in emotional fusion that paradoxically calls into embodiment a psychic corporeality vouched for in readers' own bodily responses (Babb; Vermeule; Warhol, *Having*; Walsh, "Why We Wept"). With the exception of some rhetorical narrative theory (especially Phelan's indefatigable theorizing on the topic, in *Reading People, Reading Plots*; *Experiencing Fiction*; and *Living to Tell about It*) and recent empirical studies in discourse processing (Bortolussi and Dixon; Miall, *Literary*), actual readers' behavior as a response to fictional character has rarely been addressed by narratology. Placed under a tacit ban, the unruly behavior of real readers often undermines critical consensus about the functions of textual configurations and the limits of textual cues.

As teachers, we can keep the most flagrant of readerly engagements with character out of the realm of the analytical essay, sending them along to the zone of creative writing (where they thrive!), but nothing will stop readers (ourselves included) from lending extra characteristics, borrowed from the real world or from other fictions, to the matrix of character. The cognitivists suggest that we bring along and contribute knowledge structures to our reading of character; indeed, we do far more than that, when as embodied readers we rehearse our own temperaments in our responses to fictional character. Studying narrative empathy has persuaded me that there is neither an inherent hierarchy of values invested in narrative techniques, nor a right or predictable set of responses to those techniques. The situation is kaleidoscopic: a theory of temperamental character does not simplify matters. It validates the variable, fluctuating, and irregular experiences of real readers in their encounters with character. This variety should serve as a starting point for future theorizing, not as an embarrassment to be bracketed by narratological models that look the other way.

9

FROM NOVEL READERS AND THE EMPATHETIC ANGEL OF OUR NATURE

In *Empathy and the Novel* I posed dozens of questions about which I could discover little or no empirical research at the time, or about which existing studies pointed in contradictory directions. I summarized these in a series of hypotheses (see above 6–7). This chapter does not attempt to catch up on all of the questions, many of which have been pursued—and taken in new directions—by other researchers in a variety of disciplines.

Instead, I zero in on the application of the empathy-altruism hypothesis to narrative empathy in response to novel reading. In *Empathy and the Novel* I contested the moral sentimental claim that novel reading inevitably works to form a more altruistic and peaceable citizenry. Martha Nussbaum [in *Cultivating Humanity* and other works], … evokes psychology's empathy-altruism hypothesis in the context of reading fictional narratives (Batson, "Altruism"). Nussbaum promises a beneficial civic and moral yield from novel reading, a view that has also been embraced by philosophers of moral development and developmental psychologists (Blum, *Friendship*; Hoffman). This essay updates the debate by offering some comments on recent work by another influential voice, Steven Pinker, in his important recent book *The Better Angels of Our Nature: Why Violence has Declined* (2011). It is to Pinker that I allude in my title, "Novel Readers and the Empathetic Angel of our Nature." His nuanced account of change from a more violent to a more peaceable human species (over the long term) includes a cultural shift towards empathy and altruism but does not place undue causal emphasis on novel reading.

Whether narrative empathy and other feelings evoked by fiction reading actually result in moral improvement has been questioned, not only by me—the history of this suspicion goes back at least to the eighteenth century (*Empathy and the Novel* 37–64) A version of it appears in Saint Augustine's lament that he was wasting

DOI: 10.4324/9781003264071-12

his time feeling with Vergil's fictional creations. Among moral philosophers, the debate about the status of emotional responsiveness to narrative typically centers on the question of whether it should be cultivated (to encourage recognition of other minds, enhance comprehension, or form morality) or distrusted, as a potentially misleading capitulation to a frame of reference warped by bias or as an incitement to unruly behavior (Plato). Ironically, the argument in favor of aesthetic emotions (cultivation through narrative) results in a more proscriptive, narrower list of valued narratives, while the suspicious argument (advocating dispassion) more willingly admits the potentially deleterious impact of narrative as encouraging escapism, time-wasting, and vicious habits. This latter side admits a broader range of narrative, including comic books, video games, and romance novels, but does so to warn against the dangers of emotionally-engaged reading practices. The stress marks between the two positions about narrative impact reveal different attitudes to reading itself, one admitting a broad range of narrative in an array of media (and fearing the impact of reading on people and society) and the other emphasizing the special benefits of reading canonical or at least celebrated and complex literary narratives (and promising the development of good world citizens and improved societies). Which is it to be? To approach these questions requires reference to research far afield from philosophy and literary studies.

[The year] 2013 marked the centenary of Vernon Lee's foundational work on aesthetic empathy in *The Beautiful* (published originally by Cambridge University Press): after a long hiatus, it is again a great time to be doing interdisciplinary work on empathy. I have written elsewhere on the 60 to 75 years following the first flowering of empathy research, during which scholarly and scientific conversations about literature and the emotions were rare, interdisciplinary study of aesthetic emotions scarce, and questions about what happens in real readers as they feel with imaginary worlds and their inhabitants discouraged as a disparaged "psychologizing" [See chapter 10, below, on Wimsatt and Beardsley]. Following on the cognitive turn of the 1960s and the narrative turn of the 1990s, the affective turn of recent years encourages active reading of psychology by literary theorists—psychology rather than psychoanalytic theory, a psychology that includes brain science. New interdisciplinary combinations in the sciences of brain and behavior, such as social neuroscience, give the literary student of empathy a great deal to consider. Though modern empathy research has been going on steadily since the 1980s, this recent cross-disciplinary conversation marks a change in the situation. A decade ago when I went to my college library looking for something to cite on empathy as a component of literary reading, there were some resources to be found, but very little engagement outside of the separate silos of ethics, developmental psychology, cognitive science, and what was just then a very new research program in neuroscience, on mirror neurons. The theorists of film were in the vanguard of engagement with philosophers and cognitive scientists, some of the virtue ethicists were reading some of the developmental psychologists, but on the whole there was relatively little cross-disciplinary conversation around empathy. My home field of narratology, for example, was at that time virtually innocent of developments in discourse processing or the psychology of narrative impact.

Four publications since 2007 illustrate the difference a decade makes and impress with the interdisciplinary liveliness of the field: Jean Decety and William Ickes's *Social Neuroscience of Empathy*, Amy Coplan and the late Peter Goldie's *Empathy: Philosophical and Psychological Perspectives*, Jean Decety's *Empathy: From Bench to Bedside*, and a recent issue of *Emotion Review* substantially devoted to empathy. Each of these collections of essays contains work from scholars and scientists working in diverse disciplinary homes, and even though most of them frankly acknowledge the challenges of arriving at shared vocabularies and mutually recognizable concepts, there's more evidence than ever before that the philosophers are reading the social psychologists, the cognitive scientists are reading the neuroscientists, the medical educators are considering the findings of the developmental psychologists, educational theorists, and practitioners, even that questions posed by humanists (including literary scholars like me) are getting some attention from empirical researchers. Re-evaluation of earlier theorizing in light of the new research proceeds apace.

The most salient challenges to the claims of *Empathy and the Novel* have come from psychologists and cognitivists working with literary texts in studies of narrative impact. [The Raymond Mar lab in Toronto and the Dan R. Johnson lab in Lexington, Virginia have produced some of the most important studies linking empathy in reading to other traits or subsequent pro-social behaviors.] Let me review my earlier argument against applying the well-substantiated empathy-altruism hypothesis (Batson, "Altruism") to experiences of *narrative* empathy. I doubted that fiction reading, even fiction reading of a certain elevated kind, focused on canonical works of the great tradition, produced good world citizens. I showed that it was difficult to disentangle novel reading from a host of other formative experiences that might encourage altruism or the lighter standard of prosocial behavior in individuals or whole societies. I believed that the world wars and genocidal violence of the twentieth century, a century in which many novels were written and read, argued against a causal or even correlational relation between mass consumption of narrative fiction and concern for real others in the world. Steven Pinker's redaction of the social science on declining rates of violence has made me re-evaluate that critique, as I will shortly discuss. I criticized studies that extrapolated from preschool children to predict behavior of adults. I differed with studies that claimed to show a causal link between experiences of narrative empathy and prosocial action in the world, when they confounded reading with the other activities employed with the experimental subjects. Adding a role-playing game, staging a discussion, even certain forms of solicitation to charity seemed to me to blend the reading experience with other prompts towards prosocial action. These studies primed the subjects to act prosocially, or confounded the results of reading and other incitements to emotional engagement and identification. Some studies erroneously attributed all the impact to the very short fictions or films that evoked empathy and ignored the effects of the activities involving real people on subsequent pro-social actions. The literary version of psychology's empathy-altruism hypothesis, I argued, amounts to an unsubstantiated faith tradition without robust support by empirical demonstrations. Serious work still needed to be done to demonstrate that *narrative* empathy contributes to real-world altruism, personally costly and socially significant action on behalf of others.

In narrative empathy as in other aspects of moral development, people have more influence on other people than narrative fiction by itself. Questioning the causal link between altruism and narrative empathy devalues neither narrative empathy nor the widespread hope in the socially beneficial yield of novel reading. It shifts the emphasis to what people choose to do with their reading experiences, how they share them, and how they encourage themselves and others to act on feeling responses. While I do criticize causal arguments that equate experiences of narrative empathy with real world empathy for living others, I recognize that many writers and readers believe that there *ought* to be a connection. Thus my subsequent work on narrative empathy has focused on theorizing the conditions and circumstances that permit communication of authorial empathy to different audiences by means of strategic empathizing (see above 40ff). We should not forget the important contribution made by people themselves, around shared fiction-reading, as a vital component of the transaction from author to text to reader. Parents, teachers, librarians, reading-group participants, and enthusiastic book-recommenders everywhere are too ready to erase their own contribution, giving all the credit for impact away to the books themselves. Consistent with a pedagogical ethics of care, as advocated by Nel Noddings and Michael Slote, among others, I underscore the important role played in moral development by the people who love and share novels. Scratch any story about a novel that changed someone's life, or her attitudes, or his actions, and you will find another person somewhere in there, taking a kid to a library, putting a treasured book in someone's hands, leading a discussion, modeling the notion that our fiction reading shapes who we can become. So, while novel-reading can affect our vocabulary, our knowledge of the world, and our vocations, including the rare but wonderful effect of recruiting the next generation of novelists, as humanists we should recall the impact of other human beings on our moral development. Novels can't be left to do that work on their own.

In *Empathy and the Novel* I suggested that immersion reading experiences of stories perceived as fiction, a phenomenon sometimes studied under the name "transportation," are especially likely to be involved in narrative empathy. This suggestion has received some experimental confirmation from psychologist Dan R. Johnson, who has shown that training in visualizing mental imagery, following the work of Emily Holmes, encourages immersion reading, enhances empathy, and results in increased prosocial behavior as measured by a spill test. That's a well-verified technique for measuring impulses to help, in which a collaborator "accidentally" drops a bunch of magic markers on the floor near the subjects. People whose empathetic natures had just been jogged by reading fiction immersively, after receiving mental visualizing instructions, voluntarily got up and stooped down to pick up the markers. They did so at a greater rate than less empathetic subjects. From my conversations with Dan Johnson I have learned that the subjects in the mental visualizing condition acted helpfully while those who had received perspective-taking prompts did not. Rather than overt "perspective-taking" imagining as in the social-studies version of fiction reading, which instructs a reader to "put yourself in the shoes" of the character (to enhance empathy), the related experiences of immersing oneself in an absorbing fictional world and joining a fictive community of creatures quite unlike oneself, Dan Johnson has shown, has an impact on enhanced empathy and even prosocial behavior. Being out of one's own self and in another world differs from the ethical instruction to "walk a mile in another's shoes." From another psychological study of readers of *Harry Potter* and *Twilight*, Shira Gabriel and Ariana Young have shown that escapism and fantasy empathy may be accomplishing some of the work typically attributed to perspective-taking exercised across barriers of difference. They hypothesize a "narrative collective-assimilation" theory that experiencing a narrative leads readers to be part of the collective described in the fictional world. The warm feeling of belonging, even to a tribe of vampires, may be contributing to the ethical effects of narrative usually attributed to imaginative extension of role-taking or perspective taking. Both of these research directions suggest that we ought to revise our prejudice against immersion in fantasy worlds and escapism as prominent effects of fiction reading.

Finally, in *Empathy and the Novel* I criticized narrative ethics and some philosophy for making claims about the moral effects of novel-reading while hedging the definition of "the novel" all around with barriers of canonicity, high literary style, and quality, thereby automatically ruling out all sort of narrative fiction in popular genres as if the readers' empathy felt there simply couldn't or shouldn't count. The hope that exposure to art refines emotional perceptiveness and sensitivity animates philosophical aesthetics with applications in the philosophy of education (Carroll, "Aesthetics"), but ordinarily only realistic, literary fiction gets any credit. Working from a cognitivist standpoint, philosophers Martha Nussbaum and Ronald DeSousa have advocated recognition of the rationality of emotions, in *Upheavals of Thought* (2001) and *The Rationality of Emotion* (1987), respectively. DeSousa argues that emotions are a kind of perception, possessing a dramatic structure and playing a crucial role in decision-making, beliefs, desires, and rationality. Exposure to art, according to DeSousa, helps to elaborate "paradigm scenarios" to benefit one's management of emotional experience (182). Nussbaum often writes about the cultivation of the moral imagination, positing not just personal but civic impacts to be garnered through novel reading. But which novels yield such social benefits in these theories? Not most Oprah books, despite Winfrey's evident commitment to cultivating empathy. Philosophers naturally approach literary texts differently than literary critics, concerned to make generalizations about how human beings learn from literature, rather than seeking to generate fresh interpretations of individual works. Still, by examining particular works, they commend them to our attention. Nussbaum holds that a reader's emotional involvement in a novel by Henry James or Charles Dickens engages her in processes of empathy and conjecture that make her a better citizen in the real world (*Cultivating* 90). According to Nussbaum, concern for fictional characters, their circumstances and needs, awakens moral and political interests in readers (104). Nussbaum claims that fictional narratives play a direct, shaping role in forming feeling readers into good world citizens who will make right decisions in favor of unknown others.

I have criticized this argument because of all the novel reading it leaves out: what about the vast majority of novels that real people actually read? Praise of the ethical and socially beneficial effects of The Novel rarely means all novels. To omit popular fiction is especially convenient to theorists of narrative impact who want to see only virtuous results of novel reading and want to avoid considering any vicious consequences of emotionally arousing narratives. This particular case has been vigorously and humorously pursued by both Gregory Currie and Joshua Landy. If "the novel" and "novel-reading" are to be credited with morally efficacious effects on readers, leading to prosocial or even altruistic actions in the real world, then we need to be open to the novels that readers actually read, including mass market fiction and genres associated with women readers, for to do otherwise is to introduce a biasing screen into our investigations.

Something inspires altruism, however, and as Steven Pinker reminds us, aspects of Enlightenment thinking contribute to reductions of violence if not compassion in action. In his short article, "Taming the Devil within Us," Pinker writes

> Attempts to quantify the death tolls from earlier centuries suggest that many of the collapsing empires, conquering maniacs, horse-tribe invasions, slave trades and annihilations of native peoples had individual death tolls that, adjusted for population, are comparable to those of each of the two world wars. War before civilization was even bloodier. Forensic archaeology and ethnographic demography suggest that around 15% of people living in non-state societies died violently— five times the proportion of violent deaths in the twentieth century from war, genocide and man-made famine combined.
>
> (309)

Pinker goes on to describe related declines in violence:

> The obsolescence of major war is just one of many historical declines of violence. European homicide rates have dropped at least 30-fold since the Middle Ages, from about 40 per 100,000 people per year in the fourteenth

> century to 1.3 at the end of the twentieth. Barbaric customs that were unexceptional for millennia, such as human sacrifice, the persecution of witches and heretics, chattel slavery, blood sports, punitive torture and mutilation, sadistic executions (burning, breaking, crucifixion, disemboweling, impalement) and execution for victimless crimes have been abolished in most of the world. The past 50 years have seen a cascade of rights revolutions— civil, women's, children's, gay, animal — which have demonstrably driven down rates of lynching, pogroms, rape, spousal abuse, child abuse, spanking, gay-bashing, hunting and callousness to laboratory animals.
>
> ("Taming" 309–10)

This account raises a host of questions about causation. If Pinker is right about the decline of violence, then to what does he attribute the change? How have the Better Angels of our human nature, including empathy, received the encouragement to society-wide expression? Pinker describes a changing historical climate that interacts with human dispositions to produce less violent societies on the whole. In his description of human personality, Pinker's five "inner demons"—sadism, revenge, dominance, violence in pursuit of a practical benefit, violence in pursuit of an ideology—face off against four "better angels": self-control, empathy, morality, and reason. Note that empathy isn't alone here: Pinker strongly emphasizes the self-regulating containment of the more impulsive demons by self-control and the governments to which we delegate the task of social ordering. For all his interest in the push-me/pull-you effects of our emotional natures, Pinker attributes a great deal of the reduction in violence to the elevation of *reason* and *morality* in post-Enlightenment societies, including mechanisms of social control. In an interview with the *Harvard Gazette* about the process of writing the book, he said, "*Better Angels* made me appreciate the forces of civilization and enlightenment which have made our lives so much more peaceable than those of our ancestors: the police, a court system, democracy, education, literacy, commerce, science, the Enlightenment, and the forms of secular humanism that grew out of it — which are easy to take for granted" (Sweeney). We do not see Pinker emphasizing empathy or novel-reading here; indeed, he writes "empathy cannot be the whole story…it is a fickle emotion. It is triggered by cuteness, good looks, kinship, friendship and solidarity. And it is easily shut off or converted to its opposite, schadenfreude, by competition or revenge" ("Taming" 310). To Pinker's caveats we should add that evolutionary psychologists' suggestion that human empathy has evolved in part as an aspect of Machiavellian intelligence: on the savannah, empathy with future victims, prey species, helps human hunters to anticipate their behavior and kill them more expeditiously.

In his book, Pinker does support his big-picture analysis of change in human behavior over the past millennia with several points about novel reading, and at least implicitly readers' narrative empathy. His discussion of nose cutting (a disfiguring punishment) occupies more pages of his book than novels, but Pinker does note the growth in the number of circulating libraries during the eighteenth-century, he catches the involvement of eighteenth and nineteenth century novelists in the movement toward moral sentimentalism and the education of the sympathetic imagination, and he endorses most of historian Lynn Hunt's thesis about novel-reading in the eighteenth century and what she calls "The Invention of Human Rights" (*Better Angels* 176). Hunt argues that the imaginative exercise of taking the side of a servant girl in Richardson's *Pamela* (and other popular novels of the period) introduced a perspective-taking habit of mind that ushered in a way of thinking expressed in extension of human rights. Pinker writes,

> Whether or not novels in general, or epistolary novels in particular, were the critical genre in expanding empathy, the explosion of reading may have contributed to the Humanitarian Revolution by getting people into the habit of straying from their parochial vantage points. And it may have contributed in a second way: by creating a hothouse for new ideas about moral values and the social order.
>
> (177)

Pinker is also informed by Nussbaum, Keith Oatley, Frank Hakemulder, and Raymond Mar. Pinker sees the link between real experiences and fictional experiences as similarly effective, because people "often blur the two in their memories," in confusions of fact and fiction studied by Strange (589). Yet he concedes that we do not actually know whether reading fiction makes people more empathetic or whether empathetic people are more likely to enjoy fiction. He judiciously surveys the potential downsides of empathy, including injustice. For Pinker, "The ultimate goal should be policies and norms that become second nature and render empathy unnecessary" (592). While Pinker acknowledges that perspective-taking may impel a person to act altruistically, he speculates that fiction reading, one of what he calls "technologies of vicarious experience" has expanded "our collective sense of sympathy" for others and "helped drive the Humanitarian Revolution, the Long Peace, the New Peace, and the Rights Revolution" (583). Pinker cites

> the outsourcing of deterrence and revenge to a disinterested third party, including the police and court system; the growth of commerce, which replaces zero-sum plunder with positive-sum trade and reciprocity; the forces of cosmopolitanism, such as mobility and literacy, which encourage people to take other vantage points and hence consider their interests; and the growth of education, public discourse, science, and abstract reasoning, which discourage parochial tribalism and encourage people to treat violence as a problem to be solved rather than as a contest to be won.
>
> (Sweeney)

Pinker thus bets on literacy as a driver of that training in perspective taking.

As in many of his sources, only certain genres of narrative receive credit for expanding the empathetic circle. Pinker singles out "realistic fiction," with its capacity to seduce readers into thinking and feeling like people very different from themselves (*Better Angels* 173–4). But what about the unruly reading behavior of people not governed by a syllabus or the Great Tradition? Simon Dickie, studying the same period as Lynn Hunt, the eighteenth century, in his illuminating archaeology of ordinary sadistic humor, *Cruelty and Laughter*, Dickie describes one of his book's recurring themes: "the sheer slowness with which ordinary sufferings—the unheroic miseries of poverty, the humiliations of disease, the private trauma of a rape victim—became worthy of sympathy and serious aesthetic representation" (4) and catalogs the eighteenth century love of jokes about cripples, the blind rape, and domestic abuse. If there were a dataset to mine, Pinker would undoubtedly attempt to demonstrate that our humor has changed to match our reduced appetite for violence against the handicapped, the visually-impaired, rape victims and domestic abuse sufferers. But cruel humor itself, and other vicious modes of representation, has certainly not disappeared. YouTube contains a treasure trove of "funny" injuries and humiliations. The internet has enhanced the availability of sadistic humor, just as it has encouraged a market in child pornography (or virtual-kiddie porn), once a rarity, now widely disseminated. A fair discussion of narrative impact on morality must consider diverse content, audiences, and genres. If novel-reading does have an impact on the real world, we need to be able to consider the results without deciding ahead of time what they ought to be: they may encourage vice rather than virtue. If we do find positive results of reading fiction, the booklist of real readers will be considerably more diverse than the narrow high-brow syllabi of the narrative ethicists. The readers whose lives have been changed may not be middle class to begin with.

Investigating the impact of literary reading on behavior in the real world through empirical studies is a project in its infancy. One of the most interesting experiments that does have demonstrated results employs literary reading to reduce criminal recidivism, or repeat convictions. The Changing Lives Through Literature (CLTL) programs, founded by Robert Waxler and Jean Trounstine, contends that

> Individuals who read about characters in literature may find a connection between themselves and those characters. If literature is a regular companion in our lives, this is not news. But, many adults and youth do not have access to literature and its transformative nature. CLTL participants, judges, probation officers, and instructors believe that bringing carefully selected works of literature to criminal offenders may help these men and women gain insight into their lives and behavior, while learning that they are not alone with their problems. The written word affects us far beyond the moment of reading.
>
> (*Changing Lives Through Literature*)

In brief, here's how CLTL works: judges recruited to the program sentence selected convicts to a course of reading and discussion, usually in gender-segregated groups, instead of jail time. Changing Lives through Literature began in Massachusetts in 1991 and has now spread as far as Texas and the UK. From the outset, CLTL programs have included the sentencing judge and probation officer. They join a discussion leader (usually a local professor or advanced graduate student), who guides a small group of convicted criminals in a course of reading and discussion, usually featuring contemporary short stories (though novels are sometimes used). The courses last 10–14 weeks, attendance and participation is mandatory, and the results are statistically significant: CLTL boasts a less than 20% recidivism rate compared to the 45% rate of convicts not in alternative sentencing programs (Jarjoura and Krumholz 130, 133). The personal testimony gathered in *Finding a Voice*, Trounstine and Waxler's 2005 book on CLTL, relates impressive cases of perspective taking, character identification leading to empathy, and thoughtful self-examination prompted by the imaginary experiences of fictional characters. Combine this with the proven reduction in the recidivism rate and it looks like solid evidence that reading fiction cultivates the sympathetic imagination and leads to an improvement in society: if not altruism, at least less crime. This raises the question of what prescribed reading works in such circumstances.

From the lofty heights of Nussbaum's perspective, the CLTL reading lists are quite middle-brow (there's no Henry James, George Eliot or Charles Dickens). They include some Toni Morrison at the high end (usually *The Bluest Eye*), and literary fiction by John Cheever, Joyce Carol Oates, Raymond Carver, TC Boyle, Julia Alvarez, Tim O'Brien, Willa Cather, and even Katherine Mansfield. The mode of discussion differs quite markedly from the formal, thematic, and contextual analysis of the college classroom, though many CLTL classes are held on college campuses (that's part of their formula). Instead, an Oprah-like emphasis on making personal connections guides the questioning: How do we learn to feel ugly? What does it mean to be a victim? What does it mean to be a good mother? Will you tell about a dream that you've had that is as important to you as the dream in *Of Mice and Men?* What are your possibilities in life? The discussions that ensue stem from the shared reading, but they are prompted by skilled questioning. They also take place in the presence of the three powerful figures, the professor, the judge, and the probation officer. The empowering effect of joining a discussion as an equal with the judge who sentenced you and the leveling of social status experienced by the elite participants are often commented-upon aspects of the arrangements. Apparently Changing Lives Through Literature works, and the discussions seem to work because the participants read emotionally evocative fiction.

But the jury is out about what exactly is working at the level of narrative empathy. I think that the choices of rich and interesting stories that allow discovery of alternative perspectives is certainly playing a role, but if I had to guess, I'd say the extraordinary social rearrangement that brings convicted criminals, their peers, the judges, probation officers and graduate students together in discussion drives the results. Further, the unquantifiable but evident *care* that shows when a convict joins the circle of shared humanity that we classroom teachers take for granted because we encounter it every day, that has an impact, too. Social and developmental psychologists have the tools to disentangle the confounded causes wrapped up in accounts of CLTL's results. It does not debunk the power of the book or disregard reading to remember the impact of living human beings on one another.

The explosion of interest in narrative and the emotions broadly construed shows in the variety of topics taken up recently by literary scholars encouraged by and participating in the affective turn. These include studies of narrative identification, film genres and elicitation of emotions, intersubjectivity in film and fiction, narrative faculties and emotional involvement, the role of emotional involvement in absorption and reading speed, and narrative empathy. There is still a great deal that we do not know about emotionally evocative narrative techniques. Narrative strategies have diverse or protean results and readers' different temperaments have a rarely acknowledged impact on their varied engagement with narratives. When emotions arise from makers and receivers in communication, provoked by representations and by narrativity itself, the potential interactions and crossing points dazzle us with possibilities. This should not be a discouragement to further study. To acknowledge the complications involved in studying narrative and the emotions and the impact of literary reading on the real world is to prepare a sturdier foundation for subsequent narratology, narrative ethics, philosophical aesthetics, and the psychology of narrative impact. It might change what we read. It might change the questions we ask our students and each other. Who knows, it might even change the world, if we decided it ought to.

PART III

Interdisciplinary Applications of Empathy, Affect, and Cognition

Interdisciplinary Applications of Empathy, Affect, and Cognition

When literary critics and theorists engage with colleagues in other disciplines, the effort to communicate successfully over disciplinary boundaries demands clarity about terminology, premises, and approaches. The first three essays excerpted in this section undertake such an effort. The 2011 essay, "Introduction: Narrative and the Emotions," originally written to frame an interdisciplinary double special issue of *Poetics Today*, provides both historical background and a genealogy of terms and schools of thought. For example, in a note that has since been eliminated from the essay that opens this section, I wrote:

> The best practice for clarity's sake when writing about the emotions is to declare one's assumptions. These are mine: 1) emotions arise from human beings' mammalian endowment, and basic emotions can be observed across species and cultures; 2) emotional responses are prompted by both bodily cues and cognitive appraisals, a perceptual theory (Prinz 2004) that explains the different stages of empathy better than a purely cognitive approach; 3) cognitive appraisals (judgments, evaluations, or thoughts) are often involved in emotions (Frijda 1986, 2006) but are not required for all emotional responses, such as homeostatic feelings responding to bodily states (Craig 2002) and responses to all non-referential elements and patterns encountered in language and other media; 4) emotions are more changeable than relatively durable dispositions or temperaments (Kagan and Snidman 2004); 5) emotional experience plays a profound role in human development and behavior (Bowlby 1969-80); 6) human evolution has been shaped

DOI: 10.4324/9781003264071-13

> by the emotional interactions of people, especially children and caregivers (Hrdy 1999, 2007); 7) age, gender (and aspects of identity), experience, individual memory, and the surrounding culture inflect emotional experience (Tsai 1999); 8) as for a list of emotions, I accept Ekman's (1992) list of core emotions observable from fleeting facial expressions: anger, sadness, fear, surprise, disgust, contempt, and happiness (Paul Ekman's cross-cultural fieldwork on facial expressions of emotions supports Darwin's [1998 (1872,1889)] contention that humans and animals share basic emotions showing in bodily expressions); 9) I also accept as complex emotions, besides those in Plutchik listed above, moral sentiments (empathy and compassion) and social emotions (shame, embarrassment, envy, guilt and hatred as well as the positive calm and *amae,* or comfort in belonging [Doi 1981]). avoidance, arousal and quiescence systems governing adaptive behavior), see Schulkin (2004: 20).
>
> *Keen, "Introduction" 6*

In 2011 it felt more urgent to a literary theorist attempting to engage in cross-disciplinary conversation to demonstrate bona fides through comprehensive declarations of allegiances and assumptions than it does a decade later. Perhaps the advances in interdisciplinary collaboration, along with a more habitual sharing of what we actually mean by key terms, obviates elaborate gestures such as the one I quote above.

Yet each time we enter into a discussion with interlocutors whose interests chime with ours, our pleasure at intellectual resonances may disguise profound differences in the way we understand our evidently shared area of inquiry. This can lead to confusion and even unproductive squabbling about the legitimacy of one another's approaches or conclusions. The essays collected in this section represent my effort, over time, to build bridges between rhetorical narrative theory and some of the many disciplines that have taken up my theorizing about narrative empathy. My work on empathy itself draws on research and theorizing in three distinct areas of psychology (cognitive, developmental, and social psychology), on philosophical work in ethics (moral philosophy), and on recent developments in neuroscience.

In "Empathy Studies," I discuss the debates and challenges of that interdisciplinary research context for a literary theoretical audience. Students of literature are more likely to be familiar with affect studies than with theorizing that emerges from engagement with emotion science. "Affect and Empathy Studies" considers applications of both approaches in the law and legal studies, discusses two domains of research into and theorizing about human emotions of interest to legal theorists and practitioners in the law. It offers basic definitions of the terms "empathy" and "affect," brief overviews of research areas, suggestions about the relevance of affect and empathy studies to law, and cautions about those applications' limitations and liabilities. By no means prescriptive in intention, this essay's discussion of affect and empathy studies lays bare some of the underlying assumptions and critical attitudes of work in differing fields. In it I contend that all varieties of empathy, with their affordances and limitations, are resources for the rhetorical arts of persuasion. Writers and practitioners in the law should alertly consider the roles that empathy and affect play in the law, especially when legal abstractions, doctrines, and documents that evoke strong feelings are accorded the imaginative status of persons by means of *Einfühlung*.

Essays on affect and cognition in studies of a Victorian novel, "Affective Trollope," contemporary anglophone fiction, "Twenty-First Century Experiments in Emotion and Cognition," and postcolonial literary studies round out the section. It concludes with a meditation on narrative empathy as an element of human rights discourse: "Human Rights Discourse and Universals of Cognition and Emotion" offers an elaboration of strategic narrative empathizing as a potential bridge between postcolonial literary studies and human rights discourse, which take opposing views on the notion of universal human rights.

10

FROM INTRODUCTION

Narrative and the Emotions

A Look Behind Us

Seventy-five years ago, a scholar seeking a starting point on narrative and the emotions … might have consulted colleagues in psychology and literature departments for a reading list. Quite likely the scholar would have been reminded by those colleagues of the canonical works representing several decades' worth of fruitful collaboration between their disciplines: literary theorist I. A. Richards' *Principles of Literary Criticism* (1926) and psychologist John Dewey's *Art as Experience* (1934). Not yet discouraged by the prohibitions of W.K. Wimsatt and Monroe Beardsley's 1946 *Sewanee Review* essay, "The Affective Fallacy," which disparaged discussion of elicitation of emotion as "affective relativism" (27); not yet converted to the emergent New Critical canon, which put narrative (especially those lengthy engines of sentimental response, novels) in the shade; not yet fully adopting modern theories of form in preference to older Romantic theories of the imagination (Dissanayake 142–7); not yet interpellated as either a scientist or a literary intellectual, incapable of communicating across the divide severing the "Two Cultures" (Snow): our scholar would have every reason to believe that a science of the emotions, including the study of physiological responses, could contribute to an understanding of aesthetic experience. The notion that analysis of the feelings provoked and invited by reading (and creating) narrative could illuminate the workings of mental activity would have seemed to our colleagues of 75 years ago a reasonable proposition; that the formal elements of plot arouse the emotions (in tragedy, of fear and pity) would have been axiomatic for them and their predecessors (Aristotle, chapter 14; 85–101). [The long and rich tradition of work on the emotions in the arts generally and in literary arts specifically is beyond the scope of this introduction. Needless to say, any contemporary

DOI: 10.4324/9781003264071-14

theorizing of impact that sets out its stall without exhibits from Aristotle, Plato, Horace, Longinus, Herder, Lessing, Goethe, Kant, the Romantics on estrangement and the sublime, Hume and Smith on sympathy, Brecht and Shklovsky, and so forth, risks privileging the recent over the ancient or traditional for no good reason beyond convenience. For convenience's sake, then, I refer the reader to Neal Oxenhandler . . . for a selective history of literary emotion, to Meir Sternberg for pointed critiques of cognitive poetics' omissions of their learned precursors, and to my own survey of the "Literary Career of Empathy" (Keen, *Empathy* 37–64) for starting places.]

In the work of I. A. Richards, our scholar could read, "a theory of feeling, or emotion, of attitudes and desires, of the affective-volitional aspect of mental activity, is required at all points of our analysis" (Richards, *Principles* 91). Far from banishing emotions from discussions of literature, Richards elevates them as "signs of attitudes" (132) and gives them a central place in theories of art (for Richards addresses literature, not limited to poetry or literary narrative, as one of the arts). In his definition of attitudes (of which emotions are signs), Richards' indebtedness to the psychology of his day can be discerned: attitudes, he writes, are "imaginal and incipient activities or tendencies to action" (112). These action tendencies matter to literary criticism because "all the most valuable effects of poetry" can be described in terms of "the resolution, inter-animation, and balancing of impulses" (113) as for instance in Aristotle's definition of Tragedy (chapter 6). Though it is in his discussion of rhythm and meter that Richards speaks the language of neural settings and stimuli most fluently (139), his understanding of literary narrative also has a neurological basis. For Richards, artistic communication, when efficacious and deepened by the receivers' "attitudes" (179) makes "permanent modifications in the structure of the mind" (132). Richards tacitly prefers poetry and shorter forms where coherence can be apprehended, as his emphases in his teaching and writing show. This does not rule out an application of Richards' account of reading to narrative, but the novel is conspicuous in its absence from *Principles of Literary Criticism* (Dames, *Physiology* 248–53).

Richards' work on principles of literary criticism, published in the International Library of Psychology, Philosophy and Scientific Method, indicates a tradition of interdisciplinary collaboration and conversation that had been established by an earlier generation of Victorian and turn-of-the-twentieth-century aestheticians. Examples would be Vernon Lee, who was also a novelist (Lee, *Miss Brown*; *Beautiful*) and late Victorian scientific writers who were also men of letters, such as G. H. Lewes (Lewes, *Goethe*; *Physiology*). Among the questions posed and investigated by Victorian thinkers were those about novelists' efforts to stimulate development of novel-readers' sympathetic imagination (Haight), about the nature of story-telling invention and its impact on readers' feelings (Dallas; Kreilkamp), about physiological responses to reading (Bain; Elfenbein), about empathy and *Einfühlung* (Lee, *Beautiful*), and the malleability of the reading mind, especially as regards readers' morals (Masson; Hutton; Trollope, *Autobiography*). Good guides to the overlap in

Victorians' interest in aesthetics and novel-theories on the one hand, and psychology and physiology on the other hand, can be found in the work of Rick Rylance and Nicholas Dames (Rylance; Dames, *Physiology*). The growth during and after the First World War of therapeutic psychology, including but not limited to Freudian psychoanalysis, had established a relationship between the narrative expression of emotionally charged experience and restoration of health, resting on a theory of emotions as suppressed impulses that could burst forth in a return of the repressed (Freud, "Resistance" 286–302). This reinforced psychology's faith in meliorism even in the face of the catastrophic psychic damage inflicted by the Great War, vividly documented in verse and prose. [For empirical verification of the link between improved health and expressive writing about traumatic experiences, see Pennebaker, *Opening Up: The Healing Power of Expressing Emotion* (1997). This book summarizes 25 years' worth of empirical results in narrative psychology, particularly regarding the health benefits of expressive writing...]

Even though many modernist writers expressed skepticism about the healing powers of literature, preferring to pursue aesthetics of fragmentation, alienation and anti-closure, their contemporaries in psychology remained convinced of the efficacy of narrative in restoring psychic and social equilibrium. Writing after the First World War, Richards himself still held out high hopes that psychology could sort out good or valuable experiences from bad (*Principles* 44) and correct society's "obsolete moral principles" (57). The mechanism by which human beings pass unaware "from a chaotic to a better organized state," was according to Richards "through the influence of other minds," and he named literature and the arts as "the chief means by which these influences are diffused" (57). In another work of 1926 he argued that poetry was "capable of saving us" and "a perfectly possible means of overcoming chaos" (*Science and Poetry* 82). Clearly he was underestimating the threat posed by fascism, though he would later apply his Basic English work to improved international communication on behalf of world peace (*Nations and Peace*). [Richards spent the war years at Harvard, moving there in 1939 and staying until 1974 (Storer).] In *Principles of Literary Criticism*, Richards does consider the risks of bad art and the seductive appeal of cinema, but he does not anticipate the baleful uses to which emotionality would be made in short order in an era of mass media and fascism (see also Febvre). Undisturbed by the negative possibilities of emotional arousal, Richards offers a view of reading as healthful and improving: "Everybody knows the feeling of freedom, of relief, of increased competence and sanity, that follows any reading in which more than usual order and coherence has been given to our responses. We seem to feel that our command of life, our insight into it and our discrimination of its possibilities, is enhanced, even for situations having little or nothing to do with the subject of the reading" (*Principles* 235). If this sentiment reminds the twenty-first century reader of some of the claims of contemporary literary cognitivism, it is salutary to note that Richards himself was repeating the commonplaces of Victorian defenses of (literary) reading. Our colleague of 75 years back would have found in Richards a not unfamiliar, hopeful expression of the powers of literary reading to renovate and elevate the emotions, but would have sought in vain for a thorough account of its operations.

In John Dewey's 1934 *Art as Experience*, in contrast to Richards' preference for short forms, Dewey emphasizes the lengthy duration of aesthetic experiences of narrative and drama, as well as their formal complexity. These complement his contention that emotions are not compact, simple entities: they unfold in time. In Dewey our scholar could read, "emotions are qualities, when they are significant, of a complex experience that moves and changes" (43). *Experience* is Dewey's keyword. Deweyan experience is expressed in plays and novels: "The *experience* is of material fraught with suspense and moving toward its own consummation through a connected series of varied incidents" (44). This definition throws emphasis on longer narrative forms, though ordinary experiences can also have "esthetic character" (44). Dewey writes that drama and fiction elicit aesthetic emotions, not as discrete things bearing labels ("Joy, sorrow, hope, fear, anger, curiosity" [43]), but as a unifying, "moving and cementing force" (44) that operates temporally. "The intimate nature of emotion," writes Dewey, manifests itself "in the experience of one watching a play on the stage or reading a novel" (43). Emotion "attends the development of a plot; and a plot requires...a space, wherein to develop and time in which to unfold. Experience is emotional but there are no separate things called emotion in it" (43). Our early twentieth-century scholar might well recognize patterns and structures described by Dewey as belonging to the dynamics of narrative, but in any case, he could not miss Dewey's assertion that emotional reactions "enter into the settlement of every situation, whatever its dominant nature, in which there are uncertainty and suspense" (45). Like Richards, Dewey emphasizes resolution as a goal of the unifying aesthetic experience and invests closure with importance: "the interaction [of self and object] constitutes the total experience that is had, and the close which completes it is the institution of a felt harmony" (45; cf Shusterman). As in Richards' theorizing, Dewey's emphasis appears to fall on the experiencing or reading/viewing self.

Yet the makers of art objects are not entirely eclipsed in Dewey, as they often seem to be in Richards. Not identical but closely related to natural emotions, the feelings generated by the deeds of writers prompt recognition and change in the recipients who experience them. Dewey's account of aesthetic emotion emphasizes transmission, communication, and transformation, not always pertaining to a stable subject. From the maker, for whom "expression is the clarification of turbid emotion" (80), Dewey inadvertently slides to the recipient, whose response to the expressive material and self-recognition induces transformation: "as they know themselves they are transfigured" (80). The elisions of agency in Dewey's phrasing raise questions: where does the transaction shift to the receiver, and how is the reader/viewer "transfigured" by self-recognition? Emotion and human agent seem to exist in a potent analogous relation, where "turbid emotion" receives clarification through expression and the responsive receiver gains a transfiguring self-recognition. For Dewey, "esthetic emotion is native emotion transformed through the objective material to which it has committed its development and consummation" (82), not "cut off by a chasm from … natural emotional experiences" (81). This phrasing endows emotion itself with agency and words (objective material) with transformative power, but in general Dewey returns to a human maker, at least implicitly, at the start of the expressive chain of events. Both in its creation and in its apprehension, Dewey insists, an act of expression constituting an artwork is "a construction in time, not an instantaneous emission" (62). This implies a constructor, albeit a preternaturally powerful one. When he considers the various constructors of artworks, Dewey especially notes how poets and novelists possess the double advantage of working with language, which is both referential and charged with affect. Writers work with words, characterized as "loaded dice" and "material … charged with meanings" (253). Writers build up expressions to which aesthetic emotions readily adhere (79).

Though language is an advantageous tool for writers, its powers do not extend to precise definition of emotions in Dewey's account. Dewey dismisses as unfeasible the scientific or philosophical definition of specific emotions, even as he honors fictional world-making as an art of selection and arrangement that can do what scientific descriptive terminology cannot achieve: "poet and novelist have an immense advantage over even an expert psychologist in dealing with an emotion. For the former build up a concrete situation and permit *it* to evoke emotional response. Instead of a description of an emotion in intellectual and symbolic terms, the artist 'does the deed that breeds' the emotion" (70, original italics). For Dewey, the cognitive and the affective consequences of literary composition and reception are by no means segregated, but he has little to offer when it comes to theorizing precisely how the deed that breeds is done, either in the writer or the reader. Thus our scholar of 75 years ago would have had her work cut out for her in breaking down and extending the inspirational accounts of aesthetic emotion (available in psychology and literary studies) to include specific processes, identifiable techniques, or predictable effects of formal choices on readers or viewers.

Where We Are Now

Recognition of a time in the past when scholars of literature and psychology readily conversed with one another about narrative aesthetics need not render us nostalgic, for these scientists and critics worked without the advantages of the precise vocabulary, analytical techniques, and technological advances that make interdisciplinary conversations about narrative and the emotions possible today. Yet they did possess a singular enabling condition, the late Victorian assumption that psychologists and literary theorists had something valuable to say to one another, even, as in the case of Alexander Bain, E. S. Dallas, Émile Hennequin, and G. H. Lewes, by contributing to both fields or drawing on physiological experiments to discuss narrative aesthetics (Dames, "Wave Theories"). [See for example book reviewer E. S. Dallas's call (in dialogue with G. H. Lewes) for a psychological inquiry into the nature of narrative pleasure in *The Gay Science* (Dallas 1866).] Today we shout across a ravine, never certain that those on the other side can—or want—to hear our invitations, decode our queries, or respond in language that we can comprehend. The interdisciplinarity that is our condition in the contemporary academy can result in miscommunication if we do not find strategies for discussing common interests that lead to mutual understanding: indeed, the demands of cross-disciplinary conversation should be frankly acknowledged. Today's efflorescence of interest in the emotions occurs in many disciplines: beyond the psychologists and philosophers mentioned so far, emotion researchers can be found among neuroscientists, evolutionary biologists, legal theorists, anthropologists, historians, sociologists, medical educators, linguists, and computer scientists, among others. The breadth of disciplinary home bases for research into the emotions has not invariably been recognized, but the upswell of scholarly and scientific interest in the emotions has prompted its labeling as "The Affective Turn" (Clough). The name for the present trend mirrors an earlier period's cognitive turn; it does not quite recognize the relevance of the narrative turn and theorizing of narrativity (Kreiswirth). Indeed, it is not clear that most of the emotion researchers involved in the affective turn are even alert to the work of others outside their fields.

In practice, disciplinary specialization and fragmentation have as often impeded communication about emotion research, or even awareness of work in neighboring fields, as they have stimulated cross-disciplinary conversation. Thus philosophers can write about empathy and sympathy without reference to a single contribution from literary studies (Stueber). Social theorists of affect can attribute prior explorations of the emotions to work "conducted predominantly in queer theory" (Hardt ix), an important, but surely not singular field of investigation. Historians show alertness to developments in neighboring anthropology and sociology, but not to the social psychology that is the main target of anthropology's own argumentation about the emotions (Lewis and Stearns; Rosenswein, "Worrying"). Alternatively, subjects traditionally of interest to humanists, including "cognitive, emotional, and spiritual functions, including lying, being in love, and believing in God" are the target of research in cognitive neuroscience (McCabe and Castel 344). Applications of fMRI findings, despite the known limitations in these investigative techniques (Nicholson), are often vaunted in the popular press and by leading humanists. So, for instance, novelists (Byatt) and philosophers (Churchland) both refer excitedly to developments in neuroscience. Byatt effuses: "Thought is material, according to neuroscience. I think of it in terms of Sir Charles Sherrington's description of the waking brain, the 'head-mass' as 'an enchanted loom where millions of flashing shuttles weave a dissolving pattern, always a meaningful pattern, though never an abiding one …'. The pleasure Donne offers our bodies is the pleasure of extreme activity of the brain" (Byatt). Patricia Churchland advocates for neurophilosophy, arguing that it will soon be impossible to do philosophy without recourse to evidence from neuroscience (Churchland 3). Enthusiasts for neuroscience rarely explore the reflections of their fellow humanists and professionals (Pustilnik; Illes and Racine) on the limitations of this research or the dangers of its application.

The multicolored brain scans produced by fMRI studies have an especially strong effect on the credulous; one report of several studies by cognitive scientists concludes "brain images are influential because they provide a physical basis for abstract cognitive processes, appealing to people's affinity for reductionistic explanations of cognitive phenomena" (McCabe and Castel 343). The cautions from neuroscientists themselves about what it might mean to read the human brain (Cacioppo et al.) are not often heeded by those who apply the headline versions of neuroscientific findings to their home fields. More common is extrapolation of broad significance from precise and limited neuroscientific studies, as in this recent philosophical claim about aesthetics: "advances in affective neuroscience, especially psychoneuroimmunology, suggest that beauty experiences boost the immune system and, therefore, enhance the healing process .... the persistence of beauty throughout the ages and its prevalence in various cultures may be due to its healing capacity, something known intuitively by many people but needing the sophisticated studies and technology of neuroscience to explain its impact on the body" (Vaillancourt et al. 217). The verification of humanists' intuitions by reference to scientists' sophisticated technology may induce skepticism as frequently as it persuades, but as McCabe and Castel's study of brain image illustration suggests, a colorful picture representing brain activity "associated with cognitive processes influenced ratings of the scientific merit of the reported research" compared to "identical articles including no image, a bar graph, or a topographical map." The effect was produced even by "fictional articles that included errors in the scientific reasoning" (McCabe and Castel 349).

...

What happens when we scrutinize narrative and the emotions in light of ancient and modern rhetoric, the age-old poetics of impact, empirical evidence of literary response, current cognitive, developmental, and social psychology, or recent neuroscience? In cognitive science, commitments to artificial intelligence, information processing and theories of computation have often precluded discussion of the emotions, or recast them as rational judgments. The strain of packaging affect within cognitivism has already produced reactions such as new groupings of "affective scientists," and can be seen in the citation of developmental, social, and evolutionary psychology within the work of prominent literary cognitivists such as Patrick Colm Hogan. That the narrative turn and the affective turn have coincided in the past several decades encourages a promising alternative, ... It involves re-centering the discussion of *emotions* (and narrative) in relevant subdisciplines of psychology rather than automatically foregrounding the claims of cognitivism.

...

The Affective (Re)turn

...

[T]he affective turn marks not so much a new departure but a return to questions that early twentieth-century aesthetics (and, again, earlier traditions) had opened without resolving. The next section of this essay shows what happened after the science and philosophy of aesthetics turned away from the study of emotion in the first place, eventually provoking an affective re(turn). This is of course not an isolated phenomenon. Meir Sternberg has demonstrated that an array of extraliterary fields concerned with language and text, including linguistics, semantics, pragmatics discourse analysis, conversation analysis, and their interdisciplinary blendings, have sought a scientific footing that often ignores or eschews the role of the emotions ("Universals I" and "Universals II"). Turning to literary study's recent practices, Sternberg has diagnosed a habit of hostile reading of canonical texts and suggested as an antidote recentered sympathetic reading (Sternberg, "Lakoön"), a critical practice that avoids making texts into ideoartistic battlefields (294). It so happens, moreover, that the paradigm case there is Lessing, one of the great explorers and conceptualizers of aesthetic emotion, in the line of Aristotle's poetics of impact. So the unfriendly readings of him—particularly of his *Laocoön* (1766)— in the twentieth century exhibit an affective approach to affective theorizing. As this characterization implies ..., avoidance of emotions as a subject does not strip critical, theoretical, and scholarly discourse of affect, for passionate advocacy and political stances within scholarship entail their own emotions of revision and rectitude, and accompanying gestures of anathema and scapegoating. In the humanities these show in heated contests about the status of subjects and evidence (history from below trumping the great men; literary recovery work breaking up the canon), while in the sciences they may be detected in hyper-specialization that fragments disciplines from within and, for instance, segregates affect and cognition into separate fields of study.

Since psychology took aesthetic experience as one of its core subjects early in its organization as a discipline, the eclipse of emotion in a field that understood itself as the science of mind invites comment. The rise of the behaviorist school of psychology (after 1913) de-emphasized for a half century the study of mental events and internal processes, studying instead stimuli and responses that could be recorded by objective observations in laboratories. Following John Watson and B. F. Skinner, leading practitioners had little interest in the emotions, registering subjective states and processes only as factors intervening between the environmental stimulus and the subjects' response (Mohr 84–6). Behaviorists believed that only observable behavior should be studied, and moods, emotions, and thoughts were regarded as too subjective for objective documentation. This ruled out aesthetic response for a long while. Notably, when psychologists such as Berlyne reopened questions in the new experimental aesthetics of the early 1970s (Berlyne; Machotka), this research documented and contrasted levels of physiological arousal to more and less familiar stimuli, or simpler and more complex works, studying arousal-increasing devices such as dishabituation, novelty, expectation, complexity, conflict, instability, ambiguity and multiple meanings, and arousal-moderating devices such as familiarity, exemption from inhibition and exertion, grouping and patterning (Berlyne xii–xiii). Berlyne offered a general theory of aesthetic response to the arts, including narrative—particularly novels, as vessels of subjective experience, and stories as devices employing surprising incidents. Beyond naming narratives as art objects, his work shows no awareness of the advances in narrative theory that were occurring in parallel during the 1960s and 1970s, however.

When the black box of the mind was reopened in the 1960s, internal mental states such as motivation, desires, beliefs, and unconscious promptings were once again discussed. Though language was an important ground for recovering internal operations of mind, after Noam Chomsky's critique of the limitations of Skinner's behaviorism (Chomsky), the cognitive turn did not immediately stimulate renewed interest in affect or aesthetics. A major reason for this was the computational model of mind adopted by cognitivists. Cognitive theories of narrative emphasized models of narrative communication based on artificial intelligence: computers have no emotions .... Subjective response accessed by introspection was no more a part of cognitive theories of art than it was in the new experimental aesthetics (which recorded physiological responses to art objects and performances). Emotion was downplayed in analysis of narrative springing from the encounter of cognitive psychologists with Chomskyan linguistics, when the task of elaborating story grammars emphasized the goal of comprehension and saw narrative understanding as a matter of developing cognitive skills.

Cognitive narrative theories hypothesized story grammars (or narrative rule systems), describing the elements of a story and the set order of events that facilitate understanding. [Story grammars in the main developed through study of simple oral narratives (such as folk tales), but in structuralist narratology (e.g., Pavel) they are also applied and elaborated with respect to more complex narratives.] According to story grammar theory, the mental structure of a story schema (with its constituent elements and rules for sequencing) enables storage of detail and recall on the part of a reader or listener (Mandler and Johnson). The focus is on attention, memory, and recall (or in computer terms, storage and retrieval), enabled by shaping of narratives in the so-named Canonical Story Grammar Model (CSGM): Setting / Beginning Event / Internal Reaction / Attempt / Ending (Anderson and Evans). Emotion plays a role only in the "Internal Reaction," in which a character's emotional response to the beginning event stimulates the formation of a goal. [Slightly more elaborated story grammars extend to seven categories: setting / initiating event / internal response / goal / attempt/ consequence/ and reaction (Mandler and Johnson), with emotion still limited to that experienced by the protagonist.] Neither the reader's emotional engagement with the plot or characters, nor the characters' own emotions as subjects rather than agents, nor the core affective qualities of narrativity received attention (see Sternberg, "Universals I"). Work on story grammars had narratological and pedagogical branches: in educational theory it was used to study and then to enhance comprehension in young readers. Here the emphasis on cognition is marked and the neglect of affect surprising. Obviously, comprehending written stories does require alphabetic decoding, chunking, attention, short-term processing, and recall—cognitive operations without which no print narrative could be processed. However, . . ., affective factors also contribute to understanding and the ability to learn, long before children learn to read (see Dissanayake). This is not only a matter of sympathizing with or identifying with characters, though readers' mental representation of characters' emotional states is part of the picture (Gernsbacher et al.). Psychologists have demonstrated that children with high scores for empathetic engagement better grasp the causal relations between plot events (Bourg). Examination of the role of emotion in comprehension of story schemata (Miall, "Beyond"; Kneepkens and Zwaan) came out of discourse processing work not fettered by a purely cognitive approach. . . . In the words of David Miall, inquiry had to move "beyond the schema" to get at affective comprehension (Miall, "Beyond").

Much more recent cognitive science of learning and motivation recognizes the affective element of understanding, indicating this by the phrase "hot cognition" (Kunda; van Peer, "Towards" 219). However, even though cognitive narrative poetics often claims that emotion now fits under its big tent (Stockwell 152; Hogan, *Mind*), few cognitive scientists pursue research agendas centered on emotion. It has been largely absent, deemphasized, or subsumed in cognition. Evolutionary psychologists Leda Cosmides and John Tooby speak for many scientists following Marvin Minsky [*Society of Mind* (1986); *The Emotion Machine* (2006)], asserting that "one cannot sensibly talk about emotion affecting cognition because 'cognition' refers to a language for describing all of the brain's operations, including emotions and reasoning (whether deliberative or nonconscious), and not to any particular subset of operations" (Cosmides and Tooby, "Evolutionary" 98). By this umbrella logic cognition automatically includes emotion, but it is still the case that most cognitive scientists carry out their work without regard to the emotions; basic textbooks on cognition rarely refer to emotions, and then only in passing. The field of cognitive science is still very far from conceding Meir Sternberg's point that even in processing the simplest and least artful narratives,

> emotion gets as unmistakably (if unobtrusively) twinned with comprehension as in high art's knottiest gaps. And so twinned that either dynamics of response enters into multiple relations with the other, shiftable relations at that. Affective and conceptual processing may join forces or join battle . . . or run together between the extreme junctures: now in harmony, now in disharmony, for example, or now with this balance of power, now with that. The rhetoric of narrative thrives on such protean fact/feeling interdynamics.
>
> (Sternberg, "Universals I" 364)

While some recent cognitive narrative theory takes an innate intersubjectivity as a starting point for readers' understanding of social and intermental minds in narrative (Palmer, *Fictional*), a stance that is more welcoming to discussion of the relations of affective and conceptual comprehension, mainstream cognitive science still studies intelligence, behavior, language acquisition, logic and so forth according to computational models. Even the burgeoning discussion of embodied cognition (Andy Clark; Lakoff and Johnson; Thelen and Smith) seems unlikely fundamentally to alter this disciplinary commitment.

Science truly oriented towards the study of affect has emerged from other home bases within psychology, especially developmental, social, and evolutionary psychology: in fact, literary cognitivists who have made emotion central to their enquiry … freely draw on these resources. [Amongst literary cognitivists who do not perform empirical work, Patrick Colm Hogan has most assiduously integrated emotions into his discussions of genre and literary universals. As demonstrated by his recent essay "The Brain in Love: A Case Study of Cognitive Neuroscience and Literary Theory," Hogan does not limit himself to cognitive science as a theoretical frame: indeed, he relies more heavily on research in social and affective neuroscience, with some reference to developmental and evolutionary psychology. It is a curious consequence of the indebtedness of literary study to a well-known generation of cognitivists (especially Turner, Johnson and Lakoff) that later work primarily reliant on social and affective neuroscience should continue to bear the label "cognitive."] More likely to reflect the understandings of affect and cognition as intertwined are psychology's own interdisciplinary combinations, such as affective neuroscience, social neuroscience, and the hybrid blend of social psychology and cognitive science, social cognition (Panksep, *Affective*; Hermon-Jones and Winkielman; Cacioppo et al., *Handbook*; Forgas, *Handbook*). Discussion of the emotions has begun to penetrate cognitive neuroscience, as suggested by the doubling of space dedicated to neuroscientific emotion research in the standard text, *The Cognitive Neurosciences* between the 1995 and 2004 editions (Gazzaniga). Rather than in cognitive science, in developmental psychology affect is a central concern, especially in the study of personality (Bandura) and prosocial behavior (Batson; "Altruism" Eisenberg, *Altruistic Emotion*). Evolutionary psychology sees emotions as adaptive programs with functional specializations aiding survival and successful reproduction (Cosmides and Tooby "Evolutionary"; Hrdy, *Nature; Mother*). Social psychology has also long recognized narrative as one of the types of cultural artifact possessing dynamic structuring techniques for the elicitation of emotions, and has often investigated the problem using film (Vygotsky, 5; Rottenberg et al.) Social psychology has also described emotional experience as a facet of group membership, with a bearing on bias and prejudice as well as belonging and the formation of social bonds (J. Turner). Research in social psychology has looked into positive emotions such as empathy (Davis, *Empathy*), happiness (Lyubomirsky), and love (Sternberg and Barnes), as well as negative emotions, anger (Tavris), jealousy/envy, hate (Dovidio et al., "On the Nature") and faked feelings such as false smiles and laughs (Lafrance and Woodzicka).

In a therapeutic context, shame and other consequences of trauma have been studied and theorized by psychoanalytic practitioners and clinicians (Bowlby; Tomkins). Narrative has an important role here as a fundamental method of talk therapy and with the literary expression of traumatic experience (Kacandes). I have already mentioned the narrative psychology of James Pennebaker, which employs expressive writing about emotional experiences to improve general health (Pennebaker, *Opening Up*; DeSalvo). This work grew out of Pennebaker's observation that the different varieties of talk therapy all had approximately the same success rate: he hypothesized that they had narrative expression (by the patient) in common. Pennebaker has since demonstrated in many studies that writing feelingly about emotional experiences yields improved health (Pennebaker et al.). Lengthy courses of the talking cure may indeed benefit sufferers (Levy and Ablon). Though psychoanalysis often relegates emotions to the realm of instinct, narrative can provide models for expression of unconscious anxieties according to influential applications of Freud's theories. For instance, Bruno Bettelheim writes, "the form and structure of fairy tales suggest images to the child by which he can structure his daydreams and with them give better direction to his life" (7).

Among neuroscientists, clinicians have played an important role in restoring emotion to discussions of cognition, with an emphasis on the bodily integration of emotions, moral sentiments, intuitions, and reasoning faculties. Theories of embodied minds receive elaboration from clinical observations of patients with brain injuries. When a patient cannot feel ordinary emotions, his judgments and decisions are also impaired. Damasio's scientific articles and popularizing books demonstrate this and extrapolate from clinical case studies an account of brain function that challenges the treatment of emotions and rationality as separate and dichotomous features of human experience. In Damasio's view, emotion is not extraneous to decision-making. It gains recognition as a necessary component of mental function, shaped by experience, and dependent on bodily (somatic) markers. Though its relevance to narrative studies is not immediately apparent, Antonio Damasio's work … has become a ubiquitous citation in recent literary criticism and narrative theory seeking to restore the affective to the domain of the cognitive. … Its influence is not limited to literary studies, of course. Physiologist Jay Schulkin supports Damasio's view that emotional memory lives in the body, arguing that "Visceral/autonomic information processing occurs at virtually every level of the neural axis, and what distinguishes emotional cognition from non-emotional cognition is the imposition of the visceral nervous system in decision making" (Schulkin 56). That is, as Schulkin writes, "The first part of the cognitive revolution mistakenly omitted or denigrated the importance of the visceral/autonomic system" (55). A consequence of correcting that omission, "Merging cognitive science and affective science," Schulkin suggests, would "rule out the study of a disembodied mind, a calculating mind uninformed by viscera" (55).

That emotion and cognition work together in human bodies contrasts with the age-old opposition of reason and passion (and dualistic contrasts of body and mind). Clinicians and neuroscientists have not been alone in making the case for recovering emotion, as scholars in the humanities have also made an affective (re) turn. In philosophy, for instance, work in aesthetics, ethics, and moral development builds bridges to the sciences. I have already mentioned Patricia Churchland's call to practice neurophilosophy in *Brain-Wise* (2002). More often this work has taken a cognitive direction. For instance, Nelson Goodman's *Languages of Art* (1976) breaks down the barriers between art and science in aesthetics (255), proposing *syntactic density, semantic density, syntactic repleteness,* and *exemplificationality* (252–5) as symptoms of aesthetic experience. These symptoms emphasize the cognitive role in art appreciation, but Goodman also addresses the role of the emotions in perception of art (246–8), without making any reference to Dewey's earlier theorizing. Indeed, Dewey's affective aesthetics had largely been cast aside for the better part of the twentieth century. Experimental (physiological) aesthetics had responded to Dewey's elevation of emotional experience by denigrating emotion as an accidental result of encountering an art object, not even predictable as to what emotional response would be aroused in a particular viewer or reader (Vivas, "A Note"). According to this criticism, emotional response should not be part of the definition of aesthetic appreciation (Vivas, "A Definition"). The sequestering of bodily and emotional responses from consideration has been challenged recently in Richard Shusterman's proposal of a new "somaesthetics" (*Body Consciousness*). Somaesthetics redresses philosophy's neglect of the body to benefit, among other pragmatic goals, education in the humanities (Shusterman, "Somaesthetics").

The hope that exposure to art refines emotional perceptiveness and sensitivity animates philosophical aesthetics with applications in the philosophy of education (Carroll "Aesthetics"). Working from a cognitivist standpoint, philosophers Martha Nussbaum and Ronald DeSousa have advocated recognition of the rationality of emotions, in *Upheavals of Thought* (2001) and *The Rationality of Emotion* (1987), respectively. DeSousa argues that emotions are a kind of perception, possessing a dramatic structure and playing a crucial role in decision-making, beliefs, desires, and rationality. Exposure to art, according to DeSousa, helps to elaborate "paradigm scenarios" to benefit one's management of emotional experience (182). Nussbaum often writes about the cultivation of the moral imagination, positing not just personal but civic impacts to be garnered through novel reading. [Her *Upheavals of Thought* (2001) contains an especially rich bibliography of emotions theories in ethics, even if its literary interpretations do not compel assent.] But which novels yield such social benefits? Philosophers naturally approach literary texts differently than literary critics, concerned to make generalizations about how human beings learn from literature, rather than seeking to generate fresh interpretations of individual works. Still, by examining particular works, they commend them to our attention. Nussbaum holds that a reader's emotional involvement in a novel by Henry James or Charles Dickens engages her in processes of empathy and conjecture that make her a better citizen in the real world (Nussbaum, *Cultivating* 90). Concern for fictional characters, their circumstances and needs, awakens moral and political interests in readers, according to Nussbaum (104). Nussbaum claims that fictional narratives play a shaping role in forming feeling readers as citizens who will make right decisions in favor of unknown others (cf Keen, *Empathy and the Novel* 16–26.) …

(On the empathy-altruism hypothesis, see chapter 9, above.)

Since my focus here is narrative and the emotions, I narrow the scope to those philosophers specifically interested in the aesthetics of narrative arts. Peter Goldie has explored both the philosophy of the emotions (*Emotions)* and emotions and narrative ("Remembered";"Narrative"). Gregory Currie, with his *Nature of Fiction* (1990) and Susan Feagin with her *Reading with Feeling* (1996) made important contributions to the revival of narrative aesthetics in philosophy. Gregory Currie incorporates enjoyment and pleasure into his philosophy of narrative and narrators, writing that the "experience of genuine situations of jointly attending to narrative is a formative and salient event in a person's development" (*Narratives* 97), a view that supports Ellen Dissanayake's theorizing … A recent and thorough philosophical study of the role of emotions in aesthetics is Jenefer Robinson's *Deeper Than Reason: Emotion and Its Role in Literature, Music, and Art* (2005) and her subsequent précis of her theory in "Emotion and the Understanding of Narrative." Robinson surveys research into emotion in psychology and theories of emotion in philosophy, offering her view of emotions as a process of interaction between a person and the environment (72). This process involves interconnected affective appraisals, physiological responses, and cognitive monitoring (*Deeper* 3). Robinson regards cognitive judgment theories of emotion (which assimilate emotion to cognitive appraisal of goals) as inadequate because the trigger of emotional and physiological response is not a belief or judgment allegedly, but a rapid non-conscious affective appraisal ("Emotion" 72). In her view the response is pre-linguistic at first, though cognitive monitoring may follow, confirming or denying the early impulse through reasoning (73). Reflection may modify the response, intensifying it or causing it to dissipate.

Thus Robinson sidesteps the question of the rationality or irrationality of emotions, for the process itself is always initiated by an automatic affective appraisal happening before reflection (*Deeper* 3): "When human beings have an emotional response to something in the (internal or external) environment, they make an *affective appraisal* that picks that thing out as *significant to me* (given my wants, goals, and interests) and requiring *attention*. This affective appraisal causes *physiological changes, action tendencies*, and expressive gestures, including characteristic *facial and vocal expressions*, that may be subjectively experienced (and named out of the available emotion terms in a language) as *feelings*, and the whole process is then modified by *cognitive monitoring*" (113, emphases in original). She presents this process as a universal description of human beings interacting with their environment. Robinson is attentive to cultural differences, however, which she acknowledges without stripping human emotions of their core elements that distinguish basic emotion systems (88). That is, she allows that cultural variation emphasizes different emotions and names them distinctively (80–1): these features contribute to the after-the-fact appraisal of what a person feels, according to the folk-psychological sense available in his or her culture. This labeling may indeed alter the way an emotion process unfolds in a person's experience (87). Though Robinson draws on the most up-to-date research into the emotions in psychology and neuroscience to create her description of emotions as a process, she arrives at an understanding compatible with John Dewey's views of 75 years ago, that "emotions are qualities … of a complex experience that moves and changes" (*Art as Experience* 43).

Further compatibility with Dewey (and Richards, whom she does not mention) shows in Robinson's central question, How does the engagement of the feelings in encounters with artworks contribute to their understanding? She is most interested in the sequential reading experience, not the deliberative purpose of a reader reflecting on meanings afterwards. Her Aristotle is the theorist of the emotions and the arts of persuasion (*Rhetoric* and *De Anima*), not the theorist of actions as signs of character (*Nicomachean Ethics*). Robinson makes a priority of explaining how narrative literature, particularly realistic fiction, is first understood by the reader through emotional responses. Rather than rooting the moral development of readers in their emotional reading experiences (as Nussbaum does), Robinson asserts that readers' emotional experience of novels is essential to their comprehension and plausible interpretations of them. This is a promising direction, wedding emotion and cognition in reading comprehension, without invoking the typical gendered denigration of the soppy feeling reader. Yet Robinson parts company with Dewey when she chooses *The Reef* as the text that represents not just narrative but canonical literature in her work. Dewey regarded narrative as a human art of communication and disapproved of the sequestering of art works in museums (*Art as Experience* 2–3): I infer that he would reject a narrow canon of great works of literature. He writes, disapprovingly, "When an art product once attains classic status, it somehow becomes isolated from the human conditions under which it was brought into being and from the human consequences it engenders in actual life-experience" (1). Yet choices must be made for the sake of illustration, and classics have the advantage of being well known.

Like Nussbaum, Robinson favors the realistic novelists like those of F. R. Leavis's Great Tradition (George Eliot, James and Conrad), though she includes Edith Wharton as a Jamesian psychological novelist. Indeed, *The Reef* is her sole subject of close examination, exemplifying the morally serious, character-driven realistic fiction that she regards as educating readers' emotions (*Deeper* 101). Robinson's choice of a sample novel that engages the emotions is value-laden. As she announces her selection, she dismisses lots of other kinds of narratives: good intellectual puzzles in novel form, bad didactic fiction, and genre fiction that "merely aim[s] to entertain" (159). Though her questions set aside concerns about literary merit, an investment in traditional psychological realistic fiction (over countless other options) shapes them: "*how emotion enters into our interpretation* of these works, *how we learn emotionally* from them about human nature and human motivation, and *how emotion manages and guides our responses* to them through the manipulation of form" (103, emphases in original). Would she ask the same questions about the education of the emotions by narrative if she allowed graphic novels, thrillers, and fantasies about teenaged vampires to be considered?

Although Robinson defends a reader-response theory that treats emotional responsiveness to narratives as vital data (Robinson, *Deeper* 102–6), she does not adopt the enlarged category of narrative literature—extending to the popular—that has been advanced by reader-response critics (e.g., Radway, *Reading*). Robinson's primary interest in the role of the emotions in reading comprehension makes readily understood works such as "merely entertain[ing]" popular fiction less compelling to examine (Robinson, *Deeper* 159). In any case, she does not attempt the task of explaining the role of emotional responsiveness in reading or viewing popular narratives, and she misses an opportunity to explore the emotions bound up in narrativity when she characterizes as "stock" emotions the drivers of narrative in genre fiction (136). [For efforts to understand the role of emotional response in reading of popular subgenres such as thrillers, see Gerrig *Experiencing*, on participatory responses, and Warhol, *Having a Good Cry*, on a variety of techniques employed to evoke emotion in popular narrative forms (41–50)]. Robinson allows that "It would be an unsuccessful detective story that did not make us curious and suspenseful about what is going to happen, and a failure for a Harlequin romance to arouse no feelings of satisfaction when the heroine is rescued by the mysterious dark and handsome hero" (136), but she does not pursue the possibility that similar emotions inhere in narrative in general. She finds more interesting the rarer narratives that discourage emotional involvement (137).

The avoidance of widely read popular fiction in favor of exemplary nineteenth-century realistic novels is a common flaw of philosophical defenses of novel reading as a school for the sentiments (101). Philosophy addressing the role of emotion in reading literature often avoids individuality in the form of literary studies' dedication to unique interpretations, favoring instead introspective accounts that attempt to elucidate widely shared reading experiences. [For example, see Peter H. Jones on *Middlemarch*, and Nussbaum on *The Ambassadors* (*Love's Knowledge*). An even more common emphasis among philosophers is the selection of novels containing moral dilemmas, on which see Peter Johnson.] A philosopher illustrating such reading avoids choosing a narrative that would make the examined experience appear idiosyncratic, so the desire to generalize exerts pressure in favor of canonical choices. I applaud Robinson's daring in focusing on *The Reef*, which is hardly the best known of Wharton's works; it makes a refreshing alternative to *The Ambassadors*. Yet Robinson's account of narrative emotions still depends upon dismissal of many other novels, especially ones that entertain readers (159). Why must we set aside emotional responses that contribute to enjoyment as "stock emotions" (136)? An individual reader may as readily acquire a sentimental education from an intensely emotional immersion reading experience in a formulaic romance as from an admired classic of high literary realism. Readers' tastes, cultural contexts, and emotional dispositions vary and these differences influence their responsiveness to narratives. By no means all who read narrative responsively have had their tastes formed in the Anglo-American canon of novels that loom so large in philosophers' accounts of reading and narrative impact.

To discuss the impact of emotions evoked by reading has led to a debate among philosophers about the nature of fictional emotions, or emotions evoked by reading, viewing, or hearing fictional narrative .... A number of different strategies have been employed to tackle the apparent paradox of fiction: few deny that emotional responses to imaginary beings do occur when readers or viewers immerse themselves in fictional worlds. Colin Radford initiated the modern argument that such responses are irrational, targeting the second proposition (Radford, "How"; "Tears"). Kendall Walton suggests that readers and viewers are engaging in make-believe; thus the feelings they experience in response to fiction are only "quasi-emotions" (Walton, "Fearing"), not the real emotions referred to in the first proposition, but make-believe feelings elicited in the game of pretending (Walton, *Mimesis*). Variations on counterpart theory (which presupposes possible worlds, but requires that individuals exist in only one world) suggests that readers and viewers really respond to the analogous situations of actual people, reflection upon whom receives prompting by fiction (Lewis, *Plurality*), so as to account for the first proposition. So-named "thought" theorists argue that belief in the actuality of fictional beings is not necessary to evoke emotional responses from readers (Lamarque, "How"; Carroll, *Truth*; Murray Smith). They hold that simple thoughts, without belief, can cause emotions (Carroll, *Truth*), a view that tackles the second proposition and supports the third. In research that backs up "thought" theory, Ed Tan has demonstrated that film viewers may experience the same emotional responses as witnesses, regardless of fictionality (Tan, "Film-Induced"). The research of psychologist Richard J. Gerrig and educational psychologist David N. Rapp offers support for "thought" theory. They suggest that readers must make an active effort to disbelieve the reality of fictive narratives, in contrast to Coleridge's view that readers must willingly suspend disbelief. That is, Gerrig's work argues that readers naturally experience narrative information as continuous with information gleaned from real experience and must exert themselves consciously to regard fictive narratives as fictional (Gerrig, *Experiencing*). According to the literary sociology of Janice Radway, middlebrow readers (and the publishers who cater to them) know the difference between reality and fiction, but they enjoy the feeling of surrendering to the illusion of a fictional world for the duration of a novel-reading experience and seek out narratives that invite transportation (Radway, *Feeling*).

Narrative and Emotion in Literary Studies

Middlebrow readers' feeling responses to emotionally evocative narratives and immersion in novels occurred in a separate sphere from the practices of literature professionals for most of the twentieth century. Literary studies as a discipline separated literary reading from reading for pleasure in everyday life and university-level practice by credentialed professionals from high-school-level appreciation guided by women. Thus although Dewey's theory of experiential learning influenced literature teaching in the high schools, and paved the way for reader-response criticism (an important conduit was Louise M. Rosenblatt's *Literature as Exploration* [1938]), Wimsatt and Beardsley's proscriptions of 1946 influenced generations of literary critics. These critics may have been passionate readers and teachers, but they sought to avoid the "affective fallacy" as a token of their professionalism.

Northrop Frye attempted to bring the rigor and authority of science to his descriptive taxonomies of literary genre with the enormously influential *Anatomy of Criticism* (1957), in which he briskly dispenses with "all casual, sentimental, and prejudiced value-judgments" (Frye 18). Furthermore, Frye castigated the authors of negative responses to his schematization of poetics, as revealing his critics' "strong emotional repugnance" (18). These were fighting words, dependent on the disrepute of emotionality. Frye admitted that critics have subjective backgrounds, but denied that these subjectivities were involved in critical responses to literature: "every cultivated person who is not suffering from advanced paranoia knows" that subjective pleasure and response to art "are constantly distinct" (28).

Parallel developments in New Criticism and literary formalism, disseminated by Cleanth Brooks and Robert Penn Warren's textbooks *Understanding Poetry* (1938) and *Understanding Fiction* (1943), encouraged belief in normative interpretations (rather than various readers' responses, including emotional ones), objectivity, and dispassion, under the name of critical distance employed in the interest of textual analysis. Structuralism sought to place analysis of literary texts on a scientific footing (with an emphasis on taxonomy and typology that continues to influence contemporary narratology). This entailed an official aversion to the emotive, although elements of Shklovsky's estrangement were incorporated ("radicalized" and typologized according to Sternberg, "Telling" 175]) in Genette's narratology. Simultaneously, mainstream literary criticism veered away from scientific approaches that might have integrated data from the new physiological aesthetics. Empirical evidence from the psychology laboratory was not a welcome supplement to literary critical discourse, at least until the late 1980s, when Victor Nell's *Lost in a Book: The Psychology of Reading for Pleasure* (1988) reintroduced literary critics to physiological evidence about readers. Steering a course between a distrusted empiricism on the one hand and *belles lettristic* practices of literary appreciation on the other required strict adherence on the part of literary critics to the New Critical doctrine of analyzing "the text itself."

Fashions in literary reading, particularly the academically sanctioned kinds of reading that demonstrate theories and produce interpretations, distinguished serious fiction's intellectual demands from the affective and bodily effects of popular fiction, as Janice Radway describes: "Whether cheap fiction books were to produce the skin-crawling sensations of fear, the upwelling tears of pathos, the erotic excitements of romance, or the bated breath of suspense, they were picked up precisely because they were successful at moving the body and provoking the emotions" (Radway, *Feeling* 142). Difficult modern narratives, by way of contrast, are supposed to cultivate a decoding, puzzle-solving reading style rather than extension of readerly practices of attachment, immersion, and identification. As Suzanne Clark has argued, this distinction was strongly conditioned by gender expectations (2), associating decoding of difficult texts with masculine mastery, immersion and sympathetic character identification with feminine empathy.

Academic literary critics, until the 1980s, showed scant "interest in relating their own concrete experience of a text or in appealing to the emotional responses of their readers" (Radway, *Feeling* 120). (Exceptions to the general pattern are treated below.) This left little room in criticism for reports of the individualized experiences of readers, though to be sure narratives continued to represent emotion-saturated circumstances, invite character identification, evoke responses from readers, and manipulate their feelings. Avoidance of the overt subject of affect often took the form of dodging readers' responses in theorizing of the 1970s. Roland Barthes subverts the action and the discourse sequence for estrangement, and his post-structuralist masterpiece *S-Z* deigned not to designate a code for the reader's response, though it speaks eloquently of one reader's engagement with Balzac's story. Arguably Barthes' hermeneutic code identifies units of an enigma that in practice evoke feelings of suspense, delay, and satisfaction in readers (see Sternberg, "Telling"178–96), but Barthes disallows the traditional model of communication: "writing is not the communication of a message which starts from the author and proceeds to the reader" (*S-Z* 151), renaming as "prejudice" the notion that reading is a form of reception, or "a simple psychological participation in the adventure being related" (151–2). Dissimilar in so many ways to Barthes' *S-Z*, Pierre Macherey's *A Theory of Literary Production*, shares with it a familiar dismissal of other readers' experiences. Even though Machery is officially interested in how texts communicate with readers and with the ambiguities of emotion represented by narrative and critical texts, he warns, "we must not replace a mythology of the creator by a mythology of the public" (79). Attending to other readers' experiences and opinions risks enfranchising the wrong readership, as for instance in Machery's prescription that the viewpoint of the social-democratic proletariat alone should be consulted in the appraisal of Tolstoy (343). Once "the reader" is allowed to be more than the individual critic or theorist (or the chimerical implied reader, of whose textually-initiated responses theorists may adduce virtually anything), *which* readers' responses count becomes a problem almost too large to handle.

Often the audience is left unspecified, or is implied to be those unaware of the way ideological goals work on them through manipulation of affect. For instance, the English Marxist critic Raymond Williams directed attention to "structures of feeling" in literature and life, but he does not specify who exactly lives and feels them: everyone? only the literate? all but those wise enough to detect them? It is unclear. Williams' *Marxism and Literature* (1977) explicitly employs the terms "feeling" and "affect" in defining "structures of feeling," but he does not say precisely who feels them and how often. Structures of feeling are "meanings and values as they are actively lived and felt ...characteristic elements of impulse, restraint, and tone; specifically affective elements of consciousness and relationships" (132). [On Williams' indebtedness to the traditional liberalism of F. R. Leavis, echoed in Williams' phrasing here, but also his departures from Leavisian understandings of culture, see Kanwar.] Though it is difficult to disentangle a definition of the emotional element or assign it characteristics from its place in "structures of feeling," Williams' interest in the psychological (Williams, *Culture* 246–8) as a realm of the feelings often conventionally separated from the social shows. The dividing line vanishes when Williams fuses inner experience with its outer context, directing attention to paradoxical integrations: "*not feeling against thought, but thought as felt and feeling as thought*: practical consciousness of a present kind, in a living and inter-relating continuity" (*Marxism* 132, my emphasis). Williams' critique of the politics of sensibility that allowed readers of industrial fiction to pity fictional workers while exhibiting indifference to their real-life counterparts served as an influential demonstration of the utility of his phrase "structures of feeling," even as it targeted the emotions (involved in structures of feeling) for negative criticism as a source of hypocrisy and an explanation for apathy (*Country*). Although Williams' critique of sympathy still resonates in cultural studies' approaches (Gallagher "Raymond"), his lasting influence shows in contemporary efforts to historicize and situate culturally specific experiences and narrative expression of emotions. [In an independent parallel development, in part influenced by the approaches of the Annales school, historians have also recently trained their attention on the emotions (Stearns with Stearns; Rosenwein, "Worrying"). Historian Thomas Dixon's history of the emotions as categories and his focused study of nineteenth-century altruism make substantial contributions to this young field (Dixon, *Passions* and *Invention*).] Considering this impact, it is striking that Raymond Williams's readers might search his *Keywords: A Vocabulary of Culture and Society* (1983) in vain for definitions of affect, emotions, and feelings. Between Aesthetic and Alienation, Elite and Empirical, Family and Fiction, these terms fail to appear. They are of course involved in both sensibility and sentimentalism, as glossed by Williams (*Culture and Society*). Despite the vagueness at the heart of the phrase, in combination with Williams' dynamic account of change in cultural forms (dominant, residual, and emergent forms), structures of feeling become an important target of analysis in narrative studies (Jameson, *Political*).

Fredric Jameson characterized the age of postmodernism as a period marked by a "waning of affect" (*Postmodernism* 10), but signs of positive change with respect to the emotions' place in literary-critical discourse and the literature classroom began to appear in the late 1960s and accelerated in the 1980s. Among psychoanalytic theories of narrative, Norman Holland's and Peter Brooks' contributions considered the interactions of readers' and narrative texts' drives, Holland emphasizing the defensive function of form in resistance to fantasy, and Brooks the propulsive use of desire as a dynamic of signification (Holland, *Five Readers*; Brooks). As early as 1968, Norman Holland argued in *The Dynamics of Literary Response* that readers apply meanings to literary texts as part of their defensive reactions to the works' emotional operations (Holland 104–33). The Freudian basis of Holland's early work led him to see readers as resistant to the transformations unleashed by reading: "a literary work means by reworking those rather unsavory wishful or fearful fantasies at its heart into social, moral, or intellectual themes which are consciously satisfying to the ego and unconsciously satisfying to the deep wishes being acted out by the literary work" (104). Writing many years earlier, Roman Ingarden had criticized the overshadowing of aesthetics by what he called psychologism in literary scholarship, arguing that the aesthetic values and functions are falsely "conceived either as quantities and qualities of the psychological problems occurring in the reader during his reading or as the dynamics of the perceiver's experiences of the work" (217). To shift the discussion from problems within a reader's psyche to narrative impact would turn out to entail the development of subjective criticism, the opening up of a field of research into reader responses, the revisionist work of feminists on gender and genre, and the exploration of emotion's role in rhetorical narrative studies.

David Bleich's 1969 essay, "Emotional Origins of Literary Meaning," came to the cautious conclusion that "it is not inconceivable that critical pleasure and creative pleasure are, after all, the same and.... created by identical psychological mechanisms," especially defensive responses and egoistic projections (40). Bleich's 1975 self-described "heretical" report for the National Council of the Teachers of English, *Readings and Feelings: an Introduction to Subjective Criticism*, brought emotion and narrative together by emphasizing the importance of students' emotional responses to their reading. Reader-response criticism followed Bleich's and Holland's lead in studying the responses of individual readers (Radway, *Reading*; Flynn and Schweickart; Nell), as differentiated from Wolgang Iser's reception theory, which relied on a posited implied reader (Iser, *Implied*), so idealized as to be indistinguishable from Iser himself. The focus on responses of actual readers did not yield much in the way of new insights into the interactions of narrative and the emotions *per se*, although these reports did verify that readers register their experiences of responding with feeling. Much later work in the tradition of reader-response criticism, such as Robyn Warhol's *Having a Good Cry* (2003) would make the effort of producing a narratology of emotionally-evocative devices, but the more usual situation involved invoking the word "affect" and swerving away from any precise discussion of the emotions (Fish). Iser himself noted that Holland's underlying theory of reading scarcely advanced emotive theory beyond I. A. Richards' suggestions (Iser, *Act* 44–5).

Other advances, particularly in feminist criticism, did occur as a consequence of opening up the analysis of the reading situation to hypothetically diverse readers, including women and popular fiction readers. That readings differ as much as actual readers do become a premise rather than a situation to be deplored. Feminist criticism and theory (Moi; Gallop; Butler, *Giving*) made declarations of a scholar's subject position and personal responses an acceptable academic stance, in some circles preferable to a pretended objectivity (Messer-Davidow; Miller). This change enabled the expression of emotional responses to narratives on the part of some feminist critics, while others disavowed emotionality as an imposition of patriarchy bent on confining women to second class status. An influential critique of traditional binary threefolds that put nature, woman, and emotion in opposition to culture, man, and reason (Ortner) suggested that cultural arrangements and socialization accounted for the conventional oppositions rather than innate or universal traits of the female psyche. In novel criticism, this attention to the gendering of emotionality bore fruit in many discussions of gender and genre, especially regarding sentimentality and sensation fiction (Tompkins; Tromp). Contextual and feminist narratologists enriched recent narrative theory by bringing some interest in the emotions to a structuralist endeavor that has typically ignored them (Lanser, "Are We There Yet?"; Warhol, *Having*).

Among narrative theorists, Chicago neo-Aristotelians offered new means of mediating among texts, authors, and readers that at least strongly implied a role for the emotions (Booth, *Rhetoric*; *Company*; R. S. Crane). Booth reintroduced the terms and approaches of rhetoric into narrative studies, showing the way for both rhetorical narratologists with interests in communication and ethical theorists of the novel. This has preserved a place for emotion in narrative studies as an aspect of response and elicitor of ethical engagement. This is not simply a matter of developing moral awareness through empathetic responsiveness to fictional characters (Nussbaum, *Love's Knowledge*). For instance, James Phelan's rhetorical literary ethics "conceiv[es] of the literary text as a site of a multilayered communication between author and audience, one that involves the engagement of the audience's intellect, psyche, emotions, and values" (Phelan, "Rhetorical" 630). Studies scrutinizing aspects of that multilayered communication push back against and complicate a Tolstoyan model of art as a simple transmitter of infectious feelings from author to reader (Tolstoy; Rabinowitz). Another angle focuses on effects felt by readers: Hans Robert Jauss appreciates such "communicative achievement[s] of art … as admiration, sentimental involvement, sympathetic laughter, and sympathetic tears" (Jauss, "Levels" 285) and regards this first emotional and "prereflective level of aesthetic perception" as a preparation for the reader's imaginative engagement with a narrative (287). [Jauss's hermeneutics supports Jenefer Robinson's account of emotional responses to narrative … in *Deeper Than Reason* (2005).]

That readers' appetites, aversions, and desires for fulfillment and delay—fundamental ingredients of emotional experience—receive a work-out in the temporal art of narrative brings its experiential and formal qualities closer together, without assigning limiting roles to specific narrative techniques. Meir Sternberg describes narrative's master functions (suspense, curiosity, and surprise) as the only specifically narrative emotional effects, produced by the double sequence of narrative action/communication. Though this may seem a strict limit, other feelings and other strategies of evocation of feeling are shared by narrative with other kinds of communication or are subsumed by suspense, curiosity, and surprise. Sternberg emphasizes the protean nature of correspondences among forms and their functions, allowing space for variation in individual readers' dispositions and resisting an oversimplifying formalism (Sternberg, "Telling II" 529). He challenges narrative theorists "both to mark off in sharp, principled terms the [narrative] genre's affective constants from cross-discourse variables and to systematize their flexible interrelation in generic practice," asking "How, that is, would the working of humor, anger, empathy, disgust, making strange (etc.) within narrative differ from their counterparts outside the genre?" (Sternberg, "Universals I" 379). Focusing on impact need not mean collapsing into a condition of affective relativism or gross oversimplification. The study of narrative dynamics offers fine-grained methods for analyzing emotional characteristics of genres or individual texts deploying functions such as suspense (Marie Laure Ryan; Vordere et al.), or the satisfaction of pleasure (Young, *Ordinary; Imagining*). Attending to the reading process, especially to readers' activities of framing, problem solving when confronted with gaps, and juggling previously framed, newly-corrected, and discarded but remembered hypotheses about narratives specifies key stages for the involvement of the emotions in narrative.

A Look Ahead

The explosion of interest in narrative and the emotions broadly construed shows in the variety of topics taken up recently by literary scholars encouraged by and participating in the affective turn. These include studies of narrative identification (Breger and Breithaupt; Neumann et al.), film genres and elicitation of emotions (Grodal), intersubjectivity in film and fiction (Butte), narrative faculties and emotional involvement (Walsh, "Why We Wept"), the role of emotional involvement in absorption and reading speed (Gerrig, *Experiencing*; Miall, "Foregrounding"), and narrative empathy (Fricke; Keen, "Theory")...

Clearly the recuperation of affect as a legitimate subject of study is well underway. Consolidation of inquiry into the emotions going on in many different fields may now begin. An exemplary statement of intention, The Myrifield Manifesto (Freeman), explicitly calls for study of the emotional experience of literature and the arts and nominates empathy as an underlying artistic structure. Empathy already enjoys a prominent position in theories of narrative emotion advanced by film studies experts, psychologists of mass communications, literary cognitivists, and scholars of discourse processing, so it is an especially promising research subject for cross-disciplinary discussion. The recent convening of interdisciplinary groups of scholars at symposia centered on emotions, the publication of special issues of journals dedicated to the emotions, the founding of new journals for affective science and emotion research (joining the already established *Cognition and Emotion* and *Motivation and Emotion*), and the formation of new scholarly and scientific societies as well as less formal discussion groups and listservs, all suggest the potential for an explosion of discovery, unlikely to be contained or controlled by the cognitive sciences.

The principles articulated in the Myrifield Manifesto (Freeman) suggest a way forward. The authors call for "a new emphasis," shifting scholars' focus from producing distinctive interpretations of individual texts to exploring "the experience of literature and the arts," including "their emotional aspects." While this actually represents a return to Deweyan and Richardsian commitments (a return rather than a new direction), it does endorse the reintegration of psychological aesthetics with literary studies. Recognizing that the forms of interdisciplinarity prevailing in the academy primarily involve cooperation among sister disciplines in the humanities, the Myrifield authors "propose a new interdisciplinary approach that integrates the social and biological sciences with the humanities. This proposed integration implies the readiness to become actively involved with the methodology of non-humanistic disciplines, including the development of philosophical and empirical research methodologies." (Apparently the Myrifield authors regard philosophy as a social science.) Active involvement implies a two-way conversation, including openness to critique and question, and in that spirit I make some suggestions here.

I hope that the Myrifield authors would agree that the contributions of psychology and neuroscience to the conversation about emotions and the arts extend well beyond what they characterize as "recent new developments such as embodied cognition and cognitive linguistics that have special relevance for research in literature and the arts." Empathy in particular would be far less well understood without the work of developmental and social psychologists to draw upon. Their cognitive commitments ought not to discourage collaboration with emotion researchers in the affective sciences. Reopening the aesthetic theories that address fundamentals of the various arts is a good project: doing so without the assistance of musicology, art history, dance and theater studies seems misguided, but such potential assistance is at least implied by their special welcome to "scholars in disciplines *other than* the humanities" (my emphasis). Conversation with non-humanistic disciplines should not preclude angles of approach from the humanities. In the case of "literariness" (along with empathy, a focus of the manifesto), for example, recent historical writing and genre studies should not be forgotten. Qualities of literariness almost certainly depend to some degree on the prized affects of historically situated emotional communities and changing understandings of what and how affects mean in different periods (Thomas Dixon; Rosenwein, *Emotional*). As Franco Moretti has demonstrated, narrative genres come in and out of fashion, and these trends probably also alter the valued traits of literariness in a given period (Moretti). As these suggestions imply, I think that an interest in literariness ought not to translate into a narrow range of reference to a high literary canon. Literariness ought not to mean worthiness, and its qualities should be sought in diverse exemplars. We have much to learn about emotion and narrative from a full range of texts …, unconstrained by value judgments.

…

11

FROM EMPATHY STUDIES

Current Scholarship and Debates

Understanding empathy as an aspect of readers' responses to literature, authors' creative imagining, and the textual cues that invite or repel experiences of emotional fusion with literary texts has become a lively area of literary theorizing and empirical research. Drawing on existent research in three distinct areas of psychology—cognitive, developmental, and social psychology—(see Davis, *Empathy*; Eisenberg and Strayer, ed. *Empathy*; Eisenberg, "Development"; Hoffman, *Empathy*), on philosophical work in the areas of ethics or moral philosophy (see Coplan and Goldie, ed. *Empathy*; Nussbaum, *Upheavals*; Slote, *Ethics*), and stimulated by the discovery of mirror neurons and the proposal that human beings possess a shared manifold for intersubjectivity with others (Gallese, "Roots"; Decety and Ickes, ed. *Social*), literary empathy studies has been an interdisciplinary endeavor from the outset. With roots in the German psychological aesthetics of the turn of the twentieth century, in which context the term *Einfühlung* first emerged, studies of empathy have been carried out since then by psychologists, philosophers, art and literary critics, and in recent decades by neuroscientists (sometimes working in collaboration with humanists). That richness of approach brings with it immediate challenges, starting with the terminology used to label a wide variety of empathic phenomena, many of which correlate with experiences literary theorists associate with techniques, genres, and historical periods of literature. In a literary context, novelist Vernon Lee (1913) and poetry critic Richard Harter Fogle (1949) adapted *Einfühlung* to the description of aesthetic acts and responses, but in subsequent decades literary empathy has been more squarely associated with character identification (Breger and Breithaupt, ed. *Empathie*), regarded as a version of the role-taking or perspective-taking imagination.

DOI: 10.4324/9781003264071-15

Psychologist C. Daniel Batson's 2011 article "These Things Called Empathy: Eight Related but Distinct Phenomena" usefully elaborates and describes the qualities of components of empathy, including what others have studied under the labels of cognitive empathy (and empathic accuracy), motor mimicry, emotional contagion, *Einfühlung*, Theory of Mind, perspective-taking, role-taking, putting oneself in the shoes of another, personal distress, and the older term sympathy. A limitation of Batson's list lies in his omission of fantasy empathy, involving empathic responsiveness to imaginary beings, including literary creations .... (see above 95–6).

Yet real-life empathy is subject to diminishment or even elimination from interfering biases: here-and-now biases (the tendency to favor those near us in time and place over those far away); and similarity or familiarity biases (enabling humans to connect more readily to those like ourselves or already known to us, and less well with those outside our groups or experiences). Whether the real-life empathy that human beings feel for living others work the same way and with the same limitations and benefits in *literary* empathy is a fundamental debate in empathy studies, including those carried out by scientists. Indeed, some of the most provocative and widely-publicized findings about the impact of literary reading on the empathic abilities of readers have resulted from psychological research by cognitive scientists, as for example, David Kidd and Emanuele Castano's studies showing that Theory of Mind improves as a result of reading literary (but not popular) fiction (Kidd and Castano). Humanists are not invariably convinced by the reasoning implicit in scientific studies, however, and empathy itself has its critics (Stein). For example, as philosopher Jesse Prinz suggests, empathy roused for one individual or group sometimes leads to unjust responses, regarded from a utilitarian point of view, or may be employed in a two-step process, where empathy for an in-group then paves the way for antipathy or even murderous dehumanization of an out-group (Prinz, "Against"). Among literary critics, postcolonial literary theorists in particular critique assumptions of biologically-based universal human emotions that erase differences (Keen, "Human Rights"; see chapter 15 below).

Bearing on this question are several other areas of controversy. They include: the philosophical debates about the status of fictional emotions (known as the paradox of fictional emotions in philosophy); the attribution of enhanced effectiveness to artful, literary fiction; the contention that narrative empathy leads to altruism, pro-social actions, and good world citizenship; the argument that all forms of empathy (including literary empathy) are inefficacious when false empathy, failed empathy, and personal distress intervene; and the implications of gender and other aspects of readers' intersectional identities for reception of strategic narrative empathizing on the part of authors. Cross-disciplinary stress points in empathy studies, whose interdisciplinarity involves empirical research in scientific disciplines or collaboration between and among humanists, social scientists, and natural scientists, underlie many if not all of these debates.

Narrative of the Topic

Before the neuroscience of mirror neurons emerged, late twentieth-century psychology had already recognized that human beings can and do "feel with" fictional characters in a way that resembles human empathy with real others. Batson's omission of fantasy empathy from his taxonomy of empathic phenomena should be regarded as an oversight, not an indication of a lack of interest on the part of psychologists in narrative empathy. Indeed, some developmental and social-psychological theories of empathy (e.g., Hoffman, *Empathy*) show the influence of ideas about the novel as a school for the sentiments and morality of readers. One subscale of social psychologist Mark Davis's widely adopted Interpersonal Reactivity Responsiveness test (IRI) measures subjects' fantasy empathy, which "taps respondents' tendencies to transpose themselves imaginatively into the feelings and actions of fictitious characters in books, movies, and plays" (Davis, "Multidimensional"). Keith Oatley, a cognitive psychologist and novelist, led the way in the study of emotions involved in literary response, including character identification (Oatley, "Taxonomy"), and developed a robust psychology of fiction (Oatley, *Such Stuff*). Ed S. Tan of Amsterdam, Frank Hakemulder of Utrecht, and their collaborators have been studying aspects of affect induced by film, fiction, and other media for decades. Some of this research aims at understanding how literature in a variety of media draws on human emotions to induce affects (Tan, "Film-Induced"), while other studies (e.g., Koopman and Hakemulder) investigate the effects of empathic reading or viewing experiences on a subject's subsequent emotional state, reflectiveness, and behavior. Media psychologists Melanie Green, Jeffrey Strange, David Brock, and their collaborators have studied the immersive reading referred to by the term transportation, a phenomenon that often involves experiences of empathy. David S. Miall, working in collaboration with Don Kuiken, a social and cultural psychologist, developed a sophisticated research program studying the neuroaesthetics of literary reading, including empathy and emotional engagement, in a discourse processing context.

One outcome of the efforts mentioned here, the writing of introductory guides to empirical methodologies for humanists by Sonia Zyngier, Marisa Bortolussi, Willie Van Peer, Peter Dixon, and Jemeljan Hakemulder, proves useful to empathy scholars in literary studies. A second outcome is the expansion of interdisciplinary journals in which to read about empathy from a variety of angles, as in the recent special section on Empathy in *Emotion Review* 4.1 (2012). Research about literary empathy can be found in journals such as *Scientific Study of Literature* (a publication of the society, International Society for the Empirical Study of Literature and Media [IGEL]), *Empirical Studies of the Arts* (a publication of the International Association of Empirical Aesthetics [IAEA]), and *Emotion Review* (published in association with the International Society of Research on Emotion), as well as in literary journals with an interest in cognitive poetics, such as *The Journal of Literary Theory (JLT)*, *Narrative*, *Poetics*, and *Poetics Today*.

However, the incorporation and analysis of data from empirical studies sometimes meets with resistance from humanists, especially in response to credulous, exaggerated, or inaccurate reporting of neuroscience research on empathy by non-neuroscientists. To address that concern, literary scholars should take second-hand reports in the popular press with a grain of salt, and should make every effort to read the original papers, to examine their methodology, including the constitution of the pool of research subjects, and to pay attention to the size of the effects measured. Though papers with iconic brain images in them may exert undue influence (McCabe and Castel), and neuroscientific explanations may sway some readers through "seductive allure" (Weisberg et al.), these effects are surely counteracted by humanists' judgment that neuroscience is inevitably reductive and essentializing. That dismissive position may prevent serious discussion of the results of exemplary collaborations whose findings deserve attention. Ideally, critical evaluation of neuroscientific investigations of literary reading would flow in both directions, as it does in the work of Natalie Phillips.

Some of the backlash against what is sometimes characterized as a misguided interdisciplinarity arises when speculative theorizing of evolutionary biologists and psychologists gets applied to literary studies, as if genres, styles, and literary techniques were subject to natural selection. There, too, literary scholars should engage with these theories with the skepticism and close reading skills that are the hallmarks of literary critical training: Marko Juvan's 2014 critique of literary Darwinism is exemplary in this regard. However, some of the negative response to empirical study of empathy as it bears on literary studies comes from humanists' characterization of psychologists, biologists, and neuroscientists, and cognitive scientists as engaging in universalizing descriptions of human nature that virtually all anthropologists, historians, and literary critics trained in the scrutiny of difference would reject out of hand. Perhaps the most compelling version of this critique comes from Ralph Savarese, whose call for a "neurocosmopolitanism" warns against regarding neuro-typical experience as a default version of human experience. Savarese's cautions were instigated by the medical diagnostic manuals that include an empathy deficit as a quality of autism and/or Asperger's Syndrome. Savarese suggests (and recent research supports) that an excess of empathy (verging on personal distress) rather than a lack of empathy may in fact be discovered to be the experience of autistic subjects, if one takes the trouble to ask them.

While it is certainly true that the psychological sciences emphasize empirical evidence to understand how the brain and body participate in human (and animal) behavior, these disciplines also recognize that subjects' responses distribute across ranges, revealing more and less typical possibilities. So while excellent work has been done to develop understanding of the underlying physical mechanisms and neural substrate of empathy, neuroscientists, cognitive scientists, and psychologists expect variation in both physiological empathic responses (as measured by heart rate and palm sweat as well as by suggestive brain images of blood flow in key brain areas) as well as in the conscious experience of research subjects (as elicited by querying them or observing them in an experimental setting). Since an individual person's experience of empathy (real or literary) requires both human cognition and affect, the burgeoning knowledge about how thinking and feeling interact in our responses to real and imagined others should be pertinent to theorizing about empathy. It certainly does not follow that all differences among people, differences that stem from our highly variant intersectional identities and experiences, should be erased just because psychological, neuroscientific, and cognitive studies inform the discussion. An awareness of findings about empathy emerging from empirical disciplines enriches current theorizing about literary empathy.

The career of literary empathy reaches back at least to the eighteenth century, when many of the phenomena described by Batson were theorized by Adam Smith and David Hume under the term sympathy (Keen, *Empathy and the Novel*). In keeping with later parsing of the distinctive phenomena of empathy out of sympathy (Wispé), I differentiate narrative empathy from sympathy by defining the former as a version of the *same* feeling: When Dorothea Brooke feels trapped and frustrated by her marriage to Casaubon, I feel trapped and frustrated—empathy—but my feeling of pity for her deluded and impotent husband is sympathy, because I don't share the beliefs and feelings of Casaubon. Both Smith and Hume, whose descriptions of sympathy include illustrations that we would identify as either affective or cognitive forms of empathy such as motor mimicry, emotional contagion, role-taking, and perspective taking, were read with care by literary authors. The English poetry, drama, and fiction of the eighteenth and nineteenth centuries reveals an interest on the part of these authors in evoking shared feelings, whether in the sensationalist invitations of gothic, offering thrills and chills, or in the more sober education of the sympathetic imagination that George Eliot theorized and implemented in her novels. The novel of sentiment, a genre that enjoyed popularity during a period of social change, has been understood as a school for the emotions (Richter 74–8). In *Empathy and the Novel*, I show that the argument between moral sentimentalists and their critics about the efficacy of literary empathy as a spur to morality (or a waste of the feelings on nonexistent beings and a moral dead-end) has been restaged many times since the eighteenth century. Some of the points in that debate still inform research in empathy studies today. However, before tackling what experiencing narrative empathy might result in for those who feel it, a more fundamental philosophical debate about the status of fictional emotions should be considered.

(See above 161)…

Since narrative empathy depends upon the sensation of shared feeing or emotional fusion, somehow the fictions that evoke it transcend, albeit temporarily, the barriers of nonexistence and illogic. Need "nonexistence" pose a problem, though? Samuel Johnson observed in 1756 that "imitations produce pain or pleasure, not because they are mistaken for realities, but because they bring realities to mind" ("Preface" 78). Writing about the emotional impact of drama, Johnson suggested,

> the reflection that strikes the heart is not, that the evils before us are real evils, but that they are evils to which we ourselves may be exposed. If there be any fallacy, it is not that we fancy the players, but that we fancy ourselves unhappy for a moment.... The delight of tragedy proceeds from our consciousness of fiction; if we thought murders and treasons real, they would please no more.
>
> (78)

Theorists of fictional emotions offer alternatives to Colin Radford's "irrationality" charge, in the form of "make-believe" theory, "counterpart" theory, and "thought" theory. Kendall Walton argues that readers and viewers are not irrational: they are playing a game of *make-believe*. But the feelings fiction evokes are for Walton only quasi-emotions, not the real emotions referred to in Yanal's first proposition, but make-believe feelings elicited in a game involving pretend play. *Counterpart* theory offers a different work-around of the irrationality charge. It acknowledges the existence of possible worlds, but requires that people exist in only one world. Their responses to fictional persons in secondary worlds are understood as caused by making analogies to the situations of actual people. The fictional beings, by this argument, cause the reader or viewer to think about real beings that share their real world (D. Lewis).

Cognitive theories of empathy, especially those emphasizing perspective-taking and role-taking imagining, can be seen as compatible with the restrictions of counterpart theory. The quick, seemingly involuntary emotional experiences of narrative empathy that occur during reading or viewing literary texts are more difficult to explain by make-believe or counterpart theories, however. Philosophical "thought" theorists argue that thoughts without belief in the actuality of fictional beings can still evoke emotional responses from readers (Lamarque, "How," *Truth*; Carroll, *Philosophy*; M. Smith), accounting for Yanal's second proposition and supporting his third contention, that "No emoter who takes the object of his emotion to be fiction believes that the object of the emotion exists and exhibits any emotion inducing properties" (Yanal 11). This avoidance of the irrationality charge doesn't interfere with the reader or viewer's feelings, which may after all be involuntary. Psychologists Richard J. Gerrig and David N. Rapp provide in their research on the mechanisms of narrative impact support for "thought" theory. They confute "make-believe" theory, tackling it at its source in Samuel Taylor Coleridge's *Biographia Literaria* (1817). In contrast to Coleridge's view that readers must willingly *suspend* disbelief to procure poetic faith in fictions, "these shadows of imagination" (chapter 14: 6), Gerrig and Rapp argue that readers must effortfully and actively work to disbelieve the reality of fictive narratives. Our default state is gullible, not skeptical: readers ordinarily receive narrative information as continuous with information gleaned from real experience. We have to exert ourselves consciously to think of fictional narratives as fictional, especially while we are experiencing them (Gerrig, *Experiencing*). The metaleptic gestures of metafiction, breaking the frame and reminding readers of a text's fictionality, plays with this habit of readers. Media psychologist Ed S. Tan has shown that movie viewers may experience the same emotional responses as witnesses, regardless of fictionality, in research that backs up "thought" theory.

The status of fictional emotions debate intersects in empathy studies with controversies about Theory of Mind, a branch of cognitive science that is informed by philosophies of mind (Marraffa). With regards to empathy, philosophers, cognitive scientists, and psychologists still debate whether "theory-theory" or simulation theory provides the most persuasive account of how humans share and understand the mental states and emotions of others through mindreading. Theory-theory holds that human subjects develop as children "theories" about how and why others behave the way they do. They apply these folk-psychological beliefs, which they have developed through observation as they mature cognitively, to their interpretations of others' behavior (Gopnik). Theory-theory can accommodate some innate responses, but it emphasizes the formation, testing, and revision of theories as part of a cognitive process, including theories of others' minds (ToM). Simulation theory suggests that human beings simulate, through mental modeling, others' experiences in order to arrive at an understanding of their thoughts and feelings (Goldman). This process can happen rapidly (as in reading facial expressions) and without conscious exertion. The validity of simulation theory has received a boost from the discovery of mirror neurons, which in turn suggests the existence of a physiological mechanism for a shared manifold for intersubjectivity (Gallese, "Roots"). Simulation theory places empathic behavior, *Einfühlung*, at the center of its processes (leading either to role-taking or perspective-taking). Though each of these schools of thought—simulation theory and theory-theory—represents groups of theories, some of whose adherents vehemently denounce interpretations from the other side, common sense suggests that an individual subject's empathy may be partly driven by automatic mental simulations and supported by folk theories or ideas derived by observation about how others behave. Indeed, as philosopher of science Massimo Marraffa points out, "a consensus seems to be emerging that mindreading involves both" theory-theory and simulation theory (Marraffa).

...

Many readers experience fictional emotions intensely, remembering them for years in some cases, and seeking out their repetition through more reading and viewing. Narrative empathy certainly fuels a fictional-consumption habit. My reading of the developmental psychology of personality convinces me that fiction-reading alone is unlikely permanently to shift a reader's disposition at the level of the big five personality traits, but it is certainly demonstrable that experiences of narrative empathy can change attitudes about outgroups, reduce bias, and translate into real-world sympathy for others outside of books. The link between narrative empathy and altruism (prosocial action) is still more tenuous, though psychologist Dan R. Johnson has demonstrated increases in both empathy and prosocial helping behavior as a result of immersive reading primed by mental visualizing exercises (Johnson, "Transportation"). Altruism is in itself a controversial subject in evolutionary biology, psychology, and philosophy, and whether or not it is reliably inspired by empathic feelings induced by literary works is only the first problem. Narrative empathy, like its real-world counterpart, has been criticized for evoking mistaken, false empathy (that misgauges the feelings of the other) or for inefficacious, failed empathy (that simply stalls out), sometimes as a result of the overly intense, aversive response known in the psychological literature as personal distress. When narrative empathy does stimulate emotion fusion, no moral guarantees exist. Literary works can set about to arouse empathy for morally suspect subjects, such as white supremacists, and if action arises from such emotion, it can be antisocial or even an instance of what has been described as pathological altruism (Oakley et al.). The mechanisms employed in literary texts to evoke the emotional fusion and even physiological responses characteristic of narrative empathy can be bent to amoral or vicious ends as readily as to the laudable projects of civic virtue. In my opinion understanding how narrative empathy works outside a value-laden expectation that it *ought* to be morally improving leads to a better understanding of both empathy and narrative techniques.

Narratives evoking empathy may be nonfictional or fictional. Readers, listeners, and viewers have the capacity to immerse themselves in (lose themselves in, or feel transported into) both fictional worlds, where they experience emotions more appropriate to the situations or circumstances imaginary denizens of those worlds than to themselves, and nonfictional accounts, where at least hypothetically for factual narratives of the present day, they might cross-check their empathic accuracy with real people or corroborating sources.

Suggestions for Further Research

Empathy, sympathy, and affects related to the experience of literature have been theorized for over a century. For example, narrativity's core affects, inhering in the temporal asymmetries of story and discourse, have been identified as curiosity, surprise, and suspense (Sternberg, *Expositional*). Metrical verse has been related to breathing and walking, with attributed physiological effects on heart rate and blood pressure (Richards, *Principles*). Immersion reading has been linked not only to the phenomenon of feeling "lost in a book" (Nell), but also to both positive and negative effects on the morality of readers. Immersed readers have more commonly been understood as indulging in deleterious escapism, but recently narrative immersion or transportation has been positively associated with improved empathy and prosocial behavior (Johnson, "Transportation"). From the opposite direction, working against empathy, Bertolt Brecht famously advocated that dramatic art should seek not an empathic response as a result of illusionary theater, but should instead seek an impact of estrangement (*Verfremsdungeffekt*), sometimes rendered as alienation effect (Brecht). Within the theories concerning each major mode of literature, including emergent transmedial or hybrid forms such as graphic narratives or hypertext fictions, one finds assumptions about the cognitive demands and affective impacts on readers.

As I have suggested above, the empirical study of these contentions (or assumptions) is still in its very early stages. Illuminating work has been accomplished in fine-grained neuroscientific or psychonarratological studies of the impact of particular narrative techniques, such as free indirect discourse, on aspects of narrative impact (e.g., Fletcher and Monterosso). The most difficult sorts of study to carry out are large ones, with thousands of participants, and long ones, measuring effects over time. The benefit of large studies, for example involving thousands of college-aged students as they enter and leave university, would be the ability to verify the lofty ambitions often expressed in the student learning outcomes associated with literary studies or diversity requirements. These wished-for outcomes often include improved perspective taking and increased empathy. As it is, educators often undertake large-scale shifts in curricular recommendations speculatively. The benefit of longitudinal studies would be to understand better how reading habits inform life choices and even health outcomes over the lifespan. If literary experiences of empathy do contribute to the development of civic virtues, longitudinal studies that remove confounding elements of education, experience, and identity would go a long way towards convincing the skeptical, among whom I number.

12

FROM AFFECT AND EMPATHY STUDIES

This chapter discusses two domains of research into and theorizing about human emotions, which may be of interest to legal theorists and practitioners in the law. Written by a non-lawyer with expertise in English literature, narrative theory, and interdisciplinary empathy studies, it offers basic definitions of terms, brief overviews of research areas, suggestions about the relevance of affect and empathy studies to law, and cautions about those applications' limitations and liabilities (on compassion, see Feenan, ed.). By no means prescriptive in intention, this discussion of affect and empathy studies seeks to lay bare some of the underlying assumptions and critical attitudes of work in these differing fields, so that a legal reader might navigate the burgeoning literature in affect studies and empathy studies with some awareness of the key differences in emphasis.

Both areas possess interdisciplinary reach, arising from theories and empirical study in social sciences, humanities, and (in the case of empathy) cognitive science and social neuroscience. Affect studies has the greatest purchase for humanists who share commitments to psychoanalysis or social constructionist views arising from the sociology of knowledge—that is, the belief that human behavior and identity are best understood as socially situated, and that knowledge comes from interaction with others (Hacking). Whether affect itself is innate or relational depends on your source, for to a constructivist there are few, if any, inborn aspects of human nature. However, some affect theorists following Silvan Tomkins would see human emotions as part of an evolved system of motivation ("Affects Evolved"), though they would still see affects, as Ruth Leys puts it, as "only contingently related to objects in the world" (437). Empathy studies as it interacts with the humanities (particularly in philosophy and literary studies) also has an interest in intersubjectivity (sharing between/of the minds of subjects who are inherently social creatures), but due to its conversation with social neuroscience and cognitive

DOI: 10.4324/9781003264071-16

science, empathy studies tends to rely on the following ideas: that at least some limited set of basic human emotions exist independent of cultural differences; that our brains and those of other primates possess a neural manifold for shared intersubjective perceptions (mirror neurons); that human consciousness derives some predictable features from our embodied nature; and that emotion-sharing and mind-reading among humans can occur with a reliable degree of empathic accuracy (Ickes, "Empathic Accuracy").

Though scholars in the area of empathy studies give credence to psychological and neuroscientific emotion science that their peers in affect studies might discount, there are similarities and overlaps between these disparate approaches. This means that the terms of discussion occur with different emphases in each realm. Both center on emotional experiences, and neither waves away emotion as entirely inimical to reason or cognition. Both involve forms of idealism—about interpersonal empathy and altruism on the one hand, or about political or social reorganization or other utopian potentialities, on the other hand—and both exhibit skepticism about the efficacy of empathy as a driver of moral or prosocial action. Despite these points of commonality, affect studies and empathy studies researchers are relatively infrequently found in conversation with one another, and their differences are marked. They belong to separate intellectual traditions, and rare are the migrations from one camp to the other.

For the most part affect studies pays no mind to emotion science outside the psychoanalytic tradition, and there are only a few efforts on the part of cognitive studies to grapple with the ideas of affect theorists. Patrick Colm Hogan describes the state of affairs accurately:

> There are critics and theorists who draw on both traditions equally (as in Donald Wehrs's use of sources ranging from Julia Kristeva's poststructural psychoanalysis to Antonio Damasio's neuroscience). Moreover, a number of writers associated with affect theory make selective use of affective science, while critics associated with affective science have taken up political and cultural topics. There is nonetheless a broad tendency toward a bifurcation of this sort. For example, the *Affect Theory Reader* includes no index entries for such towering affective science researchers as Antonio Damasio, Nico Frijda, Joseph LeDoux, Keith Oatley, or Jaak Panksepp. In contrast, there are particularly numerous index entries for Gilles Deleuze, Lawrence Grossberg, Félix Guattari, and Brian Massumi, who do not appear at all in a work such as *The Oxford Companion to Emotion and the Affective Sciences*. Even a figure such as Michel Foucault, prominent in *The Affect Theory Reader*, has only a very limited presence in *The Oxford Companion*.
>
> (Hogan, "Affect Studies" 5)

Because of the lack of conversation between the two areas, it is more helpful to think of degrees of commonality than agreement; disagreements stem from the deep distinctions in philosophical underpinnings (mainly concerning constructivist versus universalizing beliefs about human nature) rather than from (much) overt argument.

A sampling of areas of difference include the intra-philosophical debates about the status of fictional emotions (known as the paradox of fictional emotions); the moral sentimental view that empathy leads to altruism, prosocial actions, and good world citizenship (or its skeptical confutation with reference to the disappointments of history); the argument that all forms of shared emotion (including literary empathy) are inefficacious when false empathy, failed empathy, and personal distress intervene (vs. the insistence on a shared psychobiological humanity); and the implications of gender and other aspects of readers' intersectional identities on both affect and emotion (in which difference is either a barrier or an invitation to solidarity with outgroups). In interdisciplinary conversations about empathy, misunderstanding are rife, and they usually stem from the phenomenon of shared vocabulary that masks different political and philosophical commitments. The various ideas circulating about the importance, usefulness, dangers, or lamentable dearth of empathy in contemporary society suffer from similar obscurations ironically caused by shared vocabulary. In both affect and empathy studies, a wide array of stances toward empathy can be discovered, concerning its desirability or undesirability, its cultivation through exposure to literature or its resistance to educative processes, its relation to prosocial action on behalf of others (Hein and Singer, "Neuroscience") and morality (Eisenberg, "Development"), or to unjust allocation of resources (Batson et al., "Benefits"), and its efficacy or its failures (among other controversies).

Though a chapter of this length cannot delve into all these areas of contention, it does focus on questions and hypotheses of the greatest likely interest to lawyers and legal scholars. As the following discussion of definitions of terms will shortly reveal, there is a great deal of variation even among researchers who believe, for example, in the positive possibility of empathy in the way they define it, theorize about it, and study it empirically. Theorists employing both approaches—affect studies and empathy studies—have entered into conversation with legal studies, but from very different angles and to disparate ends. While on the one hand theorists of affect often have intellectual commitments that align with Critical Legal Studies (CLS), analyzing manifestations (often nonverbal) of subjective experiences within existing power structures in a fashion that may question the norms, forms, and politics of institutions, on the other hand advocates for the cultivation of empathy more often contribute ideas relevant to practitioners seeking to sway jurors through the arts of persuasion, to combat criminal recidivism through educational interventions, or to advocate for reparations for victims or clemency for perpetrators who have themselves been victims of earlier abuse.

Unfortunately, the ordinary words that both approaches employ—affect, emotion, empathy, sympathy, compassion, altruism, and their many common synonyms—have specific valences within their critical arenas that could unintentionally evoke, just to suggest a few of the myriad possibilities, moral sentimental assumptions (as for instance when empathy is linked to altruism), psychoanalytic principles (e.g., when using "affect" signals an allegiance to Silvan Tomkins's ideas about resonance in communication [Mühlhoff]), or Marxist critiques of hierarchical authority, political structures, or institutions. One might easily use a term that has an everyday meaning, and run headlong into resistance that arises from a commitment or belief based in one, but not all, of these arenas. For example, some scholars firmly believe that "altruism" does not exist, or has pathological impacts (Oakley et al.); others find "sympathy" unacceptably condescending; "empathy" may be regarded negatively as the cause of drive-by feeling or ill-informed projection; "compassion" itself may be invoked only to lament its inevitable fatigue; "emotion" may suggest the absence of reason or the very basis of cognition depending on the audience.

Affect and Emotion

The first term, the noun "affect," has a scientific valence that distinguishes it from ordinary terminology of feelings, emotions, and moods, as well as from the usual (verb) meaning in a legal context: bear upon, cause to alter or vary, change, conduce, exert influence, impress, or induce (Burton). Although in the field of psychology, "affect" indicates an instinctive response to a stimulus that evokes a feeling or an emotion in a subject, in affect theory an "affect" is not synonymous with a personal feeling. An influential affect theorist, Brain Massumi, writes in his gloss on Deleuze and Guattari, "L'affect (Spinoza's *affectus*) is an ability to affect and be affected. It is a prepersonal intensity corresponding to the passage from one experiential state of the body to another and implying an augmentation or diminution in that body's capacity to act. *L'affection* (Spinoza's *affectio*) is each such state considered as an encounter between the affected body and a second, affecting, body" ("Notes" xvi). As Eric Shouse lays out the distinctions, "Feelings are *personal* and *biographical*, emotions are *social*, and affects are *prepersonal*" (Shouse). The definition of "affect" in affect theory is complicated by the fact that its seminal usage by Spinoza is often glossed as synonymous with (and is translated from his Latin *affectus* as) "emotion," conflating what subsequent commentators have sought to distinguish, as they seek to understand aspects of experience that cannot readily be accounted for using dominant forms of representation. In psychological science, however, "affective" studies indicate a complement to cognitive studies, and they do concern the emotions. For affective scientist, the "affect" under study includes "a class or category of mental states that includes emotions, moods, attitudes, interpersonal stances, and affect dispositions" (Frijda and Scherer 10).

Using the term "emotion" does not necessarily indicate an intellectual allegiance to emotion science, however. Some prominent affect theorists, such as Sara Ahmed, eschew the term "affect" in favor of "emotion" (*Cultural Politics*). For

Ahmed, the move to "emotion" does not enable the universalizing move of identifying core or basic emotion sets but instead authorizes a historicizing approach that considers context:

> I actually wanted to disrupt the idea of emotion coming from within and then moving out towards objects and others.... What was interesting to me was not just how is the body affecting and being affected, but how is it that certain kinds of things are given value over time? Affects tended to be used a little bit too much at the level of an encounter between bodies. I wanted to talk about histories that preceded and directed this encounter and emotion, as a word, let me do that.
>
> ("Affect/Emotion" 97)

Clearly, emotion in Ahmed's sense has very little in common with the six or eight basic emotions theorized in psychological science (such as Robert Plutchik's fear, anger, sadness, joy, disgust, surprise, trust, and anticipation [169–200]). Ahmed's emotion instead belongs in the tradition of Raymond Williams's description "structures of feeling," or "meanings and values as they are actually lived and felt" (*Marxism and Literature* 132), which can be discerned in residual, dominant, and emergent forms (132–3). In Ahmed's conception, emotion does not indicate one of a fixed set of basic emotions. Instead, emotion places bodies inside or outside communities and forges social relationships of inclusion or exclusion: "emotions align some bodies with others, as well as stick different figures together, by the way they move us" (*Cultural Politics* 195). This kind of emotion is both contextual and ideological. In this, Ahmed sees emotionally charged naming in an Althusserian light, where, for example, a victim of hate-speech is interpellated as one who is hated: "the important question is: What effects do such encounters have on the bodies of others who become transformed into objects of hate?"(60). Given these highly relevant impacts, affect theory should be of interest to legal theorists, and perhaps also to practitioners concerned with both the flow of emotion as a regulatory force that shapes our experiences of culture, institutions, and processes (including the law), and with the potential damage inflicted on targets of repetitive or systemic emotion-driven exclusion or denigration. Employing affect theory may provide a way of bringing to light the centrality of emotional experience to all lived experience, and not only as a driver of bias, imperfect perceptions, or motivation to harm. Less clear is how precisely legal theory could usefully take up these contested terms from affect theory, given their strong ordinary meanings in everyday language.

This foray into defining two evidently contested concepts, affect and emotion, shows that profound disagreements about the location, dynamics, innateness, and shaping by culture of both affect and emotion exist, even among the most commonly cited affect theorists. This derives in part from their multiple and diverse intellectual allegiances. According Patrick Colm Hogan,

> Writers in affect theory draw on a range of psychological, social, linguistic, and other theories, most often in the service of political analysis. The psychological principles of affect theory have tended to derive from the tradition of psychoanalysis, often through its radical revision or critique by such theorists as Jacques Lacan and Gilles Deleuze. Affect theorists have also drawn extensively, sometimes more centrally, on a range of theorists outside of psychology, principally poststructuralists, such as Michel Foucault and Jacques Derrida.
>
> (Hogan, "Affect Studies" 1)

When it comes to empathy studies, we must once again straddle separate arenas. Most empirical empathy research (since the 1980s) has been done by psychologists, in developmental, social, and cognitive psychology: C. Daniel Batson, Nancy Eisenberg, Martin Hoffman, and William Ickes led the way. The related interdisciplinary field of social neuroscience has had a profound impact on our understanding of empathy, especially after the discovery of mirror neurons in humans. (Fadiga et al., 2608–11; Winerman 48)). This work shows that a physiological substrate for aspects of human empathy exists, but it does not guarantee that activation of a mirroring response in the neurons of an observer leads to the higher-order cognitive operations involved in mature empathic concern. This biological substrate is referred to as a shared manifold for intersubjectivity (Gallese, "Roots" 171); it offers a potentiality for understanding, not an inevitability of fellow feeling or compassion. The puzzle of how our shared emotional responses with others sometimes do (and sometimes *do not*) lead to concern and altruism has interested philosophers since the eighteenth century (Pinch). Indeed, the behaviors involved in motor mimicry, imitation in learning, emotional contagion, and facial and bodily mirroring that can now be attributed in part to a mirror neuron system had been observed and written about centuries earlier, under the label of sympathy. Adam Smith and David Hume also noticed the limitations imposed by barriers of distance and dissimilarity on the human expression of sympathy.

Affect theory sustains two major ways of thinking about empathy. The early psychoanalytical writers adopted the early-twentieth-century formulation of *Einfühlung* from German psychological aesthetics. Variants of empathy persist throughout psychoanalytical theory and contribute a strand to affect theory, as for example in Silvan Tomkins's terms, the experience of "affective resonance"(Nathanson xvi). Mühlhoff glosses affective resonance as "a dynamical entanglement of moving and being-moved in relation, of affecting and being-affected, which is sensitive and specific to the concrete relational and situational configuration" (1016). Though he does not use the language of intersubjectivity, Tomkins's affective resonance emphasizes that "the interaction dynamic itself creates an affective experience rather than transmitting internal feeling states between pre-existent individuals. This leads to a philosophical framework in which relationality and ontogeny are primary over separate individuals, and in which the naturalistic distinction of a fundamental physical level versus an emerging level of social processes has to be given up" (1001). Though this emphasis distances Tomkins's thinking from any kind of innate physiological substrate, Paul Ekman himself testified to the importance of Tomkins's 1964 work on the face as a fast, visible instrument that informs both others and the experiencing subject about the emotions (Ekman, "Introduction" 209–16). The second strand of thought about empathy within affect studies derives from cultural studies a deep distrust of any human universals, including universals of biology and innate nature. In its most neutral form, this critique rests on historicist assumptions, arguing, as historian of the emotions Ute Frevert does, that empathy is a modern, global, recent arrival, no more universal than out-of-favor emotions, such as honor and shame, that were more highly valued and motivating in the past (10–12) In its most critical form, empathy is suspected for imposing (likely) unjustified beliefs about others' feelings and point of view on them, in an imperious move that mimics the power structures of colonialism and racism. By this point it should be clear that what various commentators point to when they either excoriate or exult empathy may be referring to wildly different concepts, or to different aspects of the group of phenomena that fall under the term "empathy."

Empathy

In ordinary English empathy normally means the experience of sharing a feeling *with* another person. It is usually differentiated from sympathy (feeling an appropriate, congruent emotion *for* another), though in the eighteenth century, influential treatments of sympathy by Adam Smith and David Hume clearly included empathic phenomena (Wispé). In contemporary parlance, empathy is commonly understood as a beneficent moral emotion leading to good citizenship Pinker, *Better* 177; Nussbaum, *Cultivating* 90), but most scientists regard empathy as an evolved capacity that benefits human survival through mutual comprehension (including the recognition of malign intentions) that aids in successful competition for resources, through fostering of nurture (Wispé), and in cross-species perceptions that help hunters succeed in killing prey animals (Sarnecki 129–42). As John Sarnecki writes in "The Emergence of Empathy in the Context of Cross-Species Mind Reading," "A univocal definition of empathy has been notoriously difficult to pin down, but scholars typically use the term to describe shared affective or cognitive states, compassion or feeling for the distress of others, and/or imagining one's self in another's place in order to understand his or her cognitive, volitional, and affective states .... On this account, empathy allows humans to take on or imagine another individual's experiences, thoughts, drives, as well as his or her emotional responses and commitments" (130). This version of empathy incorporates most of the elements commonly attributed to the motivation, operation, and results of empathy, without limiting them to a human-to-human transaction.

Just as "affect" and "emotion" signal varying assumptions depending on the context of their usage, empathy also means different things to researchers in psychology, philosophy, and the helping professions. In his very useful article, psychologist and empathy authority C. Daniel Batson outlines a set of concepts that relate to quite different research programs in empathy studies. Concept 1, "Knowing Another Person's Internal State, Including His or Her Thoughts and Feelings," emphasizes cognitive empathy and empathic accuracy (Batson, "These Things" 4). This version of empathy may be at play whenever depositions or testimony allow a subject to explain basic things about events and circumstances. Knowing what has happened, and hearing about it from the person who knows first-hand, encourages her audience to assume they know how she feels. However, as Batson acknowledges, empathic accuracy has its limits: "you could be wrong, at least about some nuances and details" (4). Concept 2, "Adopting the Posture or Matching the Neural Responses of an Observed Other," refers to facial empathy or motor mimicry (4). It is understood to be automatic, but Batson cautions against making perception-action matching a unifying basis of all empathy: "neither humans nor other species mimic all actions of others. To find oneself tensing and twisting when watching someone balance on a tightrope is a familiar experience; it is hard to resist. Yet we may watch someone file papers with little inclination to mimic the action" (5). Batson's Concept 3, "Coming to Feel as Another Person Feels" (5), explains emotional contagion, and from a neuroscience perspective, relies on human's shared manifold for intersubjectivity (Gallese, "Roots" 171). Smith and Hume observed emotion-matching and emotion-catching, forms of affective empathy, and wrote about them under discussions of sympathy. Their observations influenced the moral-sentimental account of sympathy (and later empathy) as a moral emotion that can be cultivated through exposure to imaginative literature. As a goal of fictive representation, sympathy has had a prominent role to play in literature, with important statements in its favor by Henry Home, Lord Kames, Percy Bysshe Shelley, and George Eliot (Keen, *Empathy* 44–55).

Batson's Concept 4, "Intuiting or Projecting Oneself into Another's Situation," is the oldest concept associated with the term "empathy" specifically, as it refers to the phenomenon theorized by German psychological aesthetics at the beginning of the twentieth century, *Einfühlung* (Batson "These Things" 6). Imaginative projection into an inanimate object, such as a tumbleweed being blown across a highway, has also been theorized as an aspect of response to artworks, under the label of aesthetic empathy. Acknowledging that *Einfühlung* still has purchase in philosophical discussion of empathy (Currie "Objects"), (and he might have added, in literary applications) Batson clarifies that psychologists rarely mean *Einfühlung*'s projection into another when they refer to empathy (Batson "These Things" 6). Because Freud uses the term *Einfühlung* ("Creative Writers" 141–54), this version of empathy does turn up in Affect Studies. *Einfühlung* plays a role in reading when we attribute personalities, moods, and feelings to inanimate objects, fictional worlds, and characters. If this seems fanciful, it has long been understood as contributing to the human imagination, including in Freud's references to it as part of creative daydreaming. In literary reading, a version of *Einfühlung* may be involved in familiar phenomena: mental visualizing of spaces and movement in spaces; projection into inanimate objects and forms; indulgence in the emotional illogic of the pathetic fallacy; personification of things and landscapes; anthropomorphizing animals and natural forces; and identification with the furnishings of fictional worlds.

Einfühlung for abstract legal principles and inanimate objects such as the Constitution should interest legal scholars. The articulation of *Einfühlung* (and empathy) as concepts separate from sympathy in psychology and aesthetics (Wispé) occurred during the late nineteenth and early twentieth centuries. In German aesthetics, *Einfühlung* describes viewers' imaginative transport "into" the object, giving life to inanimate things. The spectator relates to the object analogously to the way people relate to other people, but in the late nineteenth century, *Einfühlung* had not yet acquired its meaning as a description of emotional attachment to other people. By 1913 Vernon Lee had adopted Lipps' "empathy" for *Einfühlung,* following Titchener's coinage of empathy as a translation of *Einfühlung* that chimed with but distinguished the concept from sympathy (Titchener 21). Informed by the experimental psychology of Titchener and the aesthetic psychology of Theodor Lipps, Vernon Lee's book *The Beautiful: An Introduction to Psychological Aesthetics* (1913) solidified the place of empathy (*Einfühlung*) in English-language theories of aesthetic response (66–7). Lee was especially concerned about explaining human responses to the inanimate world, in embodied responses to images, space, things, or built environments. Early twentieth-century theorists of literary empathy showed how Romantic poets conveyed oneness with nature by projecting feelings into insensate objects (Fogle 139–83).

Whenever a contract is broken, a law violated, a constitutional crisis provoked, *Einfühlung* embedded in the idioms of the language itself evokes concerned emotional projection into abstractions that take on temporary bodies subject to vivid injuries. Passionate defenses of principles and documents held to be foundational to our legal systems often evoke *Einfühlung*. For instance, *Einfühlung* for the rule of law permeates Elaine Scarry's *Rule of Law, Misrule of Men* (2010). As Scarry's work illustrates, arguments imbued with *Einfühlung* for honored texts (such as the Department of Defense's Law of War Manual or the Geneva Convention) and abstractions (such as "the rule of law" or "justice") are also often political. They can be wielded by originalists, proponents of natural law, and defenders of traditional morality. All varieties of empathy, with their affordances and limitations, are resources for the rhetorical arts of persuasion. This encourages the view that writers and practitioners in the law should alertly consider the roles that empathy and affect play in the law, especially when legal abstractions, doctrines, and documents that evoke strong feelings are accorded the imaginative status of persons by means of *Einfühlung*. Batson's dismissive treatment of *Einfühlung* under Concept 4 should not dissuade legal theorists from considering it.

Batson's Concept 5, "Imagining How Another Is Thinking and Feeling," matters to philosophers of mind (Marraffa) and psychologists interested in perspective-taking, and Theory of Mind (ToM) (Batson, "These Things 7). Though some believe it is identical to Concept 5, Batson differentiates Concept 6, "Imagining How One Would Think and Feel in the Other's Place," as role-taking, or putting oneself in the shoes of another (7). No lawyer can read that phrase without thinking of Atticus Finch's words: "You never really understand a person until you consider things from his point of view [...] until you climb into his skin and walk around in it" (H. Lee 33). Since we can never actually climb into another's skin literally (for which reason a softer version of the metaphor substitutes "shoes"), the distinction between perspective-taking and role-taking does matter. Both are versions of cognitive empathy, but in perspective-taking, the empathizer imagines the other. I know that my husband has poor night vision, so I imagine his straining to see as he drives, an effort that might trigger some anxiety in him. I am imagining him and his extra-alert and worried feelings. In role-taking, the empathizer imagines how he or she would feel in the situation of the other. What if I were behind the wheel? I have good night vision! No worries! How I would feel driving at night differs from how he feels. I don't need his glasses, with a prescription that does not correct his vision all the way to 20–20. I may share his extra-alert state but not his anxiety. Arguably, successful role-taking empathy is more effortful and more egotistical. Some theorists regard this form of empathy as more "categorical," more dependent on matches with the self and group identity, and therefore less other-directed and less likely to lead to the ethical expression of compassion than the situational focus of perspective-taking empathy. (Hogan, "Epilogue" 134–6). Indeed, role-taking as an imaginative exercise may lead to impatience or incredulity rather than sympathy if one's own imagined responses to being in other's places differ from the response they show or report. To complicate matters further, some philosophers feel quite strongly that perspective-taking is just as egotistical in its operation as role-taking, and that since only a self can perceive another, the results of an imagine-other instruction would never differ from an imagine-other instruction (Currie and Keen). As a habitual novel reader I disagree with this, for I have learned through my lifetime of fiction reading to imagine others quite unlike myself. Thus I consider Batson's treatment of the two related phenomena as offering a useful distinction, one that matters in the rhetoric of persuasion.

Concept 7, "Feeling Distress at Witnessing Another Person's Suffering," indicates an empathic response of personal distress, which usually causes aversion from the suffering subject (Batson, "These Things" 7–8). It is egotistical rather than other-directed, for it involves "feeling distressed by the state of the other" (8). In the psychological literature, personal distress responses are among the culprits for inaction or lack of sympathetic concern. Why do bystanders not intervene when they witness something going wrong? Possibly they are experiencing the phenomenon of diffusion of responsibility, where they assume others in the crowd (surely!) have already called the police, or an ambulance, or posted the video on social media. This isn't a failure of empathy but a failure to intervene. Possibly they are not feeling empathy for the victim at all, since categorical differences might prevent fellow feeling from occurring in the first place. A third possibility lies in personal distress. Unresponsive witnesses may simply be overwhelmed and even incapacitated by their empathic distress, which can even trigger traumatic flashbacks if they have been victims of similar misfortunes. The important thing to grasp about personal distress is that although it is a real and unruly kind of empathic response, it does not lead to sympathy, altruism, or positive shifts in attitudes like other forms of empathy. It leads to aversion and disengagement. Invoking it may be counterproductive in an advocacy context.

Batson's Concept 8, "Feeling for Another Person Who Is Suffering," is what remains of the capacious category of sympathy, winnowed down from the eighteenth-century concept discussed by Adam Smith and David Hume (8). It differs from contemporary understandings of empathy because it includes congruent emotions, not the matched or shared feelings of Concepts 1–3 and 5–6. As Batson puts it "empathic concern" is "felt *for* the other" (8) and its congruence "refers to the valence of the emotion—positive when the perceived welfare of the other is positive, negative when the perceived welfare is negative" (8). As Batson points out, feeling an appropriate (but different) other-oriented emotion has been identified by many names in earlier times, answering to pity, compassion, sympathetic distress, and sympathy. In my opinion much of the hope that cultural commentators place in empathy would be better invested in the cultivation of the sympathetic imagination. To feel concerned for a traumatized victim is probably a more useful state of mind than a full-blown empathic sharing of trauma, which could be incapacitating and might well lead to personal distress rather than efficacious decision-making or action on behalf of the other.

Empathy has its critics, from Edith Stein to Richard Delgado. Its limitation due to bias in the perceiver, responding to dissimilarity, unfamiliarity, or distance, makes it unreliable. Paul Bloom has criticized the "spotlight effect" of empathy (*Against* 24–6), in a critique related to Jesse Prinz's view that empathy roused for one individual or group can lead to unjust reactions or may lead to antipathy or even dehumanization of an outgroup as a result of empathy for an ingroup. Among literary critics, postcolonial literary theorists emphasize the liabilities of universalizing to critique assumptions of biologically based accounts of human emotions that occlude differences (see above 219). Critics of empathy divide on whether its most baleful effect is false empathy or failed empathy (Keen, *Empathy* 156–60).

Narrative Empathy

Batson's discussion of empathy omits not only discussion of its critics but also an important kind of empathy that has a bearing on legal applications. He leaves out what developmental psychologist Mark Davis measures as "fantasy empathy" (Davis, "Multidimensional" 85), a variety of which I theorize as "narrative empathy" (see above 8). The influential four-subscale empathy survey devised by Mark Davis, the Interpersonal Reactivity Index (IRI), is an instrument used to gauge levels of and changes in empathy among human subjects. It includes a concept of fantasy empathy, "Imagining oneself in the place of *fictitious* characters appearing in books, movies, and plays" (Davis, "Multidimensional" 85). Empathy studies in the humanities have taken a special interest in theorizing narrative empathy. Philosophers have led the investigation of the status of fictional emotions (Radford; Lamarque; Dadlez; Yanal). Not all narrative is fictional, however, and it is in this sense that the theory of narrative empathy, as elaborated in rhetorical narratology, may be of special use to the law. The rhetoric of narrative has a central role to play in the presentation of information in cases and in advocacy. Indeed, according to the *Oxford English Dictionary*, the word "narrative" enters into the English language (from the prevalent Latin *narratio*) through Scottish legal practice, meaning "1. a. A part of a legal document which contains a statement of alleged or relevant facts closely connected with the matter or purpose of the document; spec. a statement of the parties to a deed and the cause of its granting" or "1. b. An allegation made as the basis of a legal action," or "2. a. An account of a series of events, facts, etc., given in order and with the establishing of connections between them; a narration, a story, an account," with examples of all three uses dating back to the sixteenth century. Not until the mid-nineteenth century does narrative begin to be used in the literary sense, as "The part of a text, esp. a work of fiction, which represents the sequence of events, as distinguished from that dealing with dialogue, description, etc.; narration as a literary method or genre."... The intersections of narrative empathy with empathy as it may be involved in law and or legal discourse are manifold, especially when regarded in a rhetorical communication framework.

Empathy and the Law

Though dispassion and critical distance may prevail as ideals, many opportunities to share awareness of and feelings with another's situation and condition occur in the course of interactions in and around the law. The creative work of writing involves imagining an audience that one hopes to persuade. The aesthetics of production of legal writing emphasize clarity and concision, but a fine legal writer may succeed in part because of an ability to marshal empathy in the writing process. Reading depositions, hearing testimony, and rehearsing witnesses involves mental simulation not only of the narrated events but of the second-order representation of what imagined future audiences would think of the story. The aesthetics of reception can involve empathy (including personal distress) of jurors as auditors, and judges as readers, regardless of instructions about fairness. The concern that empathy and emotional responses generally are involved in unjust outcomes is involved in the Brechtian commitment to an estrangement-effect (V-Effekt) (Brecht 14–17, 91–9, 141–7, 179–205).

What techniques of narration, practitioners may reasonably inquire of narratology, most reliably invoke empathy or encourage a less emotionally charged mode of reception? The narratological categories of imaginative literature share with legal narration actants, narrative situations, pace, duration, and settings. All of these may be harnessed to evoke or impede empathetic engagement. Fictional characters and the represented persons of narrative non-fiction are perhaps the most potent formal features of narrative with respect to evocation of empathy. Though the persons of legal narratives may not reveal the rich interiority of many fictional characters, the techniques of characterization employed to describe and reveal their identity, actions, speech, and motives are not formally distinctive: they work the same way, often through metonymic shorthand that operates by inviting associations ("He was wearing a hoodie").

Empathy for persons is an aspect of persuasive rhetoric, because human beings both make and receive the communications crafted to sway their decisions. Because character identification may ensue from or invite empathy, understanding what aspects of intersectional identity (Crenshaw) or shared life experience may trigger empathy is obviously a concern for lawyers involved in jury selection. [A common assumption about gender and empathy that enters into jury selection follows on the intuition that women are more empathetic than men (Baron-Cohen, *Essential*). Eisenberg and Lennon suggested in 1983 that while self-reported measures of empathy indicated women as higher in empathy, physiological measures did not, in "Sex Differences" 100–31; Lamm, Decety, and Singer found no difference for empathy with pain, in "Meta-analytic Evidence" 2492–502. Other studies find a greater degree of emotionality in women but not overall gender difference in empathy (Rueckert, et al., "Gender Differences" 574–8).] Even judges trained in dispassionate analysis have the same shared manifold for intersubjectivity as any other human being, so they may have to learn to discipline empathetic responses. This effort may mitigate "spotlight effects" (P. Bloom 24–6) or risks of unjust allocation, but it is unlikely that it stops the involvement of empathy entirely. Throughout the communication chain, people's emotional engagement with those who communicate with them, and with the persons depicted in the narration (whether agents in a dispute, injured parties, or perpetrators), occurs to varying degrees. During the sentencing phase of a death-penalty trial, Scott Sundby has argued, advocates may succeed in getting a life sentence rather than a capital decision for a convicted criminal by narrating his life circumstances in a fashion calculated to evoke empathy. Alternative sentencing programs intended to combat criminal recidivism among non-violent offenders harness the experience of narrative empathy felt in reading and discussing imaginative literature to the project of rehabilitation. The Changing Lives Through Literature (CLTL) program, for example, uses a syllabus of literary reading and discussion (including the judge and parole officer as well as the offenders) to cultivate empathy:

> Individuals who read about characters in literature may find a connection between themselves and those characters. If literature is a regular companion in our lives, this is not news. But, many adults and youth do not have access to literature and its transformative nature. CLTL participants, judges, probation officers, and instructors believe that bringing carefully selected works of literature to criminal offenders may help these men and women gain insight into their lives and behavior, and learning that they are not alone with their problems.
>
> ("About CLTL")

Though it is not clear which elements of the CLTL philosophy drive their results, studies have shown that the course of reading and discussion, which blends role-taking and perspective-taking, does reduce recidivism ("About CLTL"). Empathy is also fundamentally involved, along with arguments about fairness, when advocates for restorative justice urge attention to the needs of victims of crimes. As legal theorists and practitioners respond to the recent discussions of affect and compassion and the law, they should attend to the separate rich literature on empathy.

13

FROM AFFECTIVE TROLLOPE

Marshaling the feelings in *Orley Farm*

This essay investigates how Anthony Trollope's fictional world-making employs representations of feelings about the self and others as construction materials. To a degree unusual among his Victorian peers, Trollope's fictive places and persons come to life in the mind of the reader within a matrix of emotions. Among the core affects of narrativity, curiosity, surprise, and suspense, Trollope privileges curiosity as a driver of his plots, but he answers narrative enigmas almost as fast as they arise. Trollope's narrator's avuncular voice reassures the reader—this is the way the world works—never troubling us with too much suspense, avoiding shocks, and consoling us that any curiosity aroused by the conundrums of the characters will soon be resolved. With Trollope as a guide readers can pleasurably surrender to the representation of others' feelings. I employ the tools of rhetorical narrative theory of fictional minds (Cohn, *Transparent*) and cognitive narratology (Fludernik; Palmer, *Fictional; Social*) to investigate Trollope's methods, specifically his use of narrated monologue (free indirect discourse) and psycho-narration (thought report) for revealing characters' feelings from the inside, and his use of externalized narration (behaviorist or objective narrative) and intermental thought (communal views) to invite readers' participation in assessing those characters' feelings. It may seem perverse to delve into the narrative techniques of a writer who is sometimes regarded as lacking a consistent or rigorous manner of world-making (Morse, *Reforming* 2–10). Cognitive narratology helps reveal the sources of Trollope's affective accomplishment, first described in detail by Henry James, to whose critique and appreciation of Trollope this essay returns in conclusion (6, 10, 168).

Trollope's novel titles convey his commitments to his characters and their feelings. Thirty of his novels are named for characters or their roles (e.g., *Rachel Ray* [1863]; *The American Senator* [1877]). Six have catchphrases as titles, half of which evoke emotionally fraught situations: *Can You Forgive Her?* (1864–65); *He*

DOI: 10.4324/9781003264071-17

Knew He Was Right (1868–69), and *An Eye for an Eye* (1879). Ten novels bear the names of places. Trollope's Barsetshire, an enduring country of the mind, is chronicled in novels named for people (*The Warden* [1855] and *Doctor Thorne* [1858]) and places: cathedral towns, a parsonage, a small house, and a county. This emphasis inclines readers to the view that Trollope creates memorable settings, as Juliet McMaster demonstrates in her readings of the emblematic valences of the settings and the allegorical uses of locations in the Palliser novels. When he describes, McMaster observes, Trollope is often "painstaking rather than vivid," or diagrammatic in his precision about properties (182). Still, detailed depiction of places and spaces is rare in the pages of Trollope's fiction. If a major use of fictional worlds is the replacement of the world of the reader with an alternative realm of story, Trollope's fictional worlds are constructed not so much out of realized spaces as out of the imagined beings that populate them and their behavior, thoughts, motives, and feelings, and their speculations about one another's feelings. *Orley Farm* (1860–61) contains within a novel named for a place Trollope's meditation on the limits of reliable knowledge about selves and the promiscuity of people's feelings about the motives of others.

In *Orley Farm*, Trollope spends more pages on describing cast iron furniture than on the actual spaces surrounding the characters, and this in a novel centrally concerned with a dispute about land. We can visualize a field and a road, an upstairs and a downstairs, but Orley Farm as a realized space is scarcely there. It has a couple of pieces of furniture, several differentiated rooms, and one contested field, the reclamation of which from a longtime renter by the impulsive heir (who wants to experiment with fertilizers) initiates the chain of events. The real meaning of Orley Farm is its money value. Orley Farm motivates a property crime carried out by forgery because it is an income-producing valuable. Even in his *Autobiography* (1883), when Trollope identifies the original for Orley Farm, a humble but Edenic retreat to which his ruined father repaired with the family, he gestures to a John Millais drawing, the frontispiece to the novel, but eschews description of the property (*Autobiography*, ch. 1). Just look at the picture, Trollope suggests, and no words will be necessary.

According to the cognitive narratologist Alan Palmer, Trollope is a great artist of *intermental thought*, "acutely attuned to the workings of social minds" (*Social Minds* 181). As Palmer has noted in his *Social Minds in the Novel*, Trollope is among those Victorian novelists whose novels are "characterized by an assumption that characters' thought processes are frequently transparent and public" (164). Just look at them and you will know what they are thinking (Wright 1122). *Orley Farm* shows Trollope examining that assumption from the reverse position, asking, as it were, what happens when a society that believes it knows others' minds is baffled by deception in the form of a calm, beautiful lady's face. Trollope employs a counterpoint technique, setting passages of externalized, behaviorist narration and communal (mis)judgments in juxtaposition with thought report that repels direct access to minds. (Trollope rarely employs quoted monologue to reveal unfiltered interiority.) Even in the climactic scene in court, when all eyes fall upon the guilty but shortly to be exonerated Lady Mason,

> she bore it all without flinching … though the state of her mind at that moment must have been pitiable. And Mrs. Orme [that is the friend who stands by the accused even though she knows her guilt], Mrs Orme who held her hand all the while, knew it was so. The hand which rested in hers was twitched as it were convulsively, but the culprit gave no outward sign of her guilt.
>
> (*Orley*, vol. 2, ch. 72)

Notice the complications here. The narrator speculates about the state of Lady Mason's mind. Mrs. Orme knows it. Everybody in the courtroom seeks to read it from Lady Mason's unflinching face. The jury has yet to be turned. We the readers know her agony though we are barred from her innermost thoughts: no consciousness represented here! Yet the passage is rich with information about thoughts and feelings. Cognitive narratology has by and large emphasized the techniques for representations of characters' knowledge about thoughts, in supplement to earlier narrative theorizing about fictional minds. For an artist dedicated to making intermentality his central subject and source of narrativity, we can observe distinct projects in Trollope's work, summed up by the following questions. What do characters *know* about the contents of others' thoughts? (Butte; Pinch). What do they believe about others' motives? What do they intuit about the state of others' feelings? How does group certainty expressed in intermental thought intersect with and complicate reports of individual thoughts and feelings? In this essay I show how Trollope rings the changes on these possibilities throughout *Orley Farm*. The source of suspense, provoker of curiosity, locus of surprise resides especially in Trollope's use of psycho-narration to report on emotions, but he gives the technique a twist by following the world's—or at least society's—judgments and feelings.

Victorian novelists employed a variety of techniques to represent intermental or communal thought in their fiction: the behaviorist or objective version, in which the group's interests, concerns, and conclusions emerge from details of speech and action; the double-cognitive implication of what a group of others *must* be thinking, conveyed through a character's certainty about social disapproval or suspicion (the certainty does not equate with correctness; right or wrong, it gains force through the character's belief in the others' attitudes); and overt thought report by the narrator about the community's opinions, ideas, and responses. The sense that Nathaniel Hawthorne had of Trollope's fiction as "solid and substantial … just as real as if some giant had hewn a great lump out of the earth and put it under a glass case, with all its inhabitants going about their daily business, and not suspecting that they were being made show of" (*Autobiography*, ch. 8) derives from Trollope's goal of offering readers characters they might recognize as "human beings like to themselves" (ch. 8). The inherent interest in Trollope's fiction, which generally speaking eschews the suspense and surprise that are the bread and butter of narrativity, lies in spurring readers' curiosity about what the characters think and feel, wrongly or rightly, about themselves and one another. As Deborah Morse writes about a different novel, Trollope's narrator shows modern consciousness as fractured: "the narrator is part of this depiction of the fissured mind, and the reader is privy to the ensuing revelations of soul" ahead of the other characters (Morse 25). Following recent work on affective experience and the techniques of fiction (Ablow; Goldie, *Mess*) and the extension of narrative theory into social modes for representation of group thoughts and feelings (Palmer, *Social*), I describe in this chapter the techniques by which means Trollope invites his readers to share the feelings and insights of his central characters and those who interact with them.

In its examination of fictional minds, cognitive narratology has established the representation of consciousness as one of the defining features of fictionality (Fludernik, "Factual" 3–6). The categories and functions of these narrative techniques have recently undergone extension. To the three modes for representing fictional minds established by Dorrit Cohn in *Transparent Minds*, cognitive narratologist Alan Palmer has recently added several other categories for techniques used by Victorian novelists. For readers unfamiliar with the narratological terminology, I review the terms, older and newer, with examples from *Orley Farm*.

Narrated Monologue

A celebrated quality of nineteenth-century novels lies in their widespread adoption of this double-voiced discourse that enables a narrator smoothly to move from presentation of externals of action and situation to glosses of the thought stream of the character(s) involved, preserving the tense and person of the narration (usually third person and past tense), but conveying the words of the character's mind. The technique variously named narrated monologue, free indirect discourse (FID), empathetic narration, or *Erlebte Rede*, carries the past-tense and third-person narration of the outer scene while reporting inwardly in words that seem to belong to the character's thought stream. This technique, by any of its theoretical labels, enjoys precedence as one of the most characteristic features of nineteenth-century narrative fiction. Jane Austen deftly deploys it; Henry James was to develop it into a mode for lavish expenditure of words in his central characters' perspectives. One can easily find examples of it in the third-person fiction of every major Victorian novelist, and its variations (spread out among many characters, as in Trollope, or limited to a single center of consciousness, as in James) have been detailed and examined by narrative theorists and literary historians of the form of the novel. [Critics of the novel after Percy Lubbock have often marked the development of techniques for the representation of consciousness as formal advances. See Auerbach; Booth; Pascal; and Watt.]

An example from early on in *Orley Farm* shows its affordances. When Lady Mason's rights to the property she has fraudulently won for her son are being challenged by a renewed lawsuit, Trollope writes, "She knew that her enemies were conspiring against her,—against her and against her son; and what steps might she best take in order that she might baffle them" (*Orley*, vol. 1, ch. 5). The tense and person of the surrounding narration preserved ("what steps might she best take in order that she might" rather than "what steps should I take to"), Trollope drops into Lady Mason's busy brain for a few phrases of thought transcript. But despite the fact that Trollope employs narrated monologue to represent the thoughts and feelings of many of his characters, not only the central ones, on this very page external cues are given priority: "Lady Mason seated herself in her accustomed chair, and all trace of the smile vanished from her face. She was alone now, and could allow her countenance to be a true index of her mind" (vol. 1, ch. 5). Lady Mason has control over whether her face reveals her mind, a quality that stands her in good stead during her courtroom appearances. Right now, in private, an external mind reader can see her agony: "She sat there perfectly still for nearly an hour, and during the whole of that time there was the same look of agony on her brow" (vol. 1, ch. 5).

Quoted Monologue

Thought transcripts of first-person, present-tense discourse that could be spoken aloud with no adjustment of tense and person constitute *quoted* or interior monologue. This mode of representation of consciousness also exists in English fiction as early as the work of Aphra Behn, but it is relatively rare in nineteenth-century fiction and appears more frequently in modern and contemporary fiction, with celebrated instances in Dorothy Richardson, James Joyce, and Virginia Woolf. It presents the thought stream of the character's mind in the present tense and implicit first person, just like dialogue, from which it is sometimes distinguished by tagging "She thought," rather than "She said." While Trollope employs a great deal of dialogue and indirect speech, quoted monologue of thoughts scarcely occurs in his fictional works. In over 800 pages of *Orley Farm* the only utterances that break into present-tense and implicit first-person address (without the quotation marks indicating dialogue) belong to the narrator, not to a character.

Psycho-narration/thought Report

Trollope relies very heavily on thought report, in which the narrator simply asserts what the character thinks or feels. As Cohn describes it, psycho-narration not only permits a narrator's characterization of states of mind but also admits generalizations about *feeling-states* of brief or long duration (Cohn 11–12). Psycho-narration often features imagistic analogies or metaphors for inner feelings, using words to catch subverbal aspects of inner experience, what Cohn calls psycho-analogies (37–44). Psycho-narration certainly cedes authority to the narrator over the character, as it can report conditions of the mind of which the character remains unaware, or it can deny access to characters' minds in what Cohn calls "evasion of an inside view" (23). Because of its tense and person, it blends readily with narrated monologue. It is the mode most often used to convey "diffuse feelings, needs, urges" (135). It blends smoothly with narrated monologue. Thought report lends itself to describing baffled efforts at mind reading among characters.

When the lawyer Mr. Furnival and Lady Mason consult about the dangers presented by the renewed lawsuit, which could drag her back into court and deprive her son of the property she has finagled for him, Trollope writes,

> By this time Mr Furnival had dropped the hand, and was sitting still, *meditating*, looking earnestly at the fire while Lady Mason was looking earnestly at him. *She was trying to gather from his face whether he had seen signs of danger*, and *he was trying to gather from her words whether there might really be cause to apprehend danger*. How was he to know what was really inside her mind; what were her actual thoughts and inward reasonings on this subject; what private knowledge she might have which was still kept back from him?
>
> (*Orley*, vol. 1, ch. 12, emphasis added)

In this passage we see how naturally psycho-narration blends back into the narrated monologue with which it ends, facilitated by the shared tense and person of both modes.

As this passage illustrates, and as cognitive narratologist Alan Palmer has demonstrated in his *Fictional Minds*, passages featuring prominent use of free indirect discourse (narrated monologue in Cohn's terms) actually include a great deal of thought report as well. This mode divulges characters' states of mind through the better-informed observations of an authorial narrator *about* his characters, and it can seem both controlling and antiquated. The time has come, however, to break the habit of interpreting changes in formal strategies as a progressive development. Abandoning a simplifying narrative of formal progress from thought report to free indirect discourse to interior monologue (or folktale to Jane Austen to Virginia Woolf) helps us first to observe how many nineteenth-century novelists incorporated all three modes in their handling of characters' internal states of mind. Despite the wide diffusion of narrated monologue, few novelists could do without thought report, and the two modes blend nicely in third-person past-tense narration. I concur with Palmer that more accurate assessments of the proportional deployment of the techniques of psycho-narration, narrated monologue, and quoted monologue will reveal that in third-person fiction, thought report dominates well into the twenty-first century. This project helps us to recognize that *many* Victorian novelists told *about* their characters' thoughts and feelings some of the time rather than presenting their inner discourse item by item all the time.

Trollope uses thought report copiously, especially for conveying the emotions of his characters, as when Lady Mason's steadfast supporter Mrs. Orme "felt much relieved" at her son's reassurance that he will accompany her to court (*Orley*, vol. 2, ch. 64) or feels her heart sink as her supportive son drives away (243). Trollope often uses thought report to disclose one character's desire to ascertain what another character thinks, feels, or knows. Furnival, the lawyer who steadfastly supports Lady Mason, is vexed by his inability to know her mind, though others can be read: "He would soon be able to ascertain what Sir Peregrine really thought—whether he suspected the possibility of any guilt; and he would ascertain also what was the general feeling in the neighborhood" (vol. 1, ch. 25), but as for asking Lady Mason directly, "It was impossible that he should ask any such question, or admit of any such confidence" (vol. 1, ch. 25). Alternatively, thought report can be used to report on what one character intuits of another's mind. This is an example of what Alan Palmer describes as a double cognitive narrative, in which one character in a fictional world gathers, from her knowledge of his disposition and the situation, what a second character *must* be thinking. So, for example, Lady Stavely feels sure that she knows her daughter's feelings about rival suitors (vol. 2, ch. 50) before Madeline knows it herself (vol. 2, ch. 50).

Externalized Narration

Behaviorist, or objective narrative, as it is sometimes labeled, eschews representation of characters' inner states and thoughts, hewing closely to the conventions of dramatic scene and relying heavily on dialogue. Externalized narration, the opposite of thought report, involves showing rather than *telling*, and it puts the reader in the position of decoding feelings and motives from external cues. In the modern period, several stories by Ernest Hemingway, such as "Hills like White Elephants" (1927) and "The Killers" (1927), are the canonical examples cited in narrative theory. In objective narration, characters know more than the narrator reveals, which shifts the "knowing" function from the narrator to the implied author and the actively decoding reader. Though rarely sustained to the length of a whole story or novel, this dramatic technique of representing minds indirectly through pure scene composed entirely of lightly tagged dialogue does occur on some pages of many nineteenth-century novels. Though the publishing circumstances of the nineteenth century encouraged expansion and even pauses for lengthy passages of description (stretching to make the length required to fill a triple-decker novel), novelists were also familiar with dramatic conventions of dialogue and group conversation. They could and did interpolate passages of objective narrative to imply qualities of mind that could be verified or enriched using narrated monologue and psycho-narration.

Trollope frequently uses externalized narration, with minimal expansions, for dialogues between lovers. In *Orley Farm* the scenes between lovers, discussions among lawyers as they strategize on both sides of the law case, and cross-examinations during the trial include passages of pure scene composed of dialogue with just a very few elaborating expansions. Trollope invites the reader to read between the lines the emotional tenor of the exchanges. For events in private, this eavesdropping mode, closely analogous to drama, invites members of an audience to come to the conclusion that if only they could hear what the characters were saying to one another, they would understand their innermost thoughts and feelings. Indeed, it comes the closest to a naturalistic representation of human mind reading (though of course fictional dialogue differs radically from transcribed real-world conversation). For the climactic public event of the trial, the same technique of transcribed dialogue points in another direction, as Trollope invites readers to imagine not just the feelings of the witnesses but also the likely responses of jury members, manipulated by the lawyers' lines of questioning.

Intermental/Communal Thought

Intermental or communal thought can be seen as the result of individual acts of mind reading, when they are pooled through gossip or shared witnessing, or it can be seen as a distinct phenomenon of group perception. Why does intermental thought, shared or communal thinking (Palmer, *Fictional* 218; *Social* 4), possess powers that intramental thought, individual thinking, cannot achieve? When it reports the conclusions of a household, village, or (in societies with newspapers) a whole class of people, intermental thought can have a socially (and narratively) amplifying effect. Beliefs held by many can be especially consequential, though the content of communal knowledge about one individual's thoughts need not be accurate. Intermental thought can be warped by prejudice and error; wrong certainties about others can be as influential as right ones. When other characters incorrectly interpret the feelings of one who shares their story world, the ensuing misunderstandings can have drastic effects. This is especially the case when a jury is involved.

Trollope represents intramental, *individual* thought using psycho-narration and narrated monologue, but he is also a great artist of intermental thought, those groups of thoughts residing in collections of characters that suggest a crowd's view. Notoriously, Trollope reveals that Lady Mason is in fact the forger of a codicil to her late husband's will very early in the novel, so all the suspense is shifted from "whodunit" to What the World Believes About Lady Mason. The phrases "The State of Public Opinion," to which Trollope dedicates an entire chapter (*Orley*, vol. 2, ch. 61), the "general sympathy of the world at large" (vol. 2, ch. 79), "the general feeling on the minds of all people" (vol. 2, ch. 53), and "a general view of the matter" (vol. 2, ch. 67) flag Trollope's reports of intermental thought. Though the professional skeptics, the lawyers, have "a very divided opinion" (vol. 2, ch. 67), society comes to its own conclusion. Eventually, everybody believes that she is guilty. Even the "last servant at The Cleeve had whispered to her fellow servant that Lady Mason had forged the will" (vol. 2, ch. 64). Subplots focused on her son and her besotted lawyer, among the last to know the truth, scrutinize the reactions of those most interested parties. Fittingly, the legal plot reveals how readily a jury can be brought to distrust the testimony of witnesses who are in fact telling the truth. In *Orley Farm* Trollope invites his reader to stop caring about the truth and to focus instead on manipulation of passionate feelings and the complex emotional aftermath (relief, grief, the pain of renunciation) in the characters closest to the guilty woman, in whom he has invested our rooting interest.

For the readers are well ahead of most of the characters. Halfway through the novel, Trollope flatters readers' mind-reading abilities:

> I venture to think, I may almost say to hope, that Lady Mason's confession at the end of the last chapter will not have taken anybody by surprise. If such surprise be felt I must have told my tale badly. I do not like such revulsions of feeling with regard to my characters as surprises of this nature must generate. That Lady Mason had committed the terrible deed for which she was about to be tried, that Mr Furnival's suspicion of her guilt was only too well founded, that Mr Dockwrath with his wicked ingenuity had discovered no more than the truth, will, in its open revelation, have caused no surprise to the reader.
>
> (*Orley*, vol. 2, ch. 45)

This writer has no interest in the usual drivers of narrativity, the feelings of reading that inhere in narrative itself: begone suspense and surprise! Instead, Trollope practices an art of manipulating feelings, as he acknowledges. Trollope's narrator steps in at the conclusion:

> I may perhaps be thought to owe an apology to my readers in that I have asked their sympathy for a woman who had so sinned as to have placed her beyond the general sympathy of the world at large. If so, I tender my apology, and perhaps feel that I should confess a fault. But as I have told her story that sympathy has grown upon myself till I have learned to forgive her, and to feel that I too could have regarded her as a friend.
>
> (vol. 2, ch. 79)

We should take this meta-narrative codicil as a rhetorical gesture, for Trollope is bragging by means of apologizing.

Trollope's pride in his mode of inviting misplaced sympathy compels interest in his technique and craft. This may seem counterintuitive to those familiar with the history of Trollope's critical reception. For some critics and theorists, Trollope condemned himself when he described his writing regime. His habit of writing without revising made him seem less than serious: "If a man knows his craft with his pen," Trollope wrote, "he will have learned to write without the necessity of changing his words or the form of his sentences" (*Autobiography*, ch. 8).

This proud statement about his bureaucratic prose, honed in reports written for the Post Office, has been regarded as the sign of an unserious writer. But consider also what Trollope says about his unedited freewriting: "It is by writing thus that a man can throw onto his paper *the exact feeling* with which his mind is impressed at the moment" (ch. 8, my emphasis). Trollope's knack for throwing onto paper those *exact feelings* make him a worthwhile object of study for rhetorical narratologists interested in the complex moves involved in the transmission of affect from author to reader(s). Trollope clearly indulged in what psychologist Marjorie Taylor [and her collaborators] have described as the illusion of independent agency (76–7), by means of which an author's imaginary creations seem to possess lives and minds of their own. Writing about his must fruitful periods of writing, when he could wander around alone in the mountains daydreaming, Trollope recalls in *An Autobiography*, "At such times I have been able to imbue myself thoroughly with the characters I have in hand. I have wandered alone among the rocks and woods, crying at their grief, laughing at their absurdities, and thoroughly enjoying their joy" (ch. 10). Taylor et al. have suggested that writers who experience this illusion of independent agency most intensely also prosper as published authors, and Trollope certainly did well in the book market. The confession of speedy composition that follows in Trollope's account, however, notoriously damaged his reputation as a craftsman. He writes, "I have been impregnated with my own creations till it has been my only excitement to sit with my pen in my hand, and drive my team before me at as quick a pace as I could make them travel" (ch. 10).

Trollope's reputation comes to us filtered through the opinions of that most rigorous early narrative theorist, Henry James. If we think of Trollope as a writer who writes fast, inviting immersion into easy, prolonged experiences of narrative transportation and lazy empathy, only to bring us up short with plot-spoiling pronouncements, we are seeing Trollope through James. James on Trollope serves as a touchstone of the emergent exacting modern writer deploring the lax form of the older generation's loose baggy monsters. Yet the artist and advocate of the center of consciousness found much to appreciate in Trollope, and James's judgment of *Orley Farm* is worth attending to (Michie). James's précis of *Orley Farm* enacts both his disdain for Trollope's management of plot and his admiration of Trollope's accomplishment as a verisimilar portraitist:

> A quiet, charming, tender-souled English gentlewoman who (as I remember the story of *Orley Farm*) forges a codicil to a will in order to benefit her son, a young prig who doesn't appreciate immoral heroism, and who is suspected, accused, tried, and saved from conviction only by some turn of fortune that I forget; who is furthermore an object of high-bred, respectful, old-fashioned gallantry on the part of a neighbouring baronet, so that she sees herself dishonoured in his eyes as well as condemned in those of her

> boy: such a personage and such a situation would be sure to yield, under Trollope's handling, the last drop of their reality.
>
> (130)

With a tip of the hat to Aristotle, James theorizes,

> There are two kinds of taste in the appreciation of imaginative literature, the taste for emotions of surprise and the taste for emotions of recognition. It is the latter that Trollope gratifies, and he gratifies it the more that the medium of his own mind, through which we see what he shows us, gives a confident direction to our sympathy.
>
> (133)

Though he does not use the term empathy (it is two decades from being coined), James's emphasis on the "emotions of recognition" and giving "direction" to sympathy suggests that Trollope is involving readers in the kind of transaction that I have described elsewhere as authorial strategic narrative empathy, which reaches out to evoke readers' empathy in audiences near and far (see above 40). The fact that we are still reading and enjoying Trollope today suggests that his strategic empathizing is of the broadcast variety, reaching, if not originally intended for, a posterity readership. James asserted quite firmly that "Trollope did not write for posterity: he wrote for the day, the moment; but these are just the writers whom posterity is apt to put into its pocket" (132).

Though he did not review the novel directly, in his *Partial Portraits* retrospective on Trollope James lumps *Orley Farm*, with *Can You Forgive Her?* (1864–65), *He Knew He Was Right* (1869), and *The Way We Live Now* (1875), as one of Trollope's "exceedingly voluminous tales" (98). James thought that Trollope's productivity would get in the way of his long-lastingness: "there is sadness in the thought that this enormous mass does not present itself in a very portable form to posterity" (133). He could not anticipate the wonderful combination of a download from Project Gutenberg and an e-reader. James acknowledges that Trollope, whose productivity and proclivity for lengthy compositions he disdains as insufficiently attuned to form and theory, nonetheless pleases his audience:

> His honest, familiar, deliberate way of treating his readers as if he were one of them, and share their indifference to a general view, their limitations of knowledge, their love of a comfortable ending, endeared him to many persons in England and America.
>
> (100)

Like a woman writer, James judges, Trollope has a knack for the texture of daily life: "And then he *felt* all daily and immediate things as well as saw them; felt them in a simple, direct, salubrious way, with their sadness, their gladness, their charm, their comicality, all their obvious and measurable meanings" (101). Unimaginative, neither pictorial, grotesque, philosophical, or even satirical, in James's view, Trollope possesses "great natural kindness" (102) toward the subjects of his representations: "There is something remarkably tender and friendly in his feeling about all human perplexities; he takes the good-natured, temperate, conciliatory view—the humorous view, perhaps, for the most part, yet without a touch of pessimistic prejudice" (102). Insofar as Trollope treats both his characters and his readers with kindness, "he has a wholesome mistrust of morbid analysis, an aversion to inflicting pain" (102) (James was perhaps not thinking of Trollope's tortured characters, Josiah Crawley and Louis Trevelyan.)

Trollope's narrative empathy is rarely empathy for suffering, making *Orley Farm* a significant anomaly among his novels. Lady Mason suffers and readers suffer with her, even though, or because, she is guilty. In admiration of his convincing but not deep-delving psychology of character, James writes that Trollope

> had no airs of being able to tell you *why* people in a given situation would conduct themselves in a particular way; it was enough for him that he felt their feelings and struck the right note, because he had, as it were, a good ear. If he was a knowing psychologist he was so by grace; he was just and true without apparatus and without effort.
>
> (105)

Ironically, James faults Trollope for showing what James would have told, at length. As a plotter, James observes, Trollope eschews what we have come to recognize as the emotional drivers of narrativity. James notes that despite their "great length," Trollope's stories "deal very little in the surprising, the exceptional, the complicated" (106). As is well known, James disapproved of Trollope's self-referential revelations and little "slaps at credulity" (116): "He took a suicidal satisfaction in reminding the reader that the story he was telling was only, after all, a make-believe" (116). This is in its way a deeply ironic observation, coming from the great artist of narrated monologue, whose fictional technique is premised on the notion that a third-person narrator can take the reader into the center of consciousness of a Strether, for instance, where without the aid of fictionality we could never go. James's criticism of Trollope has resonated in the critical history, but his appreciation of Trollope's good ear and knowing psychology should also be noted. A watchword for easy immersion experiences, for prolonged transportation into fictional worlds, and for chatty self-interruption, Trollope creates vivid fictional worlds out of the texture of feelings, as James was among the first to recognize and praise. As to why he could not have been *more* generous, James may have been inhibited in his overt recognition of Trollope's accomplishments by his unacknowledged indebtedness to this Victorian master.

14

FROM TWENTY-FIRST CENTURY FICTIONAL EXPERIMENTS WITH EMOTION AND COGNITION

Narrative Empathy and Contemporary Anglophone Novels

The invitation to co-creation that novelists extend to readers can be especially enticing when their representations invite narrative empathy, engaging readers' emotional and cognitive responses. To be sure, not all novelists aim for empathic emotional fusion with their creations, or sympathetic engagement on behalf of real people represented by fictional characters, for some invite antipathy, dispassionate judgment, or simple curiosity—there is no one right way to craft a fictional world, or to read one. However, experiments that invite fusions of feeling and meetings of minds reveal that the centuries-old ethical project of the English novel (which paradoxically invites readers to get out of this world into an imaginary one, enlarging their own humanity through a refreshing escape from reality) receives refreshing attention from contemporary novelists strategically deploying narrative empathy. At times, as in Dave Eggers's *testimonio* with Sudanese Lost Boy Valentino Achak Deng, *What is the What?* (2006) or Edwidge Danticat's picture book about the Haiti earthquake, *Eight Days* (2010), the authors' strategic appeal to empathy is directly linked to a call for social action and contributions to human-rights-related causes. Other works, such as Gillian Flynn's 2012 thriller *Gone Girl*, exercise the cognitive and affective pleasures of knowing, intuiting, or testing what another is thinking or feeling through representations of mind. Alternatively, as in the case of Lionel Shriver's *We Need to Talk About Kevin* (2003), novelists test the acuity and morality of readers by presenting inscrutable subjects, in this case a teenaged school-shooter, whose consciousness cannot be penetrated even by the narrator, his own mother, who is represented as the only character who entertains suspicions about the future murderer. Confronting the possibility of baffling mind-blindness, and the lack of self-awareness that Thomas Hardy called nescience (Keen, *Hardy's*

DOI: 10.4324/9781003264071-18

Brains 170–210), challenges many easy assumptions about the capacity of narrative fiction to improve readers' emotional and cognitive capacities. There is very little that is predictable about twenty-first-century novelists' experimentation with emotion and cognition.

In order to suggest the range of means employed by novelists to experiment with readers' human endowments of thinking and feeling about others (a practice that reaches deep into the generic heart of the novel as representing selves and societies), this essay touches on representations and techniques of narrative empathy in a wide variety of forms, including perspective-taking, empathic inaccuracy, personal distress, and *Einfühlung*. In contemporary discourse, empathy has many definitions, components, and roles to play in accounts of human emotional responsiveness, communication, social behaviour, and altruism. Most of them have a social, other-directed orientation.… [Batson's "These Things Called Empathy"] serves as a background resource for this discussion of narrative empathy, as does Lauren Wispé's "History of the Concept of Empathy" (1987) (See above 8).

. . .

[F]or each type of human empathy detailed by Batson a correlate in narrative empathy exists, and each kind of narrative empathy may in turn be evoked using a variety of techniques (see chapter 6). In a broad survey of twentieth-century Anglophone fiction one finds a plenitude of techniques involved in fictional experiments across a range of subgenres and types of novels. Unfamiliar characters, whose differences are illuminated through access to fictional consciousness; unusual narrative situations; manipulations of both pace and duration; innovations in storyworld features of setting, with new locales for interiority; and every kind of device of the discourse, including paratexts, laid bare: these foregrounding strategies contribute both to the novelty of the novel and its capacity to intrigue readers and startle them out of imaginative complacency.

While a chapter of this length cannot accomplish a full survey of either techniques or texts, I make reference to illustrative examples from a wide selection of texts, including Margaret Atwood's *Oryx and Crake* (2003), Edwidge Danticat's *The Dew Breaker* (2004), Marlon James's *A Brief History of Seven Killings* (2014), Ian McEwan's *Atonement* (2001), and Sarah Waters' *The Night Watch* (2006). Some of our most productive theorizing occurs when we enter into conversation with literary texts, so my exploration in this chapter refers glancingly to many novels before looking more closely at one text, Patrick Rothfuss's novella *The Slow Regard of Silent Things* (2014), to illustrate a variety of kinds of narrative empathy. Indeed, some rich texts evoke multiple varieties of empathy. Narrative fictions offer opportunities for readers to co-create fictional worlds, to engage imaginatively and feelingly with its human and inanimate denizens. Contemporary novelists employ and reinvent the tools and techniques of narrative fiction when they create fictional worlds, to various ends, but all aimed at reaching a readership and a global market. The vast majority of published twenty-first century fiction would not be considered experimental by most readers and critics, or at least not 'experimental' in the sense of laying bare the devices of fictional world-making and making the devices themselves subjects of invention and innovation. Yet the traditional novel as an artistic device represents a method for experimenting with human emotion and cognition, as Lisa Zunshine, Blakey Vermeule, and Keith Oatley have argued. For example, *A Gentleman in Moscow* (2016) by Amor Towles engages the core affects of narrativity—curiosity, suspense, and especially surprise—in a historical novel that evokes a richly-imagined fictional world peopled with memorable characters with whom readers develop strongly empathic rooting interests. Even on a better-informed second reading, the last hundred pages of *A Gentleman in Moscow* make the heart race and call up a lump in the throat. The highly-valued experiences of psychological realism and ingenious plotting leading to strong closure offered by this novel exemplify the rewards of traditional novelistic techniques: still going strong in the twenty-first century. Furthermore, when considering experimentation in twenty-first century fiction, a reader may discover that metafictionality and other signs of postmodernist play are so widespread that they constitute merely a contemporary style. That style of self-aware play with forms and conventions may or may not correlate with postmodernism as a philosophical commitment. Indeed, the modes of surface experimentation, such as the use of second person 'you' narration or typographical illustrations frequently coexist with contemporary themes in Anglophone world fiction, but these highly recognizable forms of experimentation do not describe the full range of innovation undertaken by novelists working in English today (Stross; Egan).

Experiments with Emotion and Cognition

Experimentation in twenty-first-century fiction can be attributed to a variety of impulses: the persistence of postmodernism or postmodern styles; the incorporation of global narrative traditions that previously lay outside the canon of English language fiction; and adaptation by way of transmediality and the blended forms that have enriched the novel with graphic and hypermedia alternatives (as in Geoff Ryman's inspired novel *253*, from 1996, and still accessible online via the Wayback Machine).

In my opinion the restoration of the resources of romance subgenres to the novel proper have played a vital role in reinvigorating the twenty-first-century novel, as I point out in a forthcoming essay on the recovery of genre in contemporary British fiction:

> Sticky mixtures and unseemly in-between-ness have much improved reputations, as the cachet of heteroglossia (Bakhtin), hybridity (Bhabha), and liminality (Turner) has improved the credibility of fiction that blends with the dominant mode of literature the devices and tropes of what Rosalie Colie long ago described as "the resources of kind." Writing about genre-theory in Renaissance literature, Colie endorsed with enthusiasm the

> literary gain to be realized in embracing the affordances of genres and in "refusing to allow generic categories to dictate or predestine the size, scope, content, and manner in any particular literary work."
>
> (Colie 103; Keen "Recovery")

Each of these reasons for experimentation in contemporary fiction (postmodernism, heteroglossic diversification through global influences, hybridity through transmediality and generic recuperation) corresponds to efforts to engage readers' emotion and cognition, as I suggest below.

Yet there is no one-to-one correspondence between a narrative technique used in fiction and a predictable readers' response. As Meir Sternberg has long argued, the possibilities inherent in narrative techniques are protean, whether those techniques are employed conventionally within traditions or experimentally in emergent forms. To assume that a specific narrative technique (such as a 'cliff-hanger' break in an instalment of a multi-part narrative) inevitably evokes a set response is to engage in metaphorical 'package-dealing' against which Sternberg cautions the careful theorist. Depending on the contents and conventions in which the cliff-hanger break interrupts the discourse, and also depending on the experiences and identity of the reader co-creating the fictional world, it may evoke anxiety, a feeling of suspense, eagerness to read on (curiosity), boredom, irritation, or empathy (among other possibilities!). Since narrative empathy is a blend of cognitive and affective responsiveness on the part of readers to authors' proffering of co-creative opportunities, the remainder of this essay employs narrative empathy as a proxy for a wider range of experiments in emotion and cognition. Consistent with my earlier work on the subject, I do not assume that there are fixed sets of empathic narrative techniques available to novelists. However, I do observe that the evocation of empathy, either as a corollary of character identification, as an effect of richly-visualized storyworlds inviting immersion reading experiences, or as a response to foregrounding effects in the language and narrative techniques, is a widespread goal of many, though not all twenty-first-century novels. How (or whether) real readers actually respond to authors' strategic narrative empathizing is subject to many variable conditions. This need not bring us to an impasse, however.

A brief review of some of the presumptions about the emotional and cognitive demands of different categories of contemporary fiction lays the groundwork for a brief consideration of some examples of experiments in this arena. Postmodern fiction is often regarded as more cognitively pleasurable than emotionally inviting, with its emphasis on ironies, parody, pastiche, and metafictional moves that draw attention to the artifice of the work. Indeed, some narrative theorists regard the frame-breaking ironies inherent in metafictional gestures as inimical to the emotional effects of empathy (see Fludernik, "Fictions"), but contemporary novels often combine surprising formal experiments that lay bare the devices of fictionality with invitations to share in the intensities of embodied experience. We need look no further than Ian McEwan's novel *Atonement* or Sarah Waters' *The Night Watch* to find exemplars of fiction that encourage empathic immersion while also inviting intellectual engagement with the affordances and limitations of conventional forms. The revelation late in *Atonement* that a novel apparently narrated by an external, overt, reliable third-person narrator bearing all the trappings of omniscience has actually been narrated all along by a motivated, truth-bending, covert narrator who exists inside the story world wherein she has the status of a major character delivers a formal shock worthy of John Barth but in no way undoes the effects of the sympathetic imagination with which McEwan endows his penitent fictional author and narrator. Even if teetering on the vertiginous edge of the reminder that she made it all up (when of course *he* always already *made it all up*!), readers have still trudged with Robbie to the beach at Dunkirk, and the richly embodied account of that experience suffers no erasure. Indeed, I know readers of *Atonement* who were so caught up in its plot that they missed the twist altogether, with no evident diminishment of their pleasure in the novel.

The backwards arrangement of the segments of Waters' *The Night Watch* certainly challenges a reader to assemble what happened to reorder an anachronous narration into a forwards story, but as the character Kay remarks of her habit of movie-going, a straight-ahead discourse is not necessarily more pleasing: "Sometimes I sit through the films twice over. Sometimes I go in half-way through, and watch the second half first. I almost prefer them that way—people's past, you know, being so much more interesting than their futures" (Waters 110). Waters binds together the out-of-order viewing pleasure, the contents of people's pasts (only gradually unspooled in the novel), and the libidinous freedoms of the cinema and (earlier) wartime experiences. Her lamentation of the consequences of the end of the war and a restored social order depends on her persuading readers that what happened before is of far more consequence than what happens next. As in these cases, some of the most effective experiments with conventions of narration also manage to deliver richly rewarding, complex depictions of characters that live up to traditional standards for canonical psychological realism. That both novels were adapted to film or television, despite their demanding narrative techniques, suggests that the novelists succeed in having it both ways, writing emotionally engaging, immersive fictions that also play significantly with the conventions of the narrative delivery system.

Hybrid forms, especially graphic narratives, are understood to be immersive and gripping, and have achieved a greater degree of critical respect than that commanded by their comic-book precursors through defamiliarizing experimentation that plays on the boundaries of what is sometimes labelled "unnatural" narratives (Alber), such as Chris Ware's *Building Stories* (2012)… Genre fiction (perhaps especially the genres of the novel associated primarily with women readers) still has a reputation of offering mindless reading experiences that deliver reliable doses of emotional experience by means of oft-repeated formulas. Yet readers of

Diana Gabaldon, Louise Penny, N. K. Jemison, and Bernard Cornwell testify to the intellectual pleasures of genre fiction even as they appreciate the expert use of conventions of historical romance, detective fiction, science fiction, and historical fiction. The presumptions detailed in the preceding sentences imply hierarchies of taste and value that have been repeatedly upended by twenty-first-century novelists, indicating that the expectations and reputations of these different kinds of fiction are often regarded as generative challenges by novelists seeking to "make it new."

Perhaps the most striking tactic of contemporary novels is the invitation to strenuous perspective-taking and/or role-taking imagining challenged by representation of extreme forms of difference. Deliberate perspective-taking, or 'imagine-other' conditions in fiction, invites attention to the other that remains aware of difference. Sometimes novelists take the reader straight into the minds and feelings of the other by locating the narrative within their perspectives. Barbara Gowdy's novel *The White Bone* (1998), narrated from the point of view of anthropomorphized elephants, may be seen as a precursor to twenty-first-century experiments more emphatic about the constructed boundaries of species difference, as in Karen Joy Fowler's *We Are All Completely Beside Ourselves* (2013), narrated by a woman whose lost twin is a chimpanzee. Fowler's novel undermines the primacy given to human language, intelligence, and communication over animal cognition, a subject that narrative theorist David Herman has recently explored in *Narratology Beyond the Human* (2018). The difference between perspective-taking and role taking is illuminated by referring to C. Daniel Batson's definitions.... (see above 93–4). Both forms are likely to be involved in readers' experiences of narrative empathy, but contemporary experiments often thwart readers' drive towards character identification by alienating the reader to different degrees, sometimes with the aim, as in Fowler's novel, of turning attention back to the self when the other's experience is revealed to be impenetrable. The possibility of narrative empathy with fictional animals emphasises the difference between perspective-taking and role-taking quite neatly: it is a different matter to be asked by a novelist to imagine what an elephant's mind, culture, feeling life, and spirituality is like (imagine other) and being asked to imagine what one's own response to the animal's circumstance would be in that position (imagine self). The most extreme challenges to the inherent anthropomorphic bias of narrative empathy are posed by radically decentered work that eschews pronouns that would assist in identifying narrative situation, as in Peter Larkin's *Leaves of Field* (2006) and other prose poetic sequences that draw the reader close to the utterly alien perspective of trees.

False and Failed Empathy

For it must be conceded that *getting it wrong* is a fundamental human experience of empathizing. Though the psychology of human empathy reinforces the sense that most people are pretty good most of the time at intuiting or judging others' thoughts and feelings, novelists experimenting against the easy assumptions of character identification exploit the possibility of empathic inaccuracy (see Keen, *Empathy and the Novel*, 136–7). It can also be thematized overtly. For example, Margaret Atwood's *Oryx and Crake* depicts a character (Jimmy/Snowman) who has grievously misunderstood every motive of his friend Crake. The reader is asked abjectly to share in Jimmy's earlier obtuseness even as Atwood sets about inviting strong rooting interest in Snowman's survival in the present-day narration. Setting aside the kind of empathic inaccuracy that occurs (sometimes because of immaturity or misunderstanding) when a reader empathizes at cross-purposes with an author's strategic narrative empathizing, we come to the experimental cases where an author deliberately courts readers' empathy only to reveal it as misjudged, misguided, over-reaching, or even a symptom of arrogant privilege. Edwidge Danticat's *The Dew Breaker*, a novel constructed of interlinked short stories set among a community of expatriate Haitians, courts empathic inaccuracy for a former torturer in order to unsettle readers' habits of connecting with others through art. The previously mentioned novel *We Need to Talk About Kevin* by Lionel Shriver may also be regarded as an exercise in empathic inaccuracy, for the mother's self-narration can be regarded as ultimately self-condemning of a chilly neglect that causes her child to become a murderer, rather than an *apologia* and appeal for sympathy. Readers can and do differ about these interpretations.

Perhaps the most striking divergence among readers of emotionally evocative fiction occurs when some readers find unbearable what others find moving and efficacious. This shows that a fictional work has the capacity to evoke personal distress. Personal distress, still an empathic reaction, focuses on one's own sensations to the point of diverting attention from the suffering other's experience. Batson describes it as "Feeling Distress at Witnessing Another Person's Suffering" ("These Things" 7). As Batson explains it, personal distress expresses not feelings *for* (sympathy) or feelings *like* the other's feelings, but "feeling distressed *by* the state of the other" (8). Personal distress can lead to cessation of the reading or viewing … (See discussion of NPD in chapter 4, above)… Left to their own devices, many readers of my acquaintance gave up on Marlon James' *A Brief History of Seven Killings* (2014) because of its representation of violence, misogyny, and homophobia; my students who hung in there until the end got past personal distress to earn the reward of comeuppance and even, in the case of one highly sympathetic victim, escape from the reach of criminality. Encouraged by the directorial style of Quentin Tarantino, and possibly also by the popularity of first-person-shooter video games, violent representations in film narrative and in the twenty-first-century novel are extraordinarily common, and it should go without saying that for some readers and viewers, these narratives evoke pleasurable excitement rather than empathic distress.

Aesthetic Empathy and *Einfühlung*

The intensities of contemporary interactions with the inanimate world as mediated by virtual reality and other electronic delivery devices makes the very oldest form of empathy to be theorized as an aspect of aesthetics freshly relevant: this survey concludes with a consideration of *Einfühlung*. Vernon Lee described *Einfühlung* as "that inference from our own inner experience which has shaped all our conceptions of an outer world, and given to the intermittent and heterogeneous sensations received from without the framework of our constant and highly unified inner experience" (*Beautiful* 68). A line of connection between Lee's *Einfühlung* and empathy exists not only in her theories but in many varieties of literary empathy. As Rae Greiner has recently argued, the "formal protocols of empathy align with those of poetry" (420), actively relating the *unalike* human perceiver and inanimate object of perception. Greiner sees empathy as operating like a metaphor, that yoking of unlikes: "With its fusion of subject and object, empathy accomplished the work of metaphor" (420). Alternatively, Greiner sees sympathy, "with its emphasis on context—one's adjacency to or distance from others with whom one does not merge—as a variety of metonymy" (421). The reader's co-creative act of reading, in a transactional model, involves something very like Lee's empathy ("that inference from our own inner experience which has shaped all our conceptions" [*Beautiful* 68]) in the imagining of the fictional worlds that a reader encounters. To zero in on the inhabitants of fictional worlds, narrative empathy felt with characters is that it appears simultaneously to invite a kind of empathy with persons and at the same time can also be regarded as an empathy with a thing—a nobody, a code for projection made out of words, a word-mass. Thus experimental writing that draws attention, through various modes of foregrounding, to words themselves, is especially suited to the estranging evocation of *Einfühlung*.

A recent lyrical novella exploits and dramatises the resources of narrative empathy in a work that explicitly thematizes *Einfühlung* through the empath Auri, a character whose strongest shared feelings are evoked by inanimate objects. Patrick Rothfuss, *New York Times* bestselling author of the well-regarded novels *The Name of the Wind* (2007) and *The Wise Man's Fear* (2011), placed his novella *The Slow Regard of Silent Things* (2014) within the fictional world of the Kingkiller Chronicle novels, extending what readers know about a secondary character, Auri. Rothfuss' treatment of Auri's *Einfühlung* enacts a Winnicottian developmental narrative as she scavenges objects willing to be collected. Her inanimate companions, including her chemical light source Foxen, are personified by Auri's perceptions of their moods and personalities. This is not at all unlike contemporary Westerners' relationships with their smartphones, but unlike our oblivious generation, Auri is aware of her environment. Her acutely sensitive *Einfühlung* helps her perceive when her surroundings are "unkilter" (Rothfuss, *Slow*, 18) and to correct them:

> So for a while he hung and swung. Auri took care not to notice any undue exuberance on his part while she gave the unnamed stairs a brisk once-over. Up and down then up again, the tight birch broom flicked and tickled the stone steps clear of fallen rocks and grit and dust. They were flattered by the attention while remaining entirely coy.
>
> (32)

This novella invites three ways of thinking about *Einfühlung*: its role in fictional representation of spaces; its attribution of personalities and moods to inanimate objects; and its experience by a character of a strongly empathic disposition. Rothfuss's *The Slow Regard of Silent Things* illuminates the specific immersive pleasure of orientation in an imagined space, as its central character Auri navigates the abandoned rooms, cellars, utility tunnels, and basement passageways that she calls "the Underthing" (6). The novella narrates the seven days of preparation that Auri undertakes as she readies herself for Kvothe's visit and it culminates in the preparation of a space and gifts for him. Kvothe is the central character of *The Name of the Wind* and *Wise Man's Fear* and an eagerly awaited third volume, *The Doors of Stone* (forthcoming). The time period of Auri's preparations occurs in temporal overlap with episodes narrated in *Wise Man's Fear* (chapters 7 through 11), so readers familiar with the fictional world will have already met Auri through Kvothe's encounters with her. Though Auri can and does go outside and ascend to rooftops, most of the narrative transpires in the Underthing, a set of linked spaces of differing degrees of antiquity, a vast underground structure that exists below the University, an ancient school of magic. Rothfuss's University and his conception of magic owe a lot to Ursula LeGuin's Wizard school on Roke and its curriculum. The University is one of the central settings of the Kingkiller Chronicles, and in addition to the expected liberal arts of such an institution, students there can study name magic, based on the folkloric or hermetic tradition of true names and the power of knowing this vocabulary. Two additional disciplines on offer at the university indicate Rothfuss's interest in empathy: studying Sympathy there introduces a form of sympathetic magic that students can learn to use to manipulate the material world, and Sygaldry is an extension of sympathetic magic involving the inscription of runes and materials science or engineering. But Auri is not a student at the university. She seems to have received a basic education in chemistry from a mentor whose underground laboratory she still visits, and she knows how to mend things. Her scavenging is on the one hand a matter of survival (she collects pine cones to extract pine nuts to eat), but on the other hand it operates by a kind of loving survey of the territory, visiting spaces, taking their emotional temperatures, addressing their lacks by bringing items to them, removing things that do not belong in them, and repairing them.

Rothfuss gives his character a kind of innate *feng shui*, which she uses to read and re-balance her surroundings. A feral survivor, she is adept at this kind of interpretation of spaces and things, reading them for threats and sympathy as she explores them. Auri's perception of the inanimate world that she patrols is ontological, imaginative, and rooted in an acutely sensitive embodied cognition: Rothfuss represents her as resonating emotionally with the objects she finds. This correlates, in terms of theories of empathy, with Hermann Lotze's 1858 conception of *Einfühlung*: "The world becomes alive to us through this power to see in forms the joy and sorrow of existence that they cannot hide: there is no shape so coy that our fancy cannot sympathetically enter into it" (qtd. in Fogle 139). Rothfuss endows Auri with heightened empathic powers and invests drama in her solitary movements by means of her *Einfühlung*. She is not lonely because the inanimate world is alive to her, but we are not accustomed to thinking of the empath as a loner (see chapter 3, above)...

Rothfuss constructs a fictional world in which *most* characters are not only *empathically inaccurate*, but obtuse: insensate to the perspectives belonging to objects and alien forces, even the adepts at sympathetic magic are clueless about their endangerment. In the larger trilogy, repression of knowledge of a malign species of predators jeopardises everybody; the main character Kvothe is an outsider, a musician, a researcher, and a storyteller who attempts to understand these predators and the threat they pose. Institutional traditions and disciplinary conventions get in the way of the trickster Kvothe's world-saving artistry. By way of contrast to this prevailing obliviousness, Rothfuss's alternative protagonist Auri, with humble skills complementing the bravura performances of Kvothe, possesses *unheimlich* empathic accuracy:

> The buckle though, it was black with bright beneath. It was a hidden thing. Might the buckle be for him? That would be a good beginning of the day. A nice thing to have settled early on, his gift all ready with his visit days away. Auri eyed the buckle sharply. Was it a proper gift for him? He *was* a tangled sort. And he was much hidden, too. Nodding, she reached out to touch the cool dark metal.
>
> But no. It didn't suit him. She should have known. He was not a one for fastening. For holding closed. Neither was he dark. Oh no. He was emberant. Incarnadine. He was bright with better bright beneath, like copper-gilded gold.
>
> (*Slow* 23)

It is also possible that descriptions of characters' disposition in space in imagined locations of prose or verse fictional storyworlds call upon readers' motor mimicry, a physiological expression of human empathy. In Rothfuss's novella, Auri navigates a vast underground structure in near darkness. She finds her way by moving through a memory map, where all the charted spaces have both names and personalities. Readers of Auri's wanderings may experience disorientation through motor mimicry; Rothfuss invites embodied responses through descriptions that emphasize sensory details:

> Then she headed down to Clinks and rinsed herself in the roiling water there. Then she washed herself, using up the slender remnant of a cake of soap that smelled of cinnas fruit and summer. After soaping and scrubbing and cleaning her hair, Auri dove into the endless black water of Clinks to rinse herself one final time. Under the surface, something brushed against her. Something slick and heavy pressed its moving weight against her leg. It did not bother her. Whatever it as, it was in its proper place and so was she. Things were just as they should be.
>
> (21)

While it is certainly true that represented emotions require real embodied audiences exercising readers' empathy to run the experiences scripted by authors in novels, it is also the case that human empathy, broadly construed, interacts with the cues of a text in co-creating far more than the human-like characters that are so often the focal point in discussions of narrative empathy. The impersonal *things* of fictional worlds—settings, clothing, spaces, places, objects, weather—involve and invite narrative empathy just as persistently as the privileged word-masses that we call characters. In literary reading, a version of *Einfühlung* may be involved in familiar phenomena: mental visualizing of spaces and movement in spaces; projection into inanimate objects and forms; indulgence in the emotional illogic of the pathetic fallacy; personification of things and landscapes, anthropomorphizing animals and natural forces, and identification with the furnishings of fictional worlds. I hazard a guess that *Einfühlung* goes a way towards explaining how the solitary exercise of our silent reading of fiction is in no way a lonely experience. Like Auri in the Underthing, we light invented worlds with the fire of our imaginations and we co-create companions out of inanimate materials. That in some cases these objects evoke our empathy and stay with us for a lifetime speaks to the animating power of aesthetic *Einfühlung*.

For a fluent reader, the mediating experience of immersion reading, or literary transportation, renders the thinginess of the novel transparent and creates an illusion of being in and sharing with the inhabitants of a fictional world. The effects of immersion and transportation are scripted by the text, and the cues in that script are written by the author, but without a co-creating reader actively imagining and indeed feeling-into the fictional world, it is inert. Novels need readers to activate them. Readers' empathy and readers' *Einfühlung* play a strong part in the creative novel-reading trance. The transactional theory of reading theory I rely on here pre-dates both reader-response criticism and reception theory, but it has become newly relevant in the twenty-first century as a consequence of neuroscientific work on attention, way-finding or spatial orientation, mental visualising, the interaction of emotion and cognition, and the system that produces what Vittorio Gallese calls a shared manifold for intersubjectivity ("Roots" 171). As Louise Rosenblatt writes, initiating the theorisation of the readers' role in the creative transaction, "a text, once it leaves its author's hands, is simply paper and ink until a reader evokes from it a literary work" (*Reader* ix). Literature comes to life in human minds, and although the words making up novels constrain the potential world-making a reader performs, novels also leave a great deal to the imagination (x). This means that the personal qualities, identities, experiences, dispositions, and tastes of individual readers contribute substantially to the novels that they read. The human capacity to attribute both Theory of Mind and emotional states to lightly sketched-in beings—often consisting of little more than a name, a characteristic, perhaps a bit of dialogue—piggybacks on our dispositional *Einfühlung*. It may be a manifestation of the way that our shared manifold for intersubjectivity scans our real and imagined surroundings, orients us in space in relation to persons and objects around our bodies, and helps us anticipate changes in our environment. This imaginative endowment, which is very difficult to stop exercising through willpower, makes it likely that narrative fictions written or scripted in the future will continue to cultivate and experiment with readers' empathy.

...

As the range of references in this essay indicates, experimentation in twenty-first-century fiction is not the sole possession of literary fiction aimed at educated readers. Some forms of experimentation can be hidden in plain sight within naturalistic novels written in a traditional manner, and they can often be discovered in genre fiction that has not always been dignified by the compliment of critical scrutiny. Anglophone fiction in the twenty-first century extends an old project of the English novel, the education of the sympathetic imagination, by employing narrative empathy strategically in a wide array of generic contexts. Cultivating the human sympathies has long been a goal associated with realistic English fiction, and although the moral sentimentalism that undergirds the purposeful use of fiction dates from the eighteenth century, it is most strongly allied with nineteenth-century realism. As George Eliot argued in a *Westminster Review* essay published in 1856, "The Natural History of German Life," novelistic art has a moral purpose, the extension of readers' sympathetic imaginations:

> The greatest benefit we owe to the artist, whether painter, poet, or novelist, is the extension of our sympathies. Appeals founded on generalizations and statistics require a sympathy ready-made, a moral sentiment already in activity; but a picture of human life such as a great artist can give, surprises even the trivial and the selfish into that attention to what is apart from themselves, which may be called the raw material of moral sentiment.
>
> (54)

Eliot implies that as participants in co-creation, readers owe artists an effort in that direction, and artists owe readers a truthful representation, so that art can act as "a mode of amplifying experience and extending our contact with our fellow man beyond the bounds of our personal lot" (54). Eliot believed these goals were best accomplished by honest representations that avoided caricature, stereotypes, and oversimplification, as well as the easy sentimentality she identified with Dickens' novels. Her judgment was an important marker in the separation (and elevation) of psychological realism and what would later be known as serious literary fiction from popular novels, sensation fiction, and what would become the 'genres' of genre fiction, or the various descendants of romance storytelling. Now that those separated streams of the great ocean of story have rejoined in the twenty-first century, critics should not be surprised to discover, widely distributed across a variety of kinds of fiction, experiments with both emotion and cognition aiming to cultivate readers' sympathetic engagement with radically different others, including the non-human beings with whom we share the planet. The novel may still be fundamentally altered by changes in its formal delivery systems and by the worlds it represents, but as long as it relies on co-creating readers to spark its illusion into realisation, we will continue to find our minds and feelings entangled in fictional worlds that entrance and startle us.

15

FROM HUMAN RIGHTS DISCOURSE AND UNIVERSALS OF COGNITION AND EMOTION

Postcolonial Fiction

In this essay, which orbits around Haitian-American writer Edwidge Danticat's work, I revisit my theory of strategic narrative empathizing with a view to considering the multiple audiences a postcolonial fiction writer such as Danticat seeks to reach and move (see above 44ff). As a practice and aim of fictional representation, narrative empathy has been a core element of postcolonial (and anti-colonial) fiction in English, capitalizing on a shared language and generic traditions (such as *bildungsroman*) to reach readers near and far (Jussawalla; Slaughter, *Human* 86–139, 270–316; Mullaney 30–46), to work on and with their feelings. The theorizing of narrative empathy can be considered an aspect of literary cognitivism's project, relying as it does on universals of cognition and emotion. Yet even as critics of the new literatures in English push back against what has been described as a "'neocolonialism' of the third world's cultural production" by postcolonial theory steeped in European sources (Jussawalla 25), their compensatory seeking of local or indigenous frames for interpretation may also rebuff cognitivism, indicting it for totalizing impulses. Recognition of writers' simultaneous or alternating outreach to multiple audiences at different removes from the representational point of origin illuminates how narrative empathy in a postcolonial text can function differently for readerships close at hand than for the world market. The literary cognitivism illustrated by a theory of narrative empathy is thus attentive to cultural contexts. Furthermore, it may point to a potential relationship between human rights discourse and literary cognitivism as an alternative to postcolonial theory and discourse.

…

From the vantage point of postcolonial theory and criticism, the Venn diagram of relationships among literary texts, empathetic techniques and effects, and the theoretical frame provided by literary cognitivism will not serve, for postcolonial

DOI: 10.4324/9781003264071-19

theory and criticism does not comfortably overlap with literary cognitivism, suspects narrative empathy, and is motivated by different aims and audiences than fiction by writers from the postcolonial Anglophone world.

A distrust on the part of many postcolonial theorists in human universals (cf Cohen 278–301)—including common human experiences, cognitive abilities enabled by human's psychobiological inheritance, and core human emotions—coexists in the contemporary literary field of practice with strategic empathizing in narratives by anti-colonial and postcolonial fiction. Some postcolonial fiction is fully in concord with postcolonial theory on the vicissitudes of fictively-elicited narrative sympathies. Yet many postcolonial poems, plays, short stories, memoirs, and novels overtly seek feeling responses and offer opportunities for readerly emotional fusion with fictional characters and their situations. That is, literary practice in a variety of genres has sought out audiences whose feelings, attitudes, and commitments it might sway by means of strategic narrative empathy. Cognitive literary study can begin to account for the functioning of narrative empathy in that narrative transaction, but the philosophical clash between postcolonial theory and criticism and cognitive literary study interferes with the application of insights from cognitivism to postcolonial literary texts. Using matters of human rights and capabilities to address the universal affordances of postcolonial letters may run afoul of postcolonial theory's distrust of the tacit neocolonialism of human rights discourse. But the shift in approach may be rewarding, for the emergent literary critical project of human rights discourse (Schaffer and Smith; Slaughter, *Human*; Bystrom) offers theoretical compatibilities with literary cognitivism, the theorizing of narrative empathy, and the rhetorical aims of much postcolonial fiction ....

This is not to suggest that human rights discourse is to be preferred to postcolonial theory simply because it conveniently embraces narrative empathy as a precursor to altruism. Human rights discourse offers just as robust a critique of real-life empathy and to a lesser degree, narrative empathy, as postcolonial theory does (Schaffer and Smith 51; Cohen 72). For instance, Schaffer and Smith write that the personal narratives they study in *Human Rights and Narrated Lives* "encourage empathetic identification, [but] that identification comes at the potential cost of reducing differences to sameness" (47). Whereas a postcolonialist might be more likely to suspect readers' empathy as an imposition of a privileged perspective on or condescension to postcolonial subjects, human rights advocates more often lament the effects of empathy fatigue, and empathy experts from the social sciences more often acknowledge barriers to empathic responding such as bias, prejudice, diffusion of responsibility and innate cruelty (DeTurk; Echols and Correll; Gernsbacher; Hollan; McFarland and Mathews). For example, evolutionary psychologist Allan Young writes that while "Mind reading, perspective-taking, hormonal responsiveness and mental time travel were likewise responsible for psychological altruism, the propensity to adjust one's desires and intentions to the perceived needs or wishes of others... Human nature [is] likewise prepared for cruel pleasures" (A. Young 32). A view that acknowledges both prosocial and antisocial impulses seems most likely to capture the push-me-pull-you representational effects that can contribute to efforts on behalf of human rights, as Lynn Hunt argues in *Inventing Human Rights* (2007), but can also impede them by indulging in cruel humor based on prejudice, as Simon Dickie has recently shown in *Cruelty and Laughter* (2011) [and Sarah Winter has thoughtfully discussed in relation to the novel]. From the outlook of postcolonial literary theory, critiques of *false* empathy dominate, whereas in the distinct approach of human rights discourse, *failed* empathy is more often described or deplored.

The resources of several disciplinary contexts assist in moving towards a workable treaty between the universalizing, generalizing aims of cognitivism and the persuasive goals of much postcolonial literature. The lens of narrative empathy focuses a review of the psychological, cognitive and affective research on attitudes towards universal human rights, cross-cultural studies of human affect, and the postcolonial critique of the limits of human universals. It reveals the usefulness of a human rights framework for apt and sensitive responding to the challenges of postcolonial novels that engage in strategic narrative empathizing to reach their various audiences. Literary cognitivism's critique of postcolonial theoretical discourse is ably analyzed by Patrick Colm Hogan ("Psychology"); I work from the opposite direction to suggest why postcolonial theory regards literary cognitivism with wariness. I juxtapose to that attitude the rhetorical aims of one postcolonial writer, Edwidge Danticat, in a preliminary case study of the appropriate place of narrative empathy in postcolonial studies. Before turning to Edwidge Danticat, I suggest how it came to be that literary cognitivists began to make inroads into a discursive field whose founding premises might seem to repel the insights of cognitivism absolutely.

Literary applications of cognitive science, affective science, and social neuroscience depend to a large degree on generalizations about how human minds and bodies work. This does not mean, as humanists sometimes suspect, that scientists seek to boil human nature down into a single data point, illustrative brain scan, or predictable behavior. Indeed, the sciences of brain and behavior more often represent ranges of response, and scales that admit high, low, or no levels of the phenomena under study. Yet humanists often judge scientists for erasing all sorts of human behavior and varieties of bodily, affective, and mental experience in the interest of discerning generalizable patterns. The concern is not limited to the humanities. Even in its own self criticism and calls for change, psychological science admits that "generalization can be insidious," as the eminent developmental psychologist Jerome Kagan puts it in an opinion piece published in *The Chronicle Review*, "Psychology's Missing Contexts." As Kagan puts it, psychology "has been woefully blind to issues of experimental context, undermining both the field's impact and its reputation" (Kagan). Of particular concern to Kagan is the overuse of male lab rats and American college students as experimental subjects in studies with fewer than 50 participants. The large numbers, diverse subjects, and long time periods favored by longitudinal medical studies set a standard that experimental psychology, let alone empirical literary study, struggles to meet. [Though the development of online participant pools for internet-based data collection in cognitive science promises to diversify participants in some psychological studies.] A postcolonial literary theorist with commitments to understanding cultural differences would be inclined to agree with Kagan's observation that "It is not at all obvious that most of the results reported in published [psychology] papers with college-age, white American participants would be the same if the same studies were done with 50-year-olds from a rural village in Ghana, the center of Beijing, a New Guinea forest, or a suburb of Quito" (Kagan). But this is not the only reason that postcolonial theory resists and distrusts the findings of psychology and cognitive science.

Postcolonial literary theorists have ardently critiqued not only the kind of hidden biases that Kagan points out, but also the very notion of human universals, including the shared set of basic emotions that apparently undergird transactions of narrative empathy. Generally speaking, postcolonial theory and criticism emerge from the world view that sees the human mind as socially constructed and regards feelings, thoughts and experiences of individuals in a given location and period as incomparable with others in different places and times. As Fredric Jameson … characterized it in a [2012] lecture at University of Helsinki, the resistance to universals is a struggle against hegemonic norms, which are thereby suppressive and exclusionary: "The Doctrine of Universal Human Rights is still a doctrine of universals" (Jameson). To the degree that postcolonial theory absorbs psychoanalytic thinking, it sees human behavior as context specific (Scheflen 269): and the relevant context from Fanon onwards includes the variable legacy of colonization, imperial dominion, resistance, and the aftermath of decolonization. Postcolonial literary studies, as distinct from the discourse of human rights and capabilities, criticizes human universals for historicist reasons. Neuroscientists and neurohumanists have taken notice: as Deborah Jensen and Marco Iacoboni observe, "Any area of human capacity celebrated as confirming what is best about the human… turns out to be involved in excluding, or dividing and conquering human populations by the measure of their circumstantial performance of this capacity cum standard" (Jensen and Iacoboni). Western political thought has occupied the default position of the universal, obscuring both its own particularity and situatedness and casting alternative understandings as provincial or barbaric. All too often have the traits of a supposedly shared humanity featured fungible binaries that leave the oppressed out of the circle of the civilized or even the human family. Literary cognitivists treating postcolonial texts run the risk of unwittingly participating in the exploitation of the colonized or condescension towards postcolonial subjects by effacing the particularity of representations of emotional experiences under what appears to postcolonialists a presumptuous and potentially damaging belief in a common human psychobiological inheritance.

Postcolonial theory's case against universalizing deserves attention, for definitions of the human and discussions of intrinsically human traits, let alone putative universals of civilization have often been used to justify exclusion, dispossession, and displacement. Even when treading carefully and evoking sensitivity to contexts and differences, few literary cognitivists can sidestep the universalizing premises of cognitivism and psychology more generally. The situation does not get simpler when we come to matters of affect and shared feeling, the physiological ground for imaginative experiences of narrative empathy. Postcolonial theorists typically regard the expression of emotions as culturally constructed and distrust assertions of biological commonalities among human beings. They rightly point out the dearth of cross-cultural comparative study in cognitive science, as in psychology overall. Cognitivism in particular has sought to theorize and verify empirically the workings of the mind by hypothesizing mental structures, internal processes, and their neurological substrates in the human species. To refer to a cognitive postcolonial literary studies implies that generalizable qualities, functions, and physiological substrates of human minds and emotions can be discerned in the writings of an extraordinarily diverse group of authors whose only experience in common may be that their forebears were at one time colonized. It may appear to expunge the differences whose elucidation and dramatization are at the heart of postcolonial literature.

The practice of cognitive postcolonial studies has centered on affect since the earliest essays of Patrick Colm Hogan, whose work on narrative universals, literary empathy, and aesthetic feelings in Sanskrit theorists and ethical emotions in the Arabic Aristotelians has established a practice of cross-cultural research for literary cognitivists. Hogan's work, exceptionally among literary cognitivists, focuses on emotion as much as cognition. Uniquely among cognitivists, Hogan draws his illustrations from world literature, ancient and contemporary, in diverse genres and languages of origin. Hogan's work is also atypical from the vantage point of postcolonial literary criticism in its pursuit of universals of form and impact. Even the very recent "turn towards the human" (as Dipesh Chakrabarty calls it) in postcolonial thinking emphasizes the local and culturally specific. Postcolonial theory and criticism rarely engages with theories of universal human traits, since universality is itself a sticking point. The emergence of a contextual cognitivism sensitive to historically contingent expressions of human experience encourages projects that could bridge the divide. Literary cognitivist work on contemporary writers of the postcolonial world deserves credit for its cross-cultural comparisons, such as that carried out by Patrick Colm Hogan, Frederick Aldama (*User's Guide*), and Shameem Black. However, as Alan Richardson warns, "this pursuit will fare badly if it becomes a matter of simplistically mapping the human universals posited by evolutionary psychology or sociobiology onto the content of fictive texts" (*Neural Sublime* 114). The handling of empathy, real and literary, illustrates the impasse. When postcolonial theorists discuss empathy, they disapprove of it: most postcolonial literary criticism distrusts narrative empathy for imposing, through perspective taking, an illusion of understanding of subaltern experience (false empathy).

While no one novel or story evokes empathy in all its readers, some texts are widely regarded as inviting empathetic responses from many readers. Several such examples can be found in *Krik? Krak!* (1996), a book of stories by the Haitian–American writer Edwidge Danticat (b. 1969). Danticat was born in Haiti and emigrated to the United States when she was 12 years old. Educated at Barnard College, where she majored in French, and Brown University, where she studied creative writing, Danticat has been publishing stories since the early 1990s. She is the author of several novels, one a hybrid novel in stories, several works of serious literary nonfiction, and a picture book for children that came out in the aftermath of the 12 January 2010 7.0 Haitian earthquake. Danticat is unusual among Haitian writers because her literary work is written in English, the language of her adoptive country, though many of her characters are represented as speakers of the French Creole of Haiti. The consciousness of multiple audiences for her work is inscribed in her stories, novels, and nonfiction.

The stories in *Krik? Krak!* explore the circumstances of Haitian individuals of a variety of ages and walks of life, and they include two stories towards the end of the volume set in the United States among immigrants from Haiti and their children. Danticat herself represents what sociologist Rubén Rumbaut has dubbed the 1.5 generation of immigrant, bringing with her knowledge and experience of her home culture in Haiti, but arriving in her new home young enough (age 12) to assimilate to its culture and complete her education here. The 1.5 generation immigrants' identity combines the cultures and traditions of both the new and old culture (Rumbaut 1166–7). Danticat self-identifies as an immigrant artist (*Create Dangerously*), but she is not confined by that label. Her work appears on the syllabi of courses in African-American literature, Caribbean fiction, postcolonial literature, memoir, and contemporary American fiction. With no one single delimiting context governing the academic discussion of Danticat, her readership is not primarily academic. Because her first novel, *Breath, Eyes, Memory* (1994) was selected for Oprah's Book Club, she has had a popular readership in the United States since the start of her career. Since that novel features three generations of Haitian women, each one traumatized in its own way, for instance by invasive virginity testing, Danticat has been criticized by Haitians for representing Haitian women in an unfavorable light—to a broad audience (*Create Dangerously* 32–3). She has not shrunk from the difficult or even dangerous representations that can evoke controversy and criticism, preferring to risk writing "dangerously, for people who read dangerously" (10). Danticat announces her vocation to write for those who take risks to read imaginative literature, perhaps far off in a posterity audience: "Somewhere, if not now, then maybe years in the future, a future that we may have yet to dream of, someone may risk his or her life to read us. Somewhere, if not now, then maybe years in the future, we may also save someone's life, because they have given us a passport, making us honorary citizens of their culture" (10).

One test for that passport that admits a writer's work into an alien culture is the work's capacity to invite narrative empathy: emotional fusion with a fictional world and its characters. Danticat uses a number of strategies and techniques that have been demonstrated to enhance the potential for empathic responses to fictional narratives. Some of these are representational choices: picking young children and vulnerable teenagers as central characters; focusing attention on the creative capacities of individuals in hopeless circumstances; telling the tales of victims of persecution or exploitation. Danticat's topics matter, and for some members of her audience, they prime empathetic responses. Yet when it comes to a world audience, relatively unfamiliar with the requirements for survival in Haiti during the Duvalier regime, for instance, the barriers of distance, lack of familiarity, and marked forms of difference (including race, ethnicity, nationality, and deficits in shared experiences) can all contribute to an unemotional, disengaged response. Aversive, disgusted reactions are rare but still possible. As a teacher I have seen Danticat's stories overcome the here-and-now and familiarity biases that reduce empathic response, so that students who are very far from the circumstances of the prostitute who narrates "Night Women," or from the teenaged refugees of "Children of the Sea," report being taken by surprise by the intensity of their shared feeling with her characters, even when they also report disapproving of the behavior of those characters. Danticat provides one avenue for narrative empathy through her use of bridge characters: literate, creative children and teenagers whose very bookishness or eloquence invites a book-reader on the other end of the narrative transaction into the story world. Yet she does not court easy sympathy through pitiable representations. Her characters are complex and often flawed. One of her most impressive accomplishments is her depiction of an escaped torturer in *The Dew Breaker* (2004). There she confronts directly the potential that the artist will improperly diagnose suffering in the subject who has actually caused others' suffering, an illustration of the grave risks of false empathy. Yet she invites not just a feeling response but humanitarian or political action: both her memoir and social criticism *Brother, I'm Dying* (2007) and her children's book *Eight Days: A Story of Haiti* (2010) position themselves as works that hope to elicit real world responses.

Efforts empirically to test the efficacy of narrative empathy's capacity to increase awareness of a group's needs and successfully solicit altruistic action on their behalf are only now in development. Narrative empathy may enhance the illusion of immersion in a fictional world by deepening the felt connection of the reader with the imaginary denizens of the narrative, without persuading that reader to take action in the real world. It is not yet known whether these two possibilities, the immersive and the other-directed responses, constitute alternatives that rarely coexist, or complementary effects that enhance narrative impact. We may hypothesize that the deeper the immersion and the stronger the empathetic connection, the greater the chance of prosocial responding. Or, we may predict the opposite—the deeper the immersion in a fictional world and the stronger the empathy for fictional characters, the weaker the connection to any real-world situation will be. Empirical verification of claims made by narratologists about narrative empathy have been investigated in collaboration with specialists in discourse processing (Maill) and psychologists who study persuasion and narrative impact (Mazzocco, Green et al.). Research into narrative empathy in cognitive science has investigated the role of emotions, including empathy, in narrative processing. Narrative empathy has also been theorized in relation to experientiality in Monika Fludernik's *Towards a 'Natural' Narratology* (1996), immersion in Marie Laure Ryan's *Narrative as Virtual Reality* (2001), and with respect to mental imaging and subsequent altruism, by cognitive scientist Dan R. Johnson (2011). Long-term effects of empathetic narratives on readers' behavior have proven more difficult to study (and to disentangle from confounding influences). An intermediary goal of changing readers' attitudes toward despised outgroups by representing them sympathetically has, however, been examined empirically; transportation, or a reader's immersion in a fictional world has been shown to enhance both empathy and subsequent prosocial behavior, at least in the short term.

Three queries about the relationship of narrative empathy and altruism persist, and trouble the effort to demonstrate a predictable link between strategic empathizing and altruistic outcomes. First, critics inquire, does every writer seek empathic responses? Clearly not. Some postcolonial writers employ strategic narrative empathy to reach distant audiences and to shift their beliefs about and behaviors toward suffering others, but not all writers pursue these persuasive goals. Some postcolonial writers work in a Brechtian tradition and prefer intellectual engagement over invitations to emotional fusion. Edwidge Danticat's strategic empathizing contrasts, for example, with Jamaica Kincaid's resolute refusal to court or cajole her readers. In novels such as *The Autobiography of My Mother* (1996) and *Mr. Potter* (2002), Kincaid rebuffs easy connections, invites disgust and dismay, pursuing antipathetic representational goals in gorgeous prose. Kincaid's work better illustrates the austerities of postcolonial literary theory, resistant to offering opportunities for ready character identification, while Danticat's work better fits a cognitivist model that (at least in its aspirations) links experiences of narrative empathy with real life altruism.

Many postcolonial writers reveal their designs on their readers' beliefs and behavior through paratextual gestures or extratextual comments. This brings me to the second query, since those announced intentions do not uniformly correlate with empathetic responses, nor with the altruistic civic behavior that is often their declared goal. A postcolonialist skeptical about narrative empathy asks whether it imposes an inaccurate and oppressive understanding of subalterns on silenced or misunderstood subjects. Unique, authentic and possibly unmatched sensations are lost. A false empathy critique would regard the sensation of shared feeling that my white affluent 19-year-old American student described in her reading of Danticat's "Night Women" as an outbreak of harmful delusion. At best such readers' empathy is an egoistic projection, calculated to make the empathizer feel virtuous for feeling with another. Even some works of *testimonio* (generally regarded as the gold standard for authenticity) are charged with evidencing a shaping hand that falsifies empathy. Postcolonial theory and criticism suspects narrative empathy of exhibiting at best patronizing "drive-by feeling" rather than genuine concern evoked by feeling with another. Distrust of emotion labels and universals of human nature undermines the possibility that writers' and readers' testimony could verify the emotional fusion of narrative empathy. False empathy critics are unpersuaded by neuroscience, by empirical study of human emotions, by laboratory demonstrations that empathy jiggers prosocial responses, or indeed by any description of human experience that could be recognized across barriers of language and culture. As for narrative empathy's potential to induce real-world altruism, an article of faith in today's varieties of moral sentimentalism, false empathy critics are aghast that anyone would fall prey to such a delusion. These views of do-gooding were the drivers of the civilizing missions that have done so much damage in the past.

The failed empathy critic offers the third challenging query. Does not a bid to evoke readers' empathy often fail or miss its mark? For example, Schaffer and Smith write, "Channeled through the interests of global capital, some sites [of storytelling] augment the coffers of advertisers; some make witnesses into spectacles of suffering; some address their audiences through emotive confrontation, setting in motion affective appeals that have a 'feel good' effect for their far-flung advocates, but may not further recognition, ethical judgment, or redress" (*Human Rights* 51). This criticism holds that narrative empathy transcending boundaries of difference *could* occur and regards prosocial outcomes favorably. It worries that narrative empathy does not work. The failed empathy critic requires evidence that my students' sensations of empathy with Danticat's Haitian refugee teenagers actually accomplished anything substantive in the world. Did my students' attitudes toward border patrols change? Did they take action by volunteering, donating, participating in advocacy, or traveling to Haiti on a human rights mission themselves? Or did they feel fleeting emotional fusion with a fictional character, shake that feeling off, and move on? The failed empathy critique typifies a human rights and capabilities orientation, discussing forthrightly varieties of empathy failure in the form of compassion fatigue, the marketing of disasters, and the ethical dilemmas of artists working with victims of human rights abuses. Possibly carers are especially vulnerable to these effects. McFarland's research into the impact of personality on support for universal human rights shows that dispositional empathy (as assessed on an empathy scale such as Mark Davis's Interpersonal Reactivity Index) correlates with supportive *attitudes* towards human rights. [The psychological study of the personality types that contribute to support for universal human rights tends to emphasize dispositional empathy of subjects and those who are prone to identify not just with family or nation but also with all humanity (McFarland 1735).] But attitudes by themselves are not actions. McFarland goes on to suggest that a subject's "identification with all humanity," a globalized form of role- and perspective-taking, correlates with active commitment to human rights. The interference that occurs between the disposition to care and the inclination to act is a matter of failed empathy.

The gravest concern for those who study commitment to human rights worldwide is the most dramatic form of "failed empathy," where fellow-feeling is displaced by disgust and disdain. This response been shown to correlate with beliefs in social dominance, authoritarianism, and nationalism. When empathy fails and disgust replaces it, Lasana Harris and Susan Fiske have shown, dehumanized perception that can facilitate perpetration of atrocities and human rights abuses becomes more likely. Though narrative ethics avoids dwelling on this possibility, preferring to focus on the cultivation of virtue rather than the attractions of vice, dehumanizing representational strategies can push readers and audiences towards disgust and even towards genocide. While false empathy critics distrust the empathy of shared humanity as a basis for concern or justice, failed empathy critics see empathy as a helpful though not always essential element of concern and commitment to improved lives around the world. This suggests that the strategic narrative empathy exercised by postcolonial writers of fiction and other literary forms may contribute to the advancement of a human rights agenda that has been subjected to critique by postcolonial literary theory. For despite empathy's theoretical disrepute among false empathy critics, postcolonial novelists and writers in literary genres have assiduously cultivated empathetic responses by employing rhetorical techniques of strategic empathizing.

The elaboration of these techniques calls upon rhetorical narrative poetics' capacity to explore the modes and dynamics of narrative situation without oversimplifying their effects. It helps to bridge the chasm between the cognitive and the postcolonial. Theorizing narrative empathy elaborates the uses to which real authors and narrative artists put their human empathy to work in imaginative character-creation and in other aspects of worldmaking, as well as accounting for varied readers' responses (Keen, "Theory"). Rhetorical narratology takes an interest in effects on readers, especially with regards to persuasion. While no narrative text consistently inspires empathy in all its readers, who vary in dispositional empathy (Keen, *Empathy* 89) and in their official and unofficial positions with respect to the text (as Goffman would have it), study of the responses of readers belonging to different audiences reveals narrative empathy in action. … (see above 44ff). Narrative empathy and the neuroscientific research into our human shared manifold for intersubjectivity deserve a place in cognitive postcolonial literary studies because many postcolonial texts cultivate empathetic responsiveness through an array of representational tactics that I have described under the terms bounded, ambassadorial, and broadcast strategic narrative empathy.

A subset of narrative empathy, *readers' empathy* leads to differentiation of readers in terms of belonging to in-groups and out-groups addressed directly by authors hoping to evoke empathy…. ("Strategic Empathizing" 478–80; see above 42, 48, and 44)….

This theory assumes that narrative fictions have multiple potential readerships, often discernible within a single text (as Brian Richardson has argued), and that different rhetorical strategies in the texts reveal this. For instance, Edwidge

Danticat's children's book *Eight Days*, narrated in first person by a boy buried in rubble, bears the dedication, "For the children of Haiti." This can and does mean children *in* Haiti, though they are more likely to speak Haitian creole and French than the text's English. The beautiful illustrations transcend language barriers and are dedicated "to all living in Haiti," not just children. The text becomes a gift *to* Haitians. Supporting that charitable direction, the publisher, Scholastic Inc., reports that it "has donated $10,000 in connection with the publication of this book to a charity that provides humanitarian aid to people all over the world in their times of need." This expands the audience to include the purchasers, and places the text's humanitarian errand within a world context: *not just* for Haitians. The first person narration, which begins with the rescue and explains what the buried boy dreams about for eight days, only addresses the narratee, *you*, a single time, in the last sentence of the story: "I tell you, I hugged them so tight I thought I would never let go." This "you" of the narratee seems equally to embrace an adult and a child audience, with different but simultaneously available emotional valences of reassurance and relief. Danticat's special concern for children shows not just in the form of the picture book, but also in the framing paratexts. A note from the author mentions the large number of children in Haiti ("Nearly half of Haiti's population is under fifteen") but redirects attention to the children of diaspora, English-speaking kids like her own who feared for relatives in Port-au-Prince. In just 14 pages of text, this austere brief narrative embeds awareness of at least five distinct audiences, and we may add the literary audience of Danticat's readers to that count. She certainly also communicates with us about her intentions and values, as underscored by her comments on being an immigrant artist in *Create Dangerously*. Danticat's *Eight Days* shows signs of all three forms of emotional invitation to engage, employing bounded, ambassadorial, and broadcast strategic empathy, with more open gestures of inclusion and embassy balancing the unusual features of the narrator's experience. This goes beyond character identification, though Danticat emphasizes the commonalities of children's embodied experiences, dispositions, and circumstances. Especially in cases where fictional appeals for sympathy dovetail with real-world campaigns for assistance, such as the response to the 2010 earthquake in Haiti, the ethics and efficacy of narrative empathy demand attention. Danticat's work fits a literary cognitivist model that (at least in its aspirations) supports narrative ethics by linking experiences of narrative empathy with real life altruism.

The disdain of many postcolonial literary theorists for any putative human universal, including empathy, is vigorously contradicted in practice by the novelists, especially those hoping to reach a readership in the large Anglophone world fiction market. An approach less inimical to the universals of human feeling implied by the Universal Declaration of Human Rights (1948) is human rights discourse, which provides an alternative theoretical frame for considering the impact of imaginative literature and the potential role of empathic responses to literary texts. Yet we should still take care in applying the empathy-altruism hypothesis to experiences of narrative empathy and the formation of good world citizens. It is difficult to disentangle *novel reading* from a host of other formative experiences that might encourage altruism or the lighter standard of prosocial behavior in individuals or whole societies.

Humanists routinely confound the impact of imaginative literature on people with the impact of people on other people. But questioning the causal link between altruism and narrative empathy—such as intense character identification, though there are other forms—devalues neither narrative empathy nor the widespread hope in the socially beneficial yield of novel-reading. It shifts the emphasis to what people choose to do with their reading experiences, how they share them, and how they encourage themselves and others to act on feeling responses. Many writers and readers, including writers such as Edwidge Danticat, believe that there ought to be a connection....

CONCLUSION

While I have been working on this collection of my previously published essays on empathy and reading, several other projects were in the works. Because they are forthcoming at the time of this writing, I describe them here to indicate the direction that my scholarship has taken, following propositions about narrative empathy, readers, and immersion reading that have interested me since the publication of *Empathy and the Novel*. These pieces concern diverse topics: the responses of far distant readers (ancient audiences of the Gospel narratives); the possibilities of stirring young readers to feel *Einfühlung* for the planet by teaching climate fiction; and the complicated set of meanings that the term "empathy" evokes, when used by scholars in the field. A fourth project also concerns *Einfühlung,* the version of empathy for inanimate objects that was theorized at the turn of the last century, in this case probed in response to an art work, artist Sarah Oppenheimer's *Sensitive Machine* (The Ruth and Elmer Wellin Museum of Art, Hamilton College, 2021). The following short account, comprised of abstracts of forthcoming work, suggests the interdisciplinary reach of topics that have grown out of my prior inquiries. As was the case from the very beginning, however, scholars in diverse fields have taken my questions much further than I could ever have done on my own. This conclusion recognizes that situation by refreshing some hypotheses about empathy that deserve further attention, and, by adding new propositions, suggests research areas that others will be in a better position to investigate than I am.

Previous inexperience in a field hasn't prevented me from venturing into unfamiliar areas, when invited! One such endeavor is my forthcoming essay, "Ancient characters and contemporary readers," a solicited response to new work on cognitive-narratological approaches to characters and characterization in New

DOI: 10.4324/9781003264071-20

Testament narratives, a project that includes analysis of represented emotions and the possibility of readers' empathy with the characters of Gospel narratives (Jan Rüggemeier and Elizabeth E. Shively, eds.). I took the opportunity in this essay to bring a narrative theorist's perspective on fictional and nonfictional contexts for character construction and characterization to an emerging conversation in cognitive Religious Studies. This essay gave me a chance to extend my thinking on the way diverse actual readers engage with characters, and to expand on my ideas about different audiences' relations to enduring texts, in this case the New Testament Gospels. I treat the Gospels as Greco-Roman lifewriting, a nonfictional genre, though one that contains fictional insets, especially in the form of exempla and parables. Because narrative empathy is explicitly part of Rüggemeier and Shively's project, I respond to the potential for both empathy and sympathy as aspects of emotional reading, applying my theory of strategic narrative empathy to the Parable of the Good Samaritan.

Lacking the ancient language training of a proper New Testament scholar, I forbore true close reading, focusing instead on what we can theorize about authorial and narrative audiences (in Peter Rabinowitz's terms) in both the ancient audiences contemporary with the text's first transmission and in audiences today. It will not be a surprise to those who have dipped into the contents of this volume that I emphasize what real readers and auditors bring to the active work of co-creation, acknowledging their differences. I also explore how their perceptions of a text's fictionality or historicity alters readers' responses, empathetic or not, to the emotional cues embedded in the Parable. Regardless of one's faith tradition or attitude towards the truth claims of the Gospels, one can see that the narrator of the Parable of the Good Samaritan, Jesus himself (performing as a secondary narrator of an inset tale) employs the story to try to teach a lesson about being a good neighbor. We are prone, he implies, to imagine that members of despised outgroups aren't likely to be good neighbors, and surprised when they outperform members of our own tribe in neighborliness.

Grappling with the imminent challenge of the climate crisis will require that we imagine distant inhabitants of our planet as neighbors. Cultivating empathy with other living beings, including faraway people, nonhuman creatures, and threatened species, has already become a project of climate fiction, sometimes called cli-fi, a term indicating its relationship to dystopian science fiction. Teachers and environmental activists worry that the grim, sometimes nihilistic narrative arcs of dystopian fiction can work against the goal of engaging younger readers in work that requires hope and determination. The potential of authors' strategic narrative empathy for imagined others representing current or imminent victims of changed weather patterns, increased storm severity, rising sea levels, and cataclysmic environmental change could be harnessed to the task. Readers' emotional responses to the plight of the planet itself also involve a kind of empathy. As Marco Caracciolo argues, "today's climate crisis calls for an expansion of our affective engagement with the nonhuman," including experiences of the "ecological sublime" rooted in human "kinesthetic resonance linking human subjects to nonhuman realities" (299). Caracciolo cautions that this kind of sublime response should "highlight our moral responsibilities vis-à-vis the natural world" (299). Climate fiction for young readers can be an instrument for stimulating that thoughtful complication and challenge. Ambassadorial strategic narrative empathy intends to stimulate shared feelings with distant others; arguably, climate fiction often employs the rhetoric of broadcast strategic empathy to bring all living creatures into the reach of its ethical and political appeal.

In an afterword to the forthcoming collection, *Literature for Change: How Educators can Prepare the Next Generation for a Climate-Challenged World*, edited by Rebecca Young, I consider the extension of the empathetic circle for faraway victims of the climate crisis, observing that "[T]he automatic fellow-feeling that undergirds empathic responses with recognition of their feelings and perspectives gets harder the further apart we are. Empathy infamously weakens with distance, dissimilarity, and unfamiliarity." This challenges our recognition of other humans as neighbors. I acknowledge that empathetic responses to fiction reading can change attitudes, but contend that converting those feelings of awareness into real alterations of settled behaviors requires more than just reading. Happily, the volume in which this afterword will appear is full of essays recommending pedagogical strategies that hold out the promise of boosting the results of empathetic reading experiences. The effort matters because it is especially difficult to rouse individuals to action in the face of enormous challenges such as the climate crisis. I offer the opinion that

> [a] major obstacle to altruistic action, prosocial intervention, and helping responses (even among those who have been awakened to the dangers of a warming planet, pollution, species loss, and so forth), lies in the psychological phenomenon known as "diffusion of responsibility." In a large crowd with many witnesses, for example, many will hang back from helping a victim under the belief that somebody else must be taking care of it. Environmental concerns suffer greatly from diffusion of responsibility. Reflective discussion and writing can address the understandable, aversive responses that push responsibility away from the self towards distant authorities, multinational corporations, or governments.
>
> ("Afterword" 241-42)

Striving to sustain longer-term reactions to empathic distress motivates those who would cultivate readers' sympathetic imagination and link their responses to action in the real world.

Can or should those imaginative experiences extend to *Einfühlung* with the inanimate world itself? Building on the foundational work on *Einfühlung* that preceded the modern science of empathy, I regard the potential of empathic "feeling-into" as encompassing the environment as a target, not only in the way that Vernon Lee described when she wrote of the empathic roots of figures of speech such as a mountain's rising. It is possible that an experience of immersive reading (or virtual reality viewing) that evokes empathy for non-human creatures and the physical homes of their ecosystems could reinforce the urgency of action. Indeed, an imaginative, even escapist experience of immersion in a fictional world could have an impact more powerful and lasting than the scientific tables, graphs, and surrounding exhortations so often employed to this end. Imaginative writing can invite the reader into the fictive perspective of a polluted body of water, an eroding cliffside, a disappearing beach, to feel with something that has no feelings. Could aesthetic empathy go so far as to stimulate the empowered participation that will be necessary to provoke real change?

Some scholars of empathy would reject the ideas in the preceding paragraph because they rely on an old-fashioned idea about empathy/*Einfühlung* as aesthetic projection (associated with Lipps and Titchener) that, in C. Daniel Batson's words, "is rarely what is meant by empathy in contemporary psychology" ("These Things" 6). Yet human responses to and interactions with the inanimate world, built and natural, and with mechanical extensions of our own bodies certainly involve *Einfühlung*, a "feeling into" sensation. In a forthcoming essay about the artist Sarah Oppenheimer's exhibit of four large interactive mechanical instruments in the Ruth and Elmer Wellin Museum's Fall 2021 exhibition, *Sensitive Machine*, I apply an understanding of empathy that includes *Einfühlung* that leads to participation. From the late nineteenth-century, the earliest theorists of psychological aesthetics understood that *Einfühlung* was involved in the human habit of anthropomorphizing inanimate objects, and long before cognitive linguists linked embodied experience with metaphor, Vernon Lee grasped that *Einfühlung* was deeply involved in our figures of speech. We bequeath imagined sensations, reactions, and even agency to objects, buildings, landscapes, and natural features. Sarah Oppenheimer's art explores the way prosthetics change the boundaries of our bodies and demand new forms of cooperation: a lengthened limb becomes part of me, but I discover that I need your help to reach an object that used to be close to me!

Studying the four instruments in the exhibit *Sensitive Machine* as I and other visitors interacted with them has evoked my empathy, responding to their scale, their stately presence, their movability and the reactive motions of lights and other instruments. I speculate that our shared manifold for intersubjectivity, the substrate of neurons that comprises the mirror-matching system (Gallese), cannot help but activate in response to the instruments, which the artist thinks of as figural. When not in motion, the four objects present as massive, solid, black and white forms, spaced apart from one another in a pristine white rectangular space. That austere impression evaporates as soon as human beings begin touching and pushing the forms. Invited to join in and move the horizontal elements of the instruments, people activate not only the works' potential motions but also playful communication, interaction, and quizzical observations of cooperative and bystanding others. *Sensitive Machine* creates nonce communities as art objects bloom into an artistic experience that hitches a ride on museum visitors' *Einfühlung*. Aesthetic empathy invites joining-in, participation, and even cooperation.

Though I maintain that narrative empathy, especially the sort mediated by reading fiction, has an intrinsic relation to *Einfühlung*, I grant that in common parlance empathy usually implies a state of emotional relation or communication between people. Difficulties of vocabulary do not end there. Even if we confine ourselves to human empathy, cognitive scientists, psychologists, neuroscientists, philosophers, emotion scientists, and those who study affect direct their attention to a disparate set of phenomena, behaviors, and their potentially related physiological substrates under the single label of empathy. I have recommended that any work on empathy make plain at the outset which definition pertains to the theorizing, empirical study, or interpretation that follows. This seems especially important when we are arguing with or taking issue with another scholar's findings or interpretations. For very often we work at cross purposes because we are not studying the same thing at all. To tackle this vocabulary problem, ideally to arrive at an agreed-upon set of specific definitions employed across all the arenas where empathy research takes place, a group of distinguished empathy scholars, led by psychologists Mark Davis and Sara Konrath have been convened. I'm honored to be a part of that conversation, especially considering that the kind of empathy I study is sometimes omitted altogether. For although narrative empathy is related not just to *Einfühlung* and aesthetic projection, but also to the rhetoric of persuasion, to mental visualizing, and to the experience of transportation out of this world into a fictional one, its relation to real-world empathy is slippery, challenging to validate, and subject to skeptical critique.

Yet narrative empathy research now burgeons in an extraordinary array of places and disciplines. In addition to empathy studies in cognitive narratology, psychology, neuroscience, philosophy, and empirical literary studies, I read with appreciation and sometimes with astonishment research drawing on narrative empathy in computer-supported information systems studies, relational international relations, ecology, diplomacy, leadership theory, environmental studies, eco-theology, peace studies, pedagogical theory, computational modeling, medical humanities, human rights studies, refugee studies, human-robot interactions, discourse analysis, music theory, art education, and occupational therapy, among others. This is a humbling state of affairs, for it is literally beyond me to keep up with, let alone master and respond to, work in such diverse fields. What these works have in common, other than an interest in narrative empathy, shines through in the authors' commitment to understanding *how* interactions work, or explaining what thwarts sympathetic communication. I have in common with other scholars in the field a desire to understand how it works, in the emotional and imaginative lives of people, between and among people when they resonate emotionally and cognitively with one another. Because many of us dream of the potential impact of increased empathy, I am also interested in the barriers to empathic understanding, and in propositions about how reading literature might lift those barriers, even if only temporarily. The impact of our fiction reading on our beliefs, feelings, and actions remains a perennial interest, especially if it could heal some of our divisions. Like other empathy skeptics, I am wary of over-promising the benefits of empathy, especially the sort that arises from encounters with unreal beings in imaginary worlds.

When I began working on the subject of narrative empathy in the early 2000s, I was fortunately situated in a great small liberal arts college with terrific library resources and generous colleagues. I was in a strong position as a mid-career scholar, with teaching that enabled me to develop deepening interests in the novel, narrative theory, and the writing of authors from the postcolonial Anglophone world. Yet the work that I have spent most of the subsequent years of my career developing, probing, and revising came from a personal place. Aspects of my identity and circumstances certainly influenced my work, especially my lifelong habit of immersive novel reading, my desire to share that experience with my students (which made me want to understand the impact of reading better), and my dismay at the nationalistic fervor that followed the 9/11 attacks.

I had begun working on empathy and the novel by the time terrorists flew their planes into the twin towers of the World Trade Center, the Pentagon, and, with the sacrificial help of the passengers, into a Pennsylvania field, murdering nearly 3000 civilians. Informed by my reading of postcolonial literature, I braced for the inevitable xenophobia and Islamophobia, likely to be evoked by the taking of so many lives. The grief was real: a childhood friend lost her older sister, and a young alum of my university died with his coworkers at Cantor Fitzgerald. The smoking earth itself seemed injured, as rescue workers picked through toxic debris. A pacifist, I worried about the war-mongering response of my nation. And I warned my students on September 13 that their civil liberties would be in jeopardy for a time, maybe for the rest of their lives. Later, I recognized that many of their educational and career choices had been altered by 9/11, as they learned languages, built skills through community-based learning, and chose lives of service. At the time I fretted about the world that they would enter when they graduated.

In 2001 I was the mother of a four and a half year old; my mind turned to the mothers of the terrorists, and contemplating what they might know or feel, I felt all over again the limitations of empathy, the ethical conundrums of what we *think* we share with other human beings, and the strong temptation, particularly when injured, to retreat to a tribal hostility to alien others. I wrote a poem about my complicated feelings:

I cut up apples

12 September 2001

the wormy ones
because they make the best pie.
I cut up apples

and a woman a world away
dips her hand in the flour and presses
the heel of her hand in the dough.

I cut up apples, imperfect,
but firm-fleshed under spotty skins.
She works from the center of the dough

to the edges. She admires her son.
She has not heard from her son.
She may no longer recognize her son.

The televisions chatter
like shocked neighbors repeating
the worst, they chatter.

She sees the same pictures
that I see. She dips her hand in the flour.
The television converts ash into flour.

The apple slips and turns.
Peel covers the nicked old two-inch blade.
I build up walls of paste, not very high.

What to tell my son,
who is not yet five?
I cannot imagine her feelings.

I cut up apples. Towards thousands
of households the mourners converge.
The women carry covered dishes.

Unwelcome knowledge makes itself
at home. It settles in. I
cut up apples. She dips her hand in the flour.
I cut up apples.

(*Milk Glass Mermaid* 53–4)

In conversation with my students, I mulled over what we thought that literary training and novel reading could do for us. Could it really help us understand the perspectives of alien others, including those who wished us harm? What would it mean to share feelings, even fleetingly, with emotions that we often seek to avoid: anger, outrage, a desire for vengeance? If we empathized instead with feelings of pain, sorrow, and grief, would that inevitably redirect our imaginative extension back to ourselves, reinforcing our sense of difference? Was empathy for distant others just a fantasy projection, mediated by the fiction we read? Stirred by a desire for authentic expression, many of my students and colleagues reached for lyric poetry instead. Escapist fiction reading, never held in particularly high esteem in the academy, seemed especially suspect, even as the lofty goals being loaded onto humanistic education piled ever higher. At the time, I found deep immersion in fictional worlds especially difficult, as what felt like an unfinished horror movie played out on the television every night. The real world demanded my attention. Like many teachers, I wondered how I could express my vocational commitments in a way that would help my students navigate a changed world.

Though I had begun my research into empathy already, the mood of the months after 9/11 made me more certain that I should undertake a project that would require several years of study before I could even start writing. Why not do something that felt a bit risky? I wanted to try to answer questions that felt clumsily outside the reach of both the theoretical and the literary analytical traditions in which I had always worked. I was not primarily motivated by a desire to celebrate the virtues of reading. Though I was convinced of the value of empathetic understanding, I had questions about the degree to which novel-reading could deliver on the promises that were being made about it. The steady drumbeat of bad news from the National Endowment for the Arts, starting in 2004 with *Reading at Risk*, emphasized the damage to our civic life of the diminishing number of readers, as tallied by the US Census. Losing readers did seem to me a real concern, but I wasn't so sure that recovering them would reverse the course of political division, susceptibility to fake news, and suspicion of one another that already characterized our times. Primarily, I wanted to understand what was actually happening when narrative fiction evoked empathy, especially for distant others. I could neither have anticipated how many more questions than answers I would find in the course of investigating empathy, nor what an extraordinary group of colleagues around the world I would join in our shared quest to understand empathy. You know who you are. The interdisciplinary conversations that I was privileged to enter taught me so much more about what we don't yet know than settling questions with certain answers. *Empathy and the Novel* ended up being a book full of questions, some of which I am still pursuing (see above 6–7). Rather than punctuating this conclusion with a full stop, then, I part company with my readers with a refreshed set of hypotheses about aesthetic empathy, derived from some of the work collected in this volume and from the forthcoming work described above:

New and Updated Proposals about Narrative Empathy

- Without readers, fictional texts are emotionally inert; readers activate the emotional potentiality of fictional worlds (co-creation);

- Readers' multiple competing axes of identity, differing temperaments, distinct cultural contexts, and individual experiences shape their co-creation of narratives;
- Authors and texts may attempt to script but do not control the emotional experience of high- or low-empathy readers (disposition-driven variation);
- A contemporary audience may be necessary to evoke narrative empathy requiring situational familiarity or a shared temporal identity (bounded strategic empathy);
- A posterity audience may respond with more skepticism or coolness than the earliest readership of a work;
- A work appealing to universal themes may sustain empathic appeal for centuries (broadcast strategic empathy);
- Empathy roused for one individual or group can lead to unjust reactions, antipathy, or even dehumanization of their antagonists or competitors (Prinz), a phenomenon that could have bearing on literary interpretations or lesson learned from fiction reading;
- Narrative empathy is not limited to feelings mirroring the represented emotions of fictional characters, extending to sensations associated with settings and to the in-built affects: curiosity, surprise, and suspense (narrativity);
- Empathic inaccuracy can arise from the gap-filling imagining of all literary reading (co-creation);
- Interpretive distinctiveness may originate with empathic inaccuracy that prompts atypical reactions to reading;
- Paratextual cues labeling a nonfiction work as lifewriting may prime readers to experience empathy akin to readers' empathy for fiction;
- *Amae*, a feeling of belonging, may facilitate empathic responses in immersion reading (Gabriel and Young);
- Narrative immersion or transportation while reading a fictional work may improve empathic responses and prosocial behavior (Dan Johnson);
- *Einfühlung* may be involved in mental visualizing of spaces and movement through settings; aesthetic projection into inanimate objects and forms; the pathetic fallacy; personification; anthropomorphizing; and identification with the furnishings of fictional worlds.

WORKS CITED

AAC&U. Association of American Colleges & Universities. "Essential learning outcomes." *The LEAP Challenge*. www.aacu.org/leap/essential-learning-outcomes. 11 Apr. 2016.

Ablow, Rachel. Ed. *The Feeling of Reading: Affective Experience and Victorian Literature*. Ann Arbor: U of Michigan P, 2010.

Achebe, Chinua. *Things Fall Apart*. London: William Heinemann, 1958.

Adamson, Sylvia. "The Rise and Fall of Empathetic Narrative: A Historical Perspective on Perspective." *New Perspectives on Narrative Perspective* Ed. Willie van Peer and Seymour Chatman. Albany, NY: SUNY P, 2001. 83–99.

Adisa, Opal Palmer. *It Begins with Tears*, Oxford and Portsmouth, NH: Heinemann, 1997.

"Affects evolved as the system of motivation for human beings." *The Tomkins Institute*, http://www.tomkins.org/what-tomkins-said/introduction/affects-evolved-so-we-could-learn-what-to-seek-and-what-to-avoid/. 16 Jan. 2018.

Ahmed, Sara. *The Cultural Politics of Emotion*. New York: Routledge, 2004.

——. "Affect/Emotion: Orientation Matters. A Conversation between Sigrid Schmitz and Sara Ahmed." *Freiburger Zeitschrift für Geschlechter Studien* 20 (2014): 97–108.

Ainslie, George and John Monterosso. "Hyperbolic Discounting Lets Empathy be a Motivated Process." *Behavioral and Brain Sciences* 25 (Feb. 2002): 20–21.

Alber, Jan. *Unnatural Narrative: Impossible Worlds in Fiction and Drama*. Lincoln: U Nebraska P, 2016.

Alber, Jan and Monika Fludernik. "Introduction." *Postclassical Narratology: Approaches and Analyses*. Columbus: The Ohio State UP, 2010. 1–31.

Aldama, Frederick Luis. *A User's Guide to Postcolonial and Latino Borderland Fiction*. Austin: U of Texas P, 2009.

Aldama, Frederick, and Herbert Lindenberger. *Aesthetics of Discomfort: Conversations on Disquieting Art*. Ann Arbor: U Michigan P, 2016.

Altmann, Ulrike, et al. "Fact versus Fiction—How Paratextual Information Shapes Our Reading Process." *Social Cognitive and Affective Neuroscience* 9. 1 (2014): 22–29.

American Library Association, "Public Library Use." www.ala.org/tools/libfactsheets/alalibraryfactsheet06. 14 Aug. 2021.

Anand, Mulk Raj. *Untouchable*. 1935. Rpt. Harmondsworth: Penguin, 1986.

Anderson, K. and C. Evans. "The Development of the Canonical Story Grammar Model and its Use in the Analysis of Beginning Reading Computer Stories." *Reading Improvement* 33 (1996): 2–15.

Anderst, Leah. "Feeling with Real Others: Narrative Empathy in the Autobiographies of Doris Lessing and Alison Bechdel." *Narrative* 23. 3 (2015): 271–90.

Andringa, Els. "Effects of 'Narrative Distance' on Readers' Emotional Involvement and Response." *Poetics* 23 (1996): 431–52.

———. "The Interface between Fiction and Life: Patterns of Identification in Reading Autobiographies" *Poetics Today* 25. 2 (2004): 205–40.

Andringa, Els, et al. "Point of View and Viewer Empathy in Film." *New Perspectives on Narrative Perspective*. Ed. Willie van Peer and Seymour Chatman. Albany, NY: SUNY, 2001. 133–57.

Appel, Markus and Barbara Malečkar. "The Influence of Paratext on Narrative Persuasion: Fact, Fiction, or Fake?" *Human Communication Research* 38. 4 (2012): 459–84.

Aristotle. *Aristotle's Poetics*. Trans. George Whalley. Ed. John Baxter and Patrick Atherton. Montreal and London: McGill-Queen's UP, 1997.

Armstrong, Paul B. *Play and the Politics of Reading: The Social Uses of Modernist Form*. Ithaca and London: Cornell UP, 2005.

Atwood, Margaret. *Oryx and Crake*. Toronto: McClelland and Stewart, 2003.

Auerbach, Erich. *Mimesis: The Representation of Reality in Western Literature*. Trans. Willard Trask. Princeton: Princeton UP, 1953.

Austen, Jane. *Mansfield Park*. 1814. Rpt. NY: Vintage Classics, 2007.

Avenanti, Alessio, et al. "Racial Bias Reduces Empathic Sensorimotor Resonance with Other-Race Pain." *Current Biology* 20 (2010): 1018–22.

Babb, Genie. "Where the Bodies are Buried: Cartesian Dispositions in Narrative Theories of Character." *Narrative* 10. 2 (Oct. 2002): 195–221.

Bailey, Merridee L. and Kimberley-Joy Knight. Eds. "Emotions in Legal History." *Journal of Legal History* 38. 2 (2017): 117–19.

Bain, Alexander. *The Emotions and the Will*. London: J. W. Parker and Son, 1859.

Bandura, Albert. *Social Foundations of Thought and Action: a Social Cognitive Theory*. Englewood Cliffs, NJ: Prentice-Hall, 1986.

Baron-Cohen, Simon. *The Essential Difference: The Truth about the Male and Female Brains*. New York: Basic Books, 2003.

Barrett, Louise. *Beyond the Brain: How Body and Environment Shape Animal and Human Minds*, Princeton: Princeton UP, 2011.

Barthes, Roland. *The Pleasure of the Text*. Trans. Richard Miller. New York: Hill and Wang, 1975.

Barthes, Roland. *S/Z: An Essay*. 1970. Trans. Richard Miller. New York: Farrar, Straus &Giroux, 1974.

Batson, C. Daniel. "Altruism and Prosocial Behavior." *The Handbook of Social Psychology*. Ed. D. T. Gilbert, S. T. Fiske, and G. Lindzey. V. 2. New York: McGraw-Hill, 1998. 282–316.

———. *The Altruism Question: Toward a Social-Psychological Answer*. Hillsdale, NJ: Erlbaum, 1991.

———. "These Things Called Empathy: Eight Related but Distinct Phenomena." *The Social Neuroscience of Empathy*. Ed. Jean Decety and William Ickes. Rpt. Cambridge: MIT P, 2011. 3–15.

Batson, C. Daniel, et al. "Benefits and Liabilities of Empathy-induced Altruism." *The Social Psychology of Good and Evil*. Ed. Arthur G. Miller. New York: Guilford P, 2004. 359–85.

Bechdel, Alison. *Fun Home: A Family Tragicomic*. New York: HarperCollins, 2006.

Berlant, Lauren. "Introduction: Compassion and Withholding." *Compassion: The Culture and Politics of an Emotion*. Ed. Lauren Berlant. London: Routledge, 2004. 1–14.

Berlyne, D. E. *Aesthetics and Psychobiology*. New York: Appleton-Century-Crofts, 1971.

Bettelheim, Bruno. *The Uses of Enchantment: the Meaning and Importance of Fairy Tales*. New York: Knopf, 1976.

Black, Shameem. *Fiction Across Borders: Imagining the Lives of Others in Late Twentieth-Century Novels*. New York: Columbia UP, 2010.

Blackford, Holly Virginia. *Out of This World: Why Literature Matters to Girls*. New York: Teachers College P, 2004.

Blakeslee, Sandra. "Cells that Read Minds." *The New York Times* (10 Jan. 2006): F1, F4.

Blankenship, Lisa. *Changing the Subject: A Theory of Rhetorical Empathy*. Logan, UT: Utah State UP, 2019.

Bleich, David. *The Double Perspective: Language, Literacy, and Social Relations*. New York: Oxford UP, 1988.

———. "Emotional Origins of Literary Meaning." *College English* 31. 1 (Oct. 1969): 30–40.

———. *Readings and Feelings: an Introduction to Subjective Criticism*. Urbana: National Council of Teachers of English, 1975.

Bloom, Harold. *A Map of Misreading*. Oxford UP, Oxford and New York, 1975.

Bloom, Paul. *Against Empathy: The Case for Rational Compassion*. New York: Ecco P, 2016.

Blum, Lawrence A. *Friendship, Altruism and Morality*. London and New York: Routledge and Kegan Paul, 1980.

Booth, Wayne C. *The Company We Keep: An Ethics of Fiction*. Berkeley: U California P, 1988.

———. "Foreword." *Literature as Exploration*, 5th ed. Louise Rosenblatt. New York: Modern Language Association of America, 1995. vii–xv.

———. *The Rhetoric of Fiction*, 2nd ed. Chicago: U Chicago P, 1983.

Bortolussi, Marisa and Peter Dixon. *Psychonarratology: Foundations for the Empirical Study of Literary Response*. Cambridge and New York: Cambridge UP, 2003.

Boucher, Abigail. Personal correspondence, 31 January 2016.

Bourg, Tammy. "The Role of Emotion, Empathy, and Text Structure in Children's and Adults' Narrative Text Comprehension." *Empirical Approaches to Literature and Aesthetics*. Ed. Roger J. Kreuz and Mary Sue MacNealy. Norwood, NJ: Ablex, 1996. 241–60.

Bowker Market Research. "Bowker updates groundbreaking consumer-focused research report for book industry." 2010. www.bowker.com/news/2010/Bowker-Updates-Groundbreaking-Consumer-Focused-Research-Report-for-Book-Industry.html. 18 September 2016.

———. "The Magic and Mystery of Book Consumer Research." 2011. www.slideshare.net/PubTrack/pubtrack-consumer-the-magic-and-mystery-of-book-consumer-research. 29 August 2021.

Bowlby, John. *Attachment and Loss*, 3 volumes. New York: Basic Books, 1969–1980.

Brecht, Bertholt. "Alienation Effects in Chinese Acting." *Brecht on Theater: The Development of an Aesthetic*. Ed. John Willett. New York: Hill and Wang, 1964. 91–99.

Breger, Claudia and Fritz Breithaupt. Ed. *Empathie und Erzählung*. Freiburg: Rombach Verlag, 2010.

Breithaupt, Fritz. *The Dark Sides of Empathy*. Trans. Ithaca: Cornell UP, 2019.

———. *Die Dunklen Seiten der Empathie*. Berlin, Germany: Suhrkamp, 2017.

———. *Kulturen der Empathie*. Frankfurt, Suhrkampf Verlag, 2009.

Brooks, Cleanth and Robert Penn Warren. *Understanding Fiction*. New York: F. S. Crofts, 1943.

———. *Understanding Poetry*. New York: Henry Holt, 1938.

Brooks, Peter. *Reading for the Plot: Design and Intention in Narrative*. New York: Knopf, 1984.

Brothers, Leslie. "A Biological Perspective on Empathy." *American Journal of Psychiatry* 146 (1989): 10–19.

Bruneau, Emile G. et al. "Distinct Roles of the 'Shared Pain' and 'Theory of Mind' Networks in Processing Others' Emotional Suffering." *Neuropsychologia* 50 (2012): 219–231.

———. "Social Cognition in members of Conflict Groups: Behavioural and Neural Responses in Arabs, Israelis and South Americans to each Other's Misfortunes." *Philosophical*.

Burton, William C. "Affect." *Burton's Legal Thesaurus*. 4th ed. McGraw Hill, 2006. https://legal-dictionary. 20 Jan. 2018.

Butler, Judith. *Gender Trouble: Feminism and the Subversion of Identity*. London: Routledge, 1990.

———. *Giving an Account of Oneself*. New York: Fordham UP, 2005.

Butte, George. *I Know That You Know That I Know: Narrating Subjects from* Moll Flanders *to* Marnie. Columbus: Ohio State UP, 2004.

Byatt, A. S. "Observe the Neurones: Between, Above, and Below John Donne." *Times Literary Supplement* (22 September 2006).

Bystrom, Kerry. "Literature and Human Rights." *Handbook of Human Rights*. Ed. Thomas Cushman. London and New York: Routledge, 2012. 637–46.

Cacioppo, John T., et al. "Just Because You're Imaging the Brain Doesn't Mean You Can Stop Using Your Head: A Primer and Set of First Principles." *Journal of Personality and Social Psychology* 85 (Oct. 2003): 650–61.

Cacioppo, John T., Louis G. Tassinary, and Gary G. Berntson. Ed. *Handbook Of Psychophysiology*. Cambridge and New York: Cambridge UP, 2007.

Cacioppo, John T. and R. E. Petty. *Social Psychophysiology*. New York: Guilford P, 1983.

Cámara Arenas, Enrique. "Causal Attribution and the Analysis of Literary Characters: A. C. Bradley's study of Iago and Othello." *Journal of Literary Semantics* 39.1 (Apr. 2010): 43–66.

Caracciolo, Marco. "Being Moved by Nature in the Anthropocene: On the Limits of the Ecological Sublime." *Emotion Review* 13.4 (Oct. 2021): 299–305.

Carrera, Pilar, et al. "I Feel So Sorry! Tapping the Joint Influence of Empathy and Personal Distress on Helping Behavior." *Motivation and Emotion*, 37 (2013): 335–45.

Carroll, Noel. "Aesthetics and the Educative Powers of Art." *A Companion to the Philosophy of Education* Ed. Randall Curren, 365–83. Malden, MA and Oxford: Blackwell, 2003.

———. *Engaging The Moving Image*, New Haven: Yale UP, 2003.

———. *The Philosophy of Horror; or, Paradoxes of the Heart*. New York: Routledge, 1990.

Chakrabarty, Dipesh. "Postcolonial Thinking and the Turn Towards the Human." The State of Postcolonial Studies, keynote address. *New Literary History* Conference. U Virginia, Charlottesville, VA, 3 Dec. 2010.

Changing Lives Through Literature. https://cltlblog.wordpress.com/about/. 14 Aug. 2021.

Character Counts. http://charactercounts. 14 Aug. 2021.

Chatman, Seymour. *Story and Discourse: Narrative Structure in Fiction and Film*. Ithaca and London: Cornell UP, 1978.

Chomsky, Noam. "A Review of B. F. Skinner's *Verbal Behavior*." *Language* 35. 1 (1959): 26–58.

Churchland, Patricia. *Brain-Wise: Studies in Neurophilosophy*. Cambridge, MA and London: MIT P, 2002.

Clark, Andy. *Being There: Putting Brain Body and World Together Again*. Cambridge, MA: MIT P, 1997.

Clark, Suzanne. *Sentimental Modernism: Women Writers and the Revolution of the Word.* Bloomington: Indiana UP, 1991.

Clough, Patricia Ticineto, with Jean Halley. *The Affective Turn: Theorizing the Social.* Durham: Duke UP, 2007.

Cohen, Stanley. *States of Denial: Knowing about Atrocities and Suffering.* Cambridge, UK: Polity P, 2001.

Cohn, Dorrit. *The Distinctiveness of Fiction.* Baltimore: Johns Hopkins UP, 1999.

———. *Transparent Minds: Narrative Modes for Presenting Consciousness in Fiction.* Princeton, NJ: Princeton UP, 1978.

Colclough, Stephen. *Consuming Texts: Readers and Reading Communities, 1695–1870.* Hampshire: Palgrave Macmillan, 2007.

Coleridge, Samuel Taylor. *Biographia Literaria.* 1817. *The Collected Works of Samuel Taylor Coleridge.* V. 7, part 2. Ed. James Engell and Walter Jackson Bate. London and Princeton: Routledge and Kegan Paul and Princeton UP, 1983.

Colie, Rosalie Littell. *The Resources of Kind: Genre-theory in the Renaissance.* Ed. Barbara K. Lewalski. Berkeley: U California P, 1973.

Collins, Suzanne. *Catching Fire.* New York: Scholastic, 2009.

———. *The Hunger Games.* New York: Scholastic, 2008.

———. *Mockingjay.* New York: Scholastic, 2010.

Connell, Jeanne M. "Aesthetic Experiences in the School Curriculum: Assessing the Value of Rosenblatt's Transactional Theory." *Journal of Aesthetic Education* 34. 1 (Spring 2000): 27–35.

Coplan, Amy, and Peter Goldie. Ed. *Empathy: Philosophical and Psychological Perspectives.* Oxford and New York: Oxford UP, 2011.

Cosmides, Leda and John Tooby. "Cognitive Adaptations for Social Exchange." *The Adapted Mind.* Ed. J. Barkow, Leda Cosmides, and John Tooby. Oxford and New York: Oxford UP, 1992. 163–228.

———. "Does Beauty Build Adapted Minds? Toward an Evolutionary Theory of Aesthetics, Fiction and the Arts." *SubStance* 30 (2001): 6–27.

———. "Evolutionary Psychology and the Emotions." *Handbook of Emotions*, 2nd ed. Ed. Michael Lewis and Jeanette M. Haviland-Jones. New York: Guilford P, 2000. 91–115.

Cosmides, Leda, John Tooby and Robert Kurzban. "Perceptions of Race." *Trends in Cognitive Sciences* 7 (2003): 173–9.

Craig, A. D. "How do you Feel? Interoception: The Sense of the Physiological Condition of theBody." *Nature Reviews Neuroscience* 3 (2002): 655–66.

Craig, K. D. "Physiological Arousal as a Function of Imagined, Vicarious, and Direct Stress Experiences." *Journal of Abnormal Psychology* 73 (1968): 513–20.

Crane, Mary Thomas. *Shakespeare's Brain.* Princeton: Princeton UP, 2001.

Crane, R. S. "The Concept of Plot and the Plot of Tom Jones." *Critics and Criticism: Ancient andModern.* Ed. R. S. Crane. Chicago: U of Chicago P, 1952.

Crenshaw, Kimberlé W. "Mapping the Margins: Intersectionality, Identity Politics, and Violence against Women of Color." *Stanford Law Review* 43. 6 (1991): 1241–99.

Currie, Gregory. "Empathy for Objects." *Empathy: Philosophical and Psychological Perspectives.* Ed. Amy Coplan and Peter Goldie. Oxford: Oxford UP, 2011. 82–98.

———. *Narratives and Narrators: a Philosophy of Stories.* Oxford and New York: Oxford UP, 2010.

———. *The Nature of Fiction.* Cambridge: Cambridge UP, 1990.

Currie, Gregory and Suzanne Keen. Discussion. Imagination and Legal Reason: History, Theory, Pedagogy. Queen Mary U London. 15 June 2016.

Dadlez, Eva M. "Fiction, Emotion, and Rationality." *The British Journal of Aesthetics* 36 (1996): 290–304.

———. *What's Hecuba to Him?: Fictional Events and Actual Emotions*. University Park: Pennsylvania State UP, 1987.

Dallas, E. S. *The Gay Science*. London: Chapman and Hall, 1866.

Damasio, Antonio R. *Descartes' Error: Emotion, Reason, and the Human Brain*. New York: Putnam, 1994.

———. *The Feeling of What Happens: Body and Emotion in the Making of Consciousness*. New York: Harcourt, 1999.

———. *Looking for Spinoza: Joy, Sorrow and the Feeling Brain*. New York: Harcourt, 2003.

Damasio, Antonio R., et al., "Somatic Markers and the Guidance of Behavior: Theory and Preliminary Testing." *Frontal Lobe Function and Disfunction*. Ed. H. S. Levin, H. M. Eisenberg, and A. L. Benton. Oxford and New York: Oxford, 1991. 217–29.

Dames, Nicolas. *The Physiology of the Novel: Reading; Neural Science, and the Form of the Victorian Novel*. Oxford and New York: Oxford UP, 2007.

———. "Wave Theories and Affective Psychologies: The Cognitive Strain in Victorian Novel Theories." *Victorian Studies* 46. 2 (Winter 2004): 206–16.

Danticat, Edwidge. *Breath, Eyes, Memory*. New York: Soho P, 1994.

———. *Brother, I'm Dying*. New York: Knopf, 2007.

———. *Create Dangerously: The Immigrant Artist at Work*. Princeton and Oxford: Princeton UP, 2010.

———. *The Dew Breaker*. New York: Knopf, 2004.

———. *Eight Days: A Story of Haiti*. Illustrated by Alix Delinois. New York: Orchard Books, 2010.

———. *Krik? Krak!* New York: Random House, 1996.

Darwin, Charles. *The Expression of the Emotions in Man and Animals*, 3rd ed. Ed. Paul Ekman. Oxford and NY: Oxford UP, 1998.

Davis, Mark H. *Empathy: a Social Psychological Approach*. Boulder, CO: Westview, 1994.

———. "Measuring Individual Differences in Empathy: Evidence for a Multidimensional Approach." *Journal of Personality and Social Psychology* 44 (1983): 113–26.

———. "A Multidimensional Approach to Individual Differences in Empathy." *JSAS Catalog of Selected Documents in Psychology*, 10 (1980): 85.

Dawes, James. *That the World May Know: Bearing Witness to Atrocity*. Cambridge, MA: Harvard UP, 2007.

Decety, Jean. Ed. *Empathy: From Bench to Bedside*. Cambridge: MIT P, 2012.

Decety, Jean and William Ickes. Ed. *The Social Neuroscience of Empathy*. Cambridge: MIT P, 2009.

Deigh, John. "Empathy and Universalizability." *Ethics* 105 (July 1995): 743–63.

Delgado, Richard. *The Coming Race War? and Other Apocalyptic Tales of America after Affirmative Action and Welfare*. New York: NYU P, 1996.

DeMan, Paul. *Allegories of Reading: Figural Language in Rousseau, Nietzsche, Rilke, and Proust*. New Haven: Yale UP, New Haven, 1979.

———. *Blindness and Insight: Essays in the Rhetoric of Contemporary Criticism*. Oxford UP, 1971.

DeSalvo, Louise. *Writing as a Way of Healing: How Telling Our Stories Transforms Our Lives*. Boston: Beacon P, 2000.

deSousa, Ronald. *The Rationality of the Emotions*. Cambridge, MA: MIT, 1987.

DeTurk, Sara. "Intercultural Empathy: Myth, Competency, or Possibility for Alliance Building." *Communication Education* 50. 4 (Oct. 2001): 374–84.

Dewey, John. 1934. *Art as Experience*. Rpt. New York: Perigee, 2005.

Dickie, Simon. *Cruelty and Laughter*. Chicago: U of Chicago P, 2011.

Diengott, Nilli. "Some Problems with the Concept of the Narrator in Bortolussi and Dixon's *Psychonarratology*." *Narrative* (Oct. 2004): 306–16.

Dissanayake, Ellen. *Homo Aestheticus: Where Art Comes from and Why*. New York: Free P, 1992.

Dixon, Peter, et al. "Literary Processing and Interpretation: Towards Empirical Foundations." *Poetics* 22 (1993): 5–33.

Dixon, Thomas. *The Invention of Altruism: Making Moral Meanings in Victorian Britain*. Oxford and New York: The British Academy and Oxford UP, 2008.

———. *From Passions to Emotions: the Creation of a Secular Psychological Category*. Cambridge and New York: Cambridge UP, 2006.

Doi, Takeo. *The Anatomy of Dependence: The Key Analysis of Japanese Behavior*, 2nd ed. Trans. John Bester. Tokyo: Kodansha International, 1981.

———. "The Concept of Amae and its Psychoanalytic Implications." *International Review of Psycho-Analysis* 16 (1989): 349–54.

Dovidio, John F., et al. "On the Nature of Prejudice: The Psychological Foundations of Hate." *The Psychology of Hate*. Ed. Robert J. Sternberg, Washington, DC: American Psychological Association, 2005. 211–34.

Echols, Stephanie and Joshua Correll. "It's More than Skin Deep: Empathy and Helping Behavior across Social Groups." *Empathy: From Bench to Bedside*. Cambridge, MA and London: MIT P, 2012. 55–71.

Egan, Jennifer. *A Visit from the Goon Squad*. NY: Knopf, 2010.

Eggers, Dave. *What is the What*. New York: McSweeney's, 2006.

Eisenberg, Nancy. *Altruistic Emotion, Cognition, and Behavior*. Hillsdale, NJ: Erlbaum, 1986.

———. "The Development of Empathy-Related Responding." *Moral Motivation through the Life Span*. Ed. Gustavo Carlo and Carolyn Pope Edwards, Lincoln: U Nebraska P, 2005. 73–117.

———. "Emotion, Regulation, and Moral Development." *Annual Review of Psychology* 51 (2000): 665–97.

Eisenberg, Nancy and Janet Strayer Ed. *Empathy and its Development*, Cambridge: Cambridge UP, 1987.

Eisenberg, Nancy and Natalie D Eggum. "Empathic Responding: Sympathy and Personal Distress." *The Social Neuroscience of Empathy*. Ed. Jean Decety and William Ickes. Cambridge: MIT P, 2009. 71–84.

Eisenberg, Nancy, et al. "Physiological Indices of Empathy." *Empathy and its Development*. Ed. Nancy Eisenberg and Janet Strayer. Cambridge and New York: Cambridge UP, 1987. 380–5.

Eisenberg, Nancy and Richard A. Fabes. "Children's Disclosure of Vicariously Induced Emotions." *Disclosure Processes in Children and Adolescents*. Ed. Ken J. Rotenberg. Cambridge and New York: Cambridge UP, 1995. 111–34.

Eisenberg, Nancy and Richard A. Fabes, et al. "The Relations of Emotionality and Regulation to Dispositional and Situational Empathy-related Responding." *Journal of Personality and Social Psychology* 66: 4 (1994): 776–97.

Ekman, Paul. "An Argument for Basic Emotions." *Cognition and Emotion* 6 (1992): 169–200.

———. *Emotions Revealed: Recognizing Faces and Feelings to Improve Communication and Emotional Life*. NY: Henry Holt, 2003.

———. "Introduction: Silvan Tomkins and Facial Expressions." *Exploring Affect: The Selected Writings of Silvan S. Tomkins* Ed. E. Virginia Demos. Cambridge: Cambridge UP, 1995. 209–16.

Elfenbein, Andrew. "Cognitive Science and the History of Reading." *PMLA* 121. 2 (2006): 484–502.

Eliot, George. "The Natural History of German Life." *Westminster Review*, XIX (1856): 51–79.

Ellmann, Richard. *James Joyce*. London: Oxford UP, 1959.

Elster, Jon. *Alchemies of the Mind: Rationality and the Emotions*. Cambridge and New York: Cambridge UP, 1999.

Evans, Dylan. *Emotion: The Science of Sentiment*. Oxford and New York: Oxford UP, 2001.

Fadiga, Luciano, et al. "Motor Facilitation during Action Observation: A Magnetic Stimulation Study." *Journal of Neurophysiology* 73 (1995): 2608–11.

Feagin, Joe R., et al. *White Racism: The Basics*. 2nd. ed. NY: Routledge, 2001.

Feagin, Susan. "Imagining Emotions and Appreciating Fictions." *The Canadian Journal of Philosophy* 18 (1988): 485–500.

———. *Reading with Feeling: The Aesthetics of Appreciation*. Ithaca: Cornell UP, 1996.

Febvre, Lucien. "La Sensibilité et L'histoire: Comment Reconstituer la Vie Affective D'autrefois?" *Annales d'histoire sociale* 3 (1941): 5–20.

Feenan, Dermot Ed. "Law and Compassion." Special Issue. *International Journal of Law in Context* 13. 2. (June 2017): 121–42.

Felski, Rita. "Suspicious Minds." *Poetics Today* 32. 2 (2011): 215–34.

———. *Uses of Literature*. Oxford and Malden, MA: Blackwell, 2008.

Feshbach, Norma D. "Studies of Empathic Behavior in Children." *Progress in Experimental Personality Research*. v. 8 Ed. Brendan A. Maher. New York Academic P, 1978. 1–47.

Fetterly, Judith. *The Resisting Reader: A Feminist Approach to American Fiction*. Bloomington: Indiana UP, 1978.

Fish, Stanley. "Literature in the Reader: Affective Stylistics." *New Literary History* 2. 1 (1970): 123–62.

Fisher, Marlene. *The Wisdom of the Heart: a Study of the Works of Mulk Raj Anand*. New Delhi, Sterling Publishers, 1985.

Fisher, Philip. *Hard Facts: Setting and Form in the American Novel*, Oxford and New York: Oxford UP, 1985.

Flack, Marjorie. *The Story about Ping*, New York, Viking, 1933.

Fletcher, Angus and John Monterosso. "The Science of Free Indirect Discourse: An Alternative Cognitive Effect." *Narrative* 24. 1 (2016): 82–103.

Fludernik, Monika. "Factual Narrative: A Missing Narratological Paradigm." *Sonderdruck aus Germanisch-Romanisch Monatsschrift* 63. 1 (2013): 117–34.

———. *The Fictions of Language and the Languages of Fiction*. London and New York: Routledge, 1993.

———. "Metanarrative and Metafictional Commentary: from Metadiscursivity to Metanarration and Metafiction." *Poetica* 35 (2003): 1–39.

———. *Towards a 'Natural' Narratology*. London and New York: Routledge, 1996.

Flynn, Elizabeth A. "Louise Rosenblatt and the Ethical Turn in Literary Theory." *College English* 70. 1 (Sept. 2007): 52–69.

Flynn, Elizabeth A. and Patrocinio P. Schweickart. Ed. *Gender and Reading: Essays on Readers, Texts, and Contexts*. Baltimore: Johns Hopkins UP, 1986.

Flynn, Gillian. *Gone Girl*. Crown, 2012.

Fogle, Richard Harter. "Empathetic Imagery." *The Imagery of Keats and Shelley: A Comparative Study*. Chapel Hill: U of North Carolina P, 1949. 139–83.

Fong, Katrina and Raymond A. Mar. "Exposure to Narrative Fiction versus Expository Nonfiction: Diverging Social and Cognitive Outcomes." *De stralende lezer; wetenschappelijk onderzoek naar de invloed van het lezen*. Ed. Frank Hakemulder. Delft, NL: Eburon Academic, 2012. 55–68.

Forgas, Joseph P. Ed. *Feeling and Thinking: The Role of Affect in Social Cognition*. Cambridge and New York: Cambridge UP; Paris: Editions de la Maison des Science de l'homme, 2000.

———. *Handbook of Affect and Social Cognition*. Mahwah, NJ: Erlbaum, 2001.

Forster, E. M. *Aspects of the Novel*. New York: Harcourt, 1927.

———. "Introduction." *Untouchable*. Mulk Raj Anand. Harmondsworth: Penguin, 1986. v–viii.

Fowler, Elizabeth. *Literary Character: The Human Figure in Early English Writing*, Ithaca: Cornell UP, 2003.

Fowler, Karen Joy. *We are All Completely Beside Ourselves*. New York: G. P. Putnam's Sons, 2013.

Freeman, Margaret H. "Manifesto." The Myrifield Institute for Cognition and the Arts. 2008. 27 Apr. 2009.

Freud, Sigmund. "Creative Writers and Daydreaming." 1907. *Standard Edition of the Complete Psychological Works of Sigmund Freud*. v. 9. Ed. James Strachey. London: Hogarth P and Institute of Psycho-Analysis, 1959. 141–54.

———. "Resistance and Repression." 1916–17. *The Standard Edition of the Complete Psychological Works of Sigmund Freud, Volume XVI. (1916–1917): Introductory Lectures on Psycho-Analysis. Part III*. Ed. and Trans. James Strachey London: Hogarth P, 1963. 286–302.

Fricke, Hannes. *Das Hört nicht auf: Trauma, Literatur und Empathie*. Göttingen: Wallstein, 2004.

Friedman, Susan Stanford. *Mappings: Feminism and the Cultural Geographies of Encounter*. Princeton, NJ: Princeton, 1998.

Frijda, Nico H. *The Emotions*. Cambridge and New York: Cambridge UP, 1986.

———. *The Laws of Emotion*. Mahwah: Lawrence Erlbaum, 2006.

Frijda, Nico and Klaus Scherer, "Affect. Psychological Perspectives." *The Oxford Companion to Emotion and the Affective Sciences*. Ed. David Sander and Klaus Scherer. Oxford: Oxford UP, 2009. 10.

Frye, Northrop. *Anatomy of Criticism: Four Essays*. Princeton UP, 1957.

Gabriel, Shira, and Ariana Young. "Becoming a Vampire Without Being Bitten." *Psychological Science* 22. 8 (2012): 990–94.

Gaines, Ernest J. *A Lesson Before Dying*, NY: Knopf, 1993.

Gallagher, Catherine. *Nobody's Story: The Vanishing Acts of Women Writers in the Marketplace, 1670–1920*. Berkeley and Los Angeles: U California P, 1994.

———. "Raymond Williams and Cultural Studies." *Social Text* 30 (1992): 79–89.

Gallese, Vittorio. "'Being Like Me': Self Other Identity, Mirror Neurons, and Empathy." *Perspectives on Imitation: From Neuroscience to Social Science. V. 1. Mechanisms of Imitation and Imitation in Animals*. Ed. Susan Hurley and Nick Chater. Cambridge, MA: MIT P, 2005. 101–18.

———. "The Roots of Empathy: The Shared Manifold Hypothesis and the Neural Basis of Intersubjectivity." *Psychopathology* 36. 4 (July–August 2003): 171–80.

Gallese, Vittorio, et al. "The Mirror Matching System: A Shared Manifold for Intersubjectivity." *Behavioral and Brain Sciences* 25 (Feb. 2002): 35–6.

———. "A Unifying View of the Basis of Social Cognition." *Trends in Cognitive Science* 8. 9 (Sept. 2004): 396–403.

Gallop, Jane. *Thinking through the Body*. New York: Columbia UP, 1988.

Gazzaniga, Michael S. *The Cognitive Neurosciences*. Cambridge, MA: MIT P, 2004.

Geer, J. H. and L. Jarmecky. "The Effect of Being Responsible for Reducing Another's Pain on Subject's Response and Arousal." *Journal of Personality and Social Psychology* (1973): 232–7.

Gernsbacher, Morton Ann. "On Not Being Human." Presidential Column. *APS Observer* 20. 2 (Feb. 2007): 5, 32.

Gernsbacher, Morton. Ann. et al. "Do Readers Mentally Represent Characters' Emotional States?" *Cognition and Emotion* 6 (1992): 89–111.

Gerrig, Richard J. "The Construction of Literary Character: a View from Cognitive Psychology." *Style* 24 (Fall 1990): 380–92.

———. *Experiencing Narrative Worlds: On the Psychological Activities of Reading.* New Haven, CT: Yale UP, 1993.

Gerrig, Richard J. and David N. Rapp. "Psychological Processes Underlying Literary Impact." *Poetics Today* 25. 2 (2004): 265–81.

Gilligan, Carol. *In A Different Voice: Psychological Theory and Women's Development.* Cambridge: Harvard UP, 1982.

Goffman, Erving. 1956. *The Presentation of Self in Everyday Life.* Rpt. Garden City: Doubleday, 1959.

Goldie, Peter. *The Emotions: A Philosophical Exploration.* Oxford: Clarendon P, 2000.

———. *The Mess Inside: Narrative, Emotion, & the Mind.* Oxford and New York: Oxford UP, 2012.

———. "Narrative, Emotion, and Perspective." *Imagination, Philosophy, and the Arts.* Ed. Matthew Kieran and Dominic Lopes. London: Routledge, 2003. 54–68.

———. "Narrative, Emotion, and Understanding." *Narrative Research in Health and Illness.* Ed. B. Hurwitz, T. Greenhalgh and V. Skultans. London: Blackwell, 2004. 156–67.

———. "One's Remembered Past: Narrative Thinking, Emotion, and the External Perspective." *Philosophical Papers* 32 (2003): 301–19.

Goldman, Alvin I. *Simulating Minds.* Oxford, Oxford UP, 2006.

Goodin, Kate. "Top 10 Girl Baby Names of 2010." *Parenting.* 30 Jan. 2012.

Goodman, Nelson. *Languages of Art: An Approach to a Theory of Symbols,* 2nd edition. Indianapolis: Hackett, 1976.

Gopnik, Alison. "The Theory Theory as an Alternative to the Innateness Hypothesis." *Chomsky and His Critics.* Ed. Louise M. Antony and Norbert Hornstein. Malden, MA: Blackwell, 2003. 238–54.

Gourevitch, Philip. *We Wish to Inform You That Tomorrow we will be Killed with our Families: Stories from Rwanda.* New York: Farrar, Straus, and Giroux, 1998.

Gowdy, Barbara. *The White Bone.* Toronto: Harper Flamingo Canada, 1998.

Gratton, Lynn M. and Paul J. Elsinger. "High Cognition and Social Behavior: Changes in Cognitive Flexibility and Empathy after Cerebral Lesions." *Neuropsychology* 3 (1989): 175–85.

Green, Melanie C., Christopher Chatham, and Marc A. Sestir. "Emotion and transportation into fact and fiction." *Scientific Study of Literature* 2. 1 (2012): 37–59.

Green, Melanie C., Jeffrey J. Strange, and Timothy C. Brock. Ed. *Narrative Impact: Social and Cognitive Foundations.* Mahwah, NJ: Lawrence Erlbaum, 2002.

Gregory, Marshall. "Ethical Criticism: What it is and Why it Matters." *Ethics, Literature, & Theory: An Introductory Reader* Ed. Stephen K. George, Lanham, MD: Rowman and Littlefield, 2005. 37–61.

Greimas, A. J. with Joseph Courtés, *Semiotics and Language: An Analytical Dictionary.* Bloomington: Indiana UP, 1982.

Greiner, Rae. "Thinking of Me Thinking of You: Sympathy versus Empathy in the Realist Novel." *Victorian Studies* 53. 3 (Spring 2011): 417–26.

Griffiths, Paul E. *What Emotions Really Are: The Problem of Psychological Categories.* Chicago, U of Chicago P, 1997.

Grodal, Torben. *Moving Pictures: A New Theory of Film Genres, Feelings, and Cognition*. Oxford and New York: Oxford UP, 1997.

Hacking, Ian. *The Social Construction of What?* Cambridge: Cambridge UP, 2001.

Haight, Gordon. *George Eliot: A Biography*. New York: Oxford UP, 1968.

Hakemulder, Jèmeljan. *The Moral Laboratory: Experiments Examining the Effects of Reading Literature on Social Perception and Moral Self-Concept*. Utrecht Publications in General and Comparative Literature 34. Amsterdam and Philadelphia: John Benjamins, 2000.

Hall, Alice E. and Cheryl C. Bracken. "'I Really Liked that Movie': Testing the Relationship Between Trait Empathy, Transportation, Perceived Realism, and Movie Enjoyment." *Journal of Media Psychology* 23. 2 (2011): 90–9.

Hallström, Lasse. Dir. *My Life as a Dog*, 1985.

Hammond, Meghan Marie. *Empathy and the Psychology of Literary Modernism*. Edinburgh: Edinburgh UP, 2014.

Hardt, Michael. "Foreward: What Affects are Good For." *The Affective Turn: Theorizing the Social*. Ed. Patricia Ticineto Clough with Jean Halley. Durham, NC: Duke UP, 2007. ix–xiii.

Harris, Lasana T. and Susan T. Fiske. "Dehumanized Perception: A Psychological Means to Facilitate Atrocities, Torture, and Genocide." *Zeitschrift für Psychologie* 219. 3 (2011): 175–81.

Hatfield, Elaine, John T. Cacioppo and Richard L. Rapson. *Emotional Contagion*. Cambridge and New York: Cambridge UP, 1994.

Hein, Grit, and Tania Singer. "I Feel How You Feel But Not Always: The Empathic Brain and Its Modulation." *Current Opinion in Neurobiology* 18. 2 (2008): 153–58.

———. "Neuroscience Meets Social Psychology: An Integrative Approach to Human Empathy and Prosocial Behavior." *Prosocial Motives, Emotions, and Behavior: The Better Angels of Our Nature*. Ed. Mario Mikulincer and Philip R. Shaver. Washington, DC: American Psychological Association, 2010. 109–125.

Herman, David. *Narratology Beyond the Human: Storytelling and Animal Life*. Oxford and New York: Oxford UP, 2018.

———. *Story Logic. Problems and Possibilities of Narrative*. Lincoln and London: U Nebraska P, 2002.

Herman, David. Ed. *The Emergence of Mind: Representations of Consciousness in Narrative Discourse in English*. Lincoln: U Nebraska P, 2011.

Hermon-Jones, Eddie and Piotr Winkielman. Ed. *Social Neuroscience: Integrating Biological and Psychological Explanations of Social Behavior*. New York: Guilford, 2007.

Hjort, Mette and Sue Laver. Ed. *Emotion and the Arts*. Oxford and New York: Oxford UP, 1997.

Hochman, Baruch. *Character in Literature*. Ithaca: Cornell UP, 1985.

Hoffman, Martin. *Empathy and Moral Development: Implications for Caring and Justice*. Cambridge and New York: Cambridge UP, 2000.

———. "The Measurement of Empathy." *Measuring Emotions in Infants and Children*. Ed. C. E. Izard. Cambridge and New York: Cambridge UP, 1982. 279–96.

Hogan, Patrick Colm. "Affect Studies and Literary Criticism." *Oxford Research Encyclopedia, Literature*. Oxford UP, literature. oxfordre.com. 2016. 11 January 2018. 5 of 33.

———. "The Brain in Love: A Case Study of Cognitive Neuroscience and Literary Theory." *Journal of Literary Theory* 1. 2 (2007): 339–56.

———. *Cognitive Science, Literature, and the Arts: A Guide for Humanists*. London and New York: Routledge, 2003.

———. "Comments on Keen: Universal Principles versus Uniformity." *Literary Universals Project*. Ed. Patrick Colm Hogan. https://literary-universals.uconn.edu/2017/10/08/universal-principles-do-not-entail-uniformity-of-individual-response-a-comment-on-suzanne-keens-narrative-empathy. 27 Sept. 2021.

———. "The Epilogue of Suffering: Heroism, Empathy, Ethics." *SubStance* 30 (2001): 119–43.

———. *Literature and Emotion*. Abingdon and New York: Routledge, 2018.

———. *The Mind and its Stories: Narrative Universals and Human Emotion*. Cambridge and New York: U Cambridge P, 2003.

———. "The Psychology of Colonialism and Postcolonialism: Cognitive Approaches to Identity and Empathy." *The Oxford Handbook of Cognitive Literary Studies*. Ed. Lisa Zunshine. NY and Oxford: Oxford UP, 2015. 329–46.

Hollan, Douglas. "Emerging Issues in the Cross-Cultural Study of Empathy." *Emotion Review* 4. 1 (January 2012): 70–78.

Holland, Norman. *The Dynamics of Literary Response*. Oxford and New York: Oxford UP, 1968.

———. *Five Readers Reading*. New Haven: Yale UP, 1975.

Howe, Stephen. *Empire: A Very Short Introduction*. Oxford and New York: Oxford, 2002.

Hrdy, Sarah Blaffer. *Nature: A History of Mothers, Infants, and Natural Selection*. NY: Pantheon Books, 1999.

———. *Mothers and Others: The Evolutionary Origins of Mutual Understanding*. Cambridge, MA: Belknap P of Harvard UP, 2007.

Hume, David. *A Treatise of Human Nature*. Ed. L. A. Selby-Bigge. Oxford: Clarendon P, 1978.

"Hunger Games Cast Subjected to Racist Attacks in Shocking Tweets." *US Weekly* (26 Mar. 2012). www. usmagazine.com/entertainment/news/hunger-games-fans-have-racist-debate-over-stars-playing-rue-thresh-2012263. 16 July 2012.

Hunt, Lynn. *Inventing Human Rights: A History*. New York and London: Norton, 2007.

Hutton, Richard Holt. *Essays on Some of the Modern Guides of English Thought in Matters of Faith*. London: Macmillan, 1887.

Iacoboni, Marco, et al. "Cortical Mechanisms of Human Imitation." *Science* 286 (1999): 2526–28.

Ickes, William. "Empathic Accuracy." *Journal of Personality* 61. 4 (1993): 587–610.

———. "Empathic Accuracy: Its Links to Clinical, Cognitive, Developmental, Social, and Physiological Psychology." *The Social Neuroscience of Empathy*. Ed. Jean Decety and William Ickes. Cambridge: MIT P, 2009. 57–70.

Ickes, William. Ed. *Empathic Accuracy*. New York: Guilford, 1997.

Ickes, William, et al. "Gender Differences in Empathic Accuracy: Differential Ability or Differential Motivation?" *Personal Relationships* 7 (2000): 95–110.

Illes, Judy and Eric Racine. "Imaging or Imagining? A Neuroethics Challenge Informed by Genetics." *American Journal of Bioethics* 5. 2 (Mar./Apr. 2005): 5–18.

Ingarden, Roman. "Psychologism and Psychology in Literary Scholarship." Trans. John Fizer. *New Literary History* 5. 2 (Winter 1974): 213–23.

Institute of Education Science. *What Works Clearinghouse: Character Education*, an evaluation of *Lessons in Character*. U. S. Department of Education, 2006. http://ies.ed.gov/ncee/wwc/reports/character_education/lic/. 12 Mar. 2010.

Iser, Wolfgang. *The Act of Reading: A Theory of Aesthetic Response*. Johns Hopkins UP, 1978.

———. *The Implied Reader: Patterns of Communication in Prose Fiction from Bunyan to Beckett*. Baltimore: Johns Hopkins UP, 1974.

———. "The Reading Process: a Phenomenological Approach." *New Literary History* 3. 2 (1972): 279–99.

Jackson, Gregory S. "'What would Jesus do?': Practical Christianity, Social Gospel Realism, and the Homiletic Novel." *PMLA* 121. 3 (May 2006): 641–61.

Jacoby, Russell and Naomi Glauberman. Ed. *The Bell Curve Debate: History, Documents, Opinions*. New York: Times Books, 1995.

James, Henry. "Anthony Trollope." *Partial Portraits*. London and New York: Macmillan, 1888. 97–133.

———. *The Art of Fiction and Other Essays*, Oxford: Oxford UP, 1948.

James, Marlon. *A Brief History of Seven Killings*. New York: Riverhead Books, 2014.

Jameson, Fredric. *The Political Unconscious: Narrative as a Socially Symbolic Act*. Ithaca: Cornell, 1981.

———. *Postmodernism, or, The Cultural Logic of Late Capitalism*. Durham, NC: Duke UP, 1995.

———. "Postmodernism Today." Lecture. Helsinki International Prose Conference: Means and Devices of Prose. Helsinki Collegium. 10 May 2012.

Jarjoura, G. R. and S. T. Krumholz. "Combining Bibliotherapy and Positive Role Modeling as an Alternative to Incarceration." Journal of Offender Rehabilitation. 28. 1–2. 1998: 127–139.

Jauss, Hans Robert. *Aesthetic Experience and Literary Hermeneutics*. Trans. Michael Shaw. Minneapolis: U Minnesota P, 1982.

———. "Levels of Identification of Hero and Audience." *New Literary History* 5. 2 (Winter 1974): 283–317.

Jensen, Deborah and Marco Iacoboni. "Literary Biomimesis: Mirror Neurons and the Ontological Priority of Representation." California Italian Studies 2. 1 (2011). https://doi.org/10.5070/C321008945. 7 Oct. 2021.

Johnson, Dan R. "Transportation into a Story Increases Empathy, Prosocial Behavior, and Perceptual Bias toward Fearful Expressions." *Personality and Individual Differences* 52 (2012): 150–55.

Johnson, Dan R., et al. "Reading Narrative Fiction Reduces Arab-Muslim Prejudice and Offers a Safe Haven from Intergroup Anxiety." *Social Cognition* (10 Sept. 2013): 578–98.

Johnson, Peter. *Moral Philosophers and the Novel: A Study of Winch, Nussbaum, and Rorty*. Houndmills and New York: Palgrave Macmillan, 2004.

Johnson, Samuel. "Preface to Shakespeare." *The Yale Edition of the Works of Samuel Johnson*, v. 7. Ed. Arthur Sherbo. New Haven: Yale UP, 1968. 59–113.

Johnson, William A. *Readers and Reading Culture in the High Roman Empire: a Study of Elite Communities. Classical Culture and Society*. Oxford and New York: Oxford UP, 2012.

Jones, Peter H. *Philosophy and the Novel*. Oxford: Clarendon P, 1975.

Jose, P. E. and W. F. Brewer. "Development of Story Liking: Character Identification, Suspense, and Outcome Resolution." *Developmental Psychology* 20 (1984): 911–24.

Joyce, James. *Ulysses*. 1922. Ed. Hans Walter Gabler. New York: Random House, 1986.

Jussawalla, Feroza. "Kim, Huck and Naipaul: Using the Postcolonial Bildungsroman to Re(define) Postcoloniality." *Links & Letters* 4 (1997): 25–38.

Juvan, Marko. "Taking Darwin Metaphorically and Literally: Genres and Sciences in a Survival Struggle." *Neohelicon* 41 (2014): 303–15.

Kagan, Jerome. "Psychology's Missing Contexts: Why Researchers should Design and Report Experiments in a More Precise Way." *The Chronicle Review*. 8 Apr. 2012. www.chronicle.com/article/psychologys-missing-contexts/.

———. *What is Emotion? History, Measures, and Meanings*. New Haven: Yale UP, 2007.

Kagan, Jerome and Nancy Snidman. *The Long Shadow of Temperament*. Cambridge, MA and London: The Belknap P of Harvard UP, 2004.

Keen, Suzanne. "Affect and Empathy Studies." *Oxford Companion to Law and the Humanities*. Ed. Simon Stern, Maksymilian Del Mar, and Bernadette Meyler. Oxford University Press, 2019. 181–97.

———. "Afterword." *Literature as a Lens for Climate Change: Using Narratives to Prepare the Next Generation*. Ed. Rebecca L.Young. Lanham, MD: Lexington Books, 2022. 239–42.

———. "'Altruism' Makes a Space for Empathy, 1852." *BRANCH: Britain, Representation and Nineteenth-Century History*. Ed. Dino Franco Felluga. Extension of Romanticism and Victorianism on the Net. 7 Nov. 2015. www.branchcollective. org/?ps_articles= suzanne-keen-altruism-makes-a-space-for-empathy-1852. 27 Sept. 2021.

———. *Empathy and the Novel*. Oxford and New York: Oxford UP, 2007.

———. "empathy so intense you stopped reading." Listserv query. VICTORIA, 31 January 2016.

———. "Fast Tracks to Narrative Empathy: Anthropomorphism and Dehumanization in Graphic Narratives." *SubStance #124* 40. 1 (2011): 135–55.

———. "Intersectional Narratology in the Study of Narrative Empathy." *Queer/ Feminist Narrative Theory*. Ed. Robyn Warhol and Susan Lanser. Columbus: Ohio State UP, 2014. 123–46.

———. "Introduction: Narrative and the Emotions." *Poetics Today* 32. 1 (Spring 2011): 1–53.

———. *Milk Glass Mermaid*. Lewiston, ID: Lewis Clark P, 2007.

———. "Narrative Empathy." *The Living Handbook of Narratology*. Ed. Peter Hühn. J. C, Meister, and J. Pier. Hamburg: Hamburg UP, 2014. v. 2. 521–30. www.lhn.uni-hamburg. de/node/42.html. 7 Oct. 2021.

———. "Narrative Empathy: A Universal Response to Fiction?" *Literary Universals Project*. Ed. Patrick Colm Hogan. https://literary-universals.uconn.edu/2017/10/07/narrative-empathy-a-universal-response-to-fiction/. 27 Sept. 2021.

———. *Narrative Form: Revised and Expanded Second Edition*. Houndsmills: Palgrave Macmillan, 2015.

———. "Readers' Temperaments and Fictional Character." *New Literary History* 42. 2 (Spring 2011): 295–314.

———. "The Recovery of Genre in Postmodern British Fiction: Return of the Romance." *The Cambridge Companion to British Postmodernism*. Ed. Bran Nichol. Cambridge and NY: Cambridge UP, forthcoming.

———. *Romances of the Archive in Contemporary British Fiction*. Toronto: U of Toronto P, 2001.

———. "Strategic Empathizing: Techniques of Bounded, Ambassadorial, and Broadcast Narrative Empathy." *Deutsche Vierteljahrs Schrift* 82. 3 (Sept. 2008): 477–93.

———. "A Theory of Narrative Empathy." *Narrative* 14. 3 (2006): 207–36.

———. *Thomas Hardy's Brains: Psychology, Neurology, and Hardy's Imagination. The Theory and Interpretation of Narrative*. Columbus: Ohio State UP, 2014.

———. "The Undergraduate Literature Classroom." *Teaching Narrative Theory*. Ed. James Phelan, Brian McHale, and David Herman. New York: MLA, 2010. 19–32.

Keysers, Christian, et al. "Demystifying Social Cognition: a Hebbian Perspective." *Trends in Cognitive Science* 8 (Nov. 2004): 501–7.

Kidd, David, and Emanuele Castano. "Reading Literary Fiction Improves Theory of Mind." *Science* 342. 6156 (2013): 377–80.

Kincaid, Jamaica. *The Autobiography of My Mother*. New York: Farrar, Straus and Giroux, 1996.

———. *Mr. Potter*. New York: Farrar Straus and Giroux, 2002.

Klemenz-Belgardt, Edith. "American Research of Response to Literature." *Poetics* 10 (1981): 357–80.

Klimaszewski, Melisa. Personal correspondence, 31 January 2016.

Kneepkens, E.W. E. M. and Rolf A. Zwaan. "Emotions and Literary Text Comprehension." *Poetics* 23. 1–2 (January 1995): 125–38.

Knights, L. C. "How Many Children Had Lady Macbeth?" *Explorations: Essays in Criticism Mainly on the Literature of the Seventeenth Century*. New York: G.W. Stewart, 1947. 15–54.

Konijn, Elly A. and Johan F. Hoorn. "Reality-based Genre Preferences Do Not Direct Personal Involvement." *Discourse Processes* 38 (2004): 219–46.

Koopman, Emy and Frank Hakemulder. "Effects of Literature on Empathy and Self-Reflection – A Theoretical-Empirical Framework." *Journal of Literary Theory* 9. 1 (2015): 79–111.

Krebs, Dennis. "Empathy and Altruism." *Journal of Personality and Social Psychology* 32 (1975): 1134–46.

Kreilkamp, Ivan. *Voice and the Victorian Storyteller*. Cambridge: Cambridge UP, 2005.

Kreiswirth, Martin. "Narrative Turn in the Humanities." *Routledge Encyclopedia of Narrative Theory*. Ed. David Herman, Manfred Jahn and Marie-Laure Ryan. Abingdon, Oxfordshire and New York: Routledge, 2005. 377–82.

Kruger, D. J. "Evolution and Altruism: Combining Psychological Mediators with Naturally Selected Tendencies." *Evolution and Human Behavior* 24 (2003): 118–25.

Kuiken, Don, et al. "Locating Self-Modifying Feelings within Literary Reading." *Discourse Processes* 38 (2004): 267–86.

Kunda, Ziva. "The Case for Motivated Reasoning." *Psychological Bulletin*, 108. 3 (1990): 480–98.

Lafrance, Marianne and Julie A. Woodzicka. "No Laughing Matter: Women's Verbal and Nonverbal Reactions to Sexist Humor." *Prejudice: The Target's Perspective*. Ed. Janet K. Swim and Charles Stangor. San Diego, CA: Academic P, 1998. 61–80.

Lakoff, George, and Mark Johnson. *Metaphors We Live By*. Chicago: U of Chicago P, 1980.

———. *Philosophy In the Flesh: The Embodied Mind And Its Challenge To Western Thought*. New York: Basic Books, 1999.

Lakoff, George, and Mark Turner. *More Than Cool Reason: A Field Guide to Poetic Metaphor*. Chicago: U of Chicago P, 1989.

Lamarque, Peter. "How Can We Fear and Pity Fictions?" *British Journal of Aesthetics* 21 (1981): 291–304.

———. "On Not Expecting Too Much from Narrative." *Mind and Language* 19 (2004). 393–408.

———. *Truth, Fiction, and Literature: A Philosophical Perspective*. Oxford: Oxford UP, 1994.

Lamm, Claus, Jean Decety, and Tania Singer. "Meta-analytic Evidence for Common and Distinct Neural Networks Associated with Directly Experienced Pain and Empathy for Pain." *NeuroImage* 54 (2011): 2492–502.

Landy, Joshua. "A Nation of Madame Bovarys: On the Possibility and Desirability of Moral Improvement through Fiction." *Art and Ethical Criticism*. Ed. Garry Hagberg. Malden, MA and Oxford: Blackwell, 2008. 63–94.

Lane, Richard D. and Lynn Nadel. Ed. *Cognitive Neuroscience of Emotion*. New York and Oxford: Oxford UP, 2000.

Lanser, Susan S. "Are We There Yet? The Intersectional Future of Feminist Narratology." *Foreign Literature Studies* 32. 4 (2010): 32–41.

———. "Negative Plotting: Or, The Shadow Knows." Handout accompanying paper presented at International Society for the Study of Narrative Plenary Session, Birmingham, England. 4–6 June 2009.

Larkin, Peter. *Leaves of Field*. Exeter: Shearsman, 2006.

"Towards a Feminist Narratology." *Style* 20. 3 (1986): 341–63.

László, János. *The Science of Stories: An Introduction to Narrative Psychology*. Hove and New York: Routledge, 2008.

Lazarus, R. S. et al. "A Laboratory Study of Psychological Stress Produced by a Motion Picture Film." *Psychological Monographs* 76 (1962): 1–35.

LeDoux, Joseph. *The Emotional Brain: The Mysterious Underpinnings of Emotional Life*. New York: Simon and Schuster, 1996.

Lee, Harper. *To Kill a Mockingbird*. Philadelphia: Lippincott, 1960. Rpt. New York: HarperCollins, 2002.

Lee, Vernon. [Violet Paget]. *The Beautiful. An Introduction to Psychological Aesthetics*. Cambridge: Cambridge UP, 1913.

———. *Miss Brown*. Edinburgh and London: Blackwood, 1884.

Lee, Vernon and C. Anstruther-Thomson. "Beauty and Ugliness." *Contemporary Review* 72 (Oct. 1897): 544–69; (Nov. 1897): 669–88.

Lennon, Randy and Nancy Eisenberg. "Gender/Age Differences in Empathy/Sympathy." *Empathy and its Development*. Ed. Nancy Eisenberg and Janet Strayer. Cambridge and New York: Cambridge UP, 1987. 195–217.

Lessing, Doris. *Under my Skin: My Autobiography, to 1949*. New York: HarperCollins, 1994.

Levenson, Robert and Anna Ruef. "Physiological Aspects of Emotional Knowledge and Papport." *Empathic Accuracy*. Ed. William Ickes. New York: Guilford P, 1997. 44–72.

Levy, Raymond A. and J. Stuart Ablon. Ed. *Handbook of Evidence-Based Psychodynamic Psychotherapy: Bridging the Gap between Science and Practice*. Totowa, NJ: Humana P, 2009.

Lewes, G. H. *The Life and Works of Goethe*. London: D. Nutt, 1855.

———. *The Physiology of Common Life*. Edinburgh: Blackwood, 1859–60.

Lewis, David. *On the Plurality of Worlds*. Oxford: Blackwell, 1986.

Lewis, Jan and Peter N. Stearns. "Introduction." *An Emotional History of the United States*. Ed. Peter N. Stearns and Jan Lewis. New York: New York UP, 1998. 1–14.

Lewis, Michael, Jeanette M. Haviland-Jones, and Lisa Feldman Barrett. Ed. *Handbook of Emotions*. New York: Guilford P, 2008.

Leys, Ruth. "The Turn to Affect: A Critique." *Critical Inquiry* 37 (2011): 434–72.

Lipps, Theodor *Äesthetik: Psycholgie des Schönen und der Kunst*. Hamburg, Germany: Voss, 1903, 1906.

———. "Das Wissen von Fremden Ichen." *Psychologische Untersuchungen* 1 (1906): 694–722.

———. *Zur Einfühlung*. Leipzig: Engleman, 1913.

Lodge, David. *Consciousness and the Novel: Connected Essays*. Cambridge, MA: Harvard UP, 2002.

Long, Elizabeth. *Book Clubs: Women and the Uses of Reading in Everyday Life*. Chicago: U of Chicago P, 2003.

Louwerse, Max and Don Kuiken. "The Effects of Personal Involvement in Narrative Discourse." *Discourse Processes* 38 (2004): 169–72.

Lubbock, Percy. *The Craft of Fiction*. London: Jonathan Cape, 1921.

Lukianoff, Greg and Jonathan Haidt. "The coddling of the American mind." *The Atlantic* (Sept. 2015): www.theatlantic.com/magazine/archive/2015/09/the-coddling-of-the-american-mind/399356/. 11 Apr. 2016.

Lyubomirsky, Sonja. *The How of Happiness: A Scientific Approach to Getting the Life You Want*. New York: Penguin, 2008.

Macherey, Pierre. *A Theory of Literary Production*. 1966. Trans. Geoffrey Wall. London and NY: Routledge, 2006.

Machotka, Pavel. "Daniel Berylne's Contributions to Empirical Aesthetics." *Motivation and Emotion* 4. 2: (1980): 113–21.

Maibom, Heidi L. Ed. *Routledge Handbook of Philosophy of Empathy*. London and New York: 2017.

Mailloux, Steven. "The Turns of Reader-Response Criticism." *Conversations: Contemporary Critical Theory and the Teaching of Literature*. Ed. Charles Moran and Elizabeth F. Penfield. Urbana: National Council of Teachers of English, 1990. 38–54.

Maltravers, Derek. *Art and Emotion*. Oxford: Oxford and London, 1998.

Mandler, Jean M. and Nancy Johnson. "Remembrance of Things Parsed: Story Structure and Recall." *Cognitive Psychology* 9 (1977): 111–51.

Mangen, Anne and Adriaan van der Weel. "The Evolution of Reading in the Age of Digitisation: An Integrative Framework for Reading Research." *Literacy* 50. 3 (Sept. 2016): 116–24.

Mangen, Anne, and Don Kuiken. "Lost in an iPad: Narrative Engagement on Paper and Tablet." *Scientific Study of Literature* 4. 2 (2014): 150–77.

Mar, Raymond A. "Stories and the Simulation of Social Experience: Neuropsychological evidence and social ramifications." U Toronto doctoral dissertation, 2008.

Mar, Raymond A. and Keith Oatley, M. Djikic, and J. Mullin. "Emotion and Narrative Fiction: Interactive Influences before, during, and after Reading. *Cognition & Emotion* 25 (2011): 818–33.

Mar, Raymond A., Keith Oatley, Jacob Hirsh, Jennifer dela Paz, and Jordan B. Peterson. "Bookworms versus Nerds: Exposure to Fiction versus Non-fiction, Divergent Associations with Social Ability, and the Simulation of Fictional Social Worlds." *Journal of Research in Personality* 40 (2006): 694–712.

Mar, Raymond A., Keith Oatley, and Jordan B. Peterson. "Exploring the Link between Reading Fiction and Empathy: Ruling Out Individual Differences and Examining Outcomes." *Communications* 34 (2009): 407–28.

Marcus, Robert F. "Somatic Indices of Empathy." *Empathy and its Development*. Ed. Nancy Eisenberg and Janet Strayer. Cambridge and New York: Cambridge UP, 1987. 374–79.

Margolin, Uri. "Character." *The Routledge Encyclopedia of Narrative Theory*. Ed. David Herman, Manfred Jahn and Marie-Laure Ryan. Abingdon and New York: Routledge, 2005. 52–7.

Marraffa, Massimo "Theory of Mind." *Internet Encyclopedia of Philosophy*. Ed. James Fieser and Bradley Dowden. 2011, https://iep.utm.edu/theomind/. 9 April 2022.

Masson, David. *British Novelists and Their Styles: Being a Critical Sketch of the History of British Prose Fiction*. Cambridge: Macmillan, 1859.

Massumi, Brian. "Notes on the Translation and Acknowledgements." *A Thousand Plateaus: Capitalism and Schizophrenia. Capitalism and Schizophrenia*. 2nd ed. Gilles Delueze and Félix Guattari, trans. Brian Massumi. Minneapolis: U Minnesota P, 1987. xvi.

———. *Parables for the Virtual: Movement, Affect, Sensation*. Durham: Duke UP, 2002.

Mazzocco, Philip J., Melanie Green, et al. "This Story is not for Everyone: Transportability and Narrative Persuasion." *Social Psychological and Personality Science* 1 (2010): 361–368.

McCabe, D. P. and A. D. Castel. "Seeing is believing: the effect of brain images on judgments of scientific reasoning." *Cognition* 107. 1 (2008): 343–52.

McCall, Leslie. "The Complexity of Intersectionality." *Signs* 30. 3 (2005): 1771–800.

McCarthy, Cormac. *Blood Meridian or the Evening Redness in the West*. New York: Random House, 1985.

McCrae, Robert R. *The Five-Factor Model of Personality Across Cultures*, New York: Kluwer Academic/Plenum, 2002.

McEwan, Ian. *Atonement*. London: Jonathan Cape, 2001.

McFarland, Sam. "Personality and Support for Universal Human Rights: A Review and Test of a Structural Method." *Journal of Personality* 78. 6 (Dec. 2010): 1735–63.

McFarland, Sam and Melissa Mathews. "Who Cares About Human Rights?" *Political Psychology* 26. 3 (2005): 365–85.

McGinn, Colin. *Ethics, Evil, and Fiction*, Oxford: Clarendon P, 1997.

McMaster, Juliet. *Trollope's Palliser Novels: Theme and Pattern*. New York and Oxford: Oxford UP, 1978.

Medina, Jennifer. "Warning: The Literary Canon Could Make Students Squirm." *The New York Times* (17 May 2014). www.nytimes.com/2014/05/18/us/warning-the-literary-canon-could-make-students-squirm.html. 20 July 2016.

Mehrabian, Albert. "Relations Among Personality Scales of Aggression, Violence, and Empathy: Validational Evidence Bearing on the Risk of Violence Scale." *Aggressive Behavior* 23 (1997): 433–45.

Melnyk, Julie. "'RE: Empathy so intense you stopped reading." Listserv discussion. VICTORIA, 1 February 2016.

Messer-Davidow, Ellen. "Philosophical Bases of Feminist Literary Criticisms." *New Literary History* 19. 1 (Autumn 1987): 65–103.

Meyer, Stephenie. *Breaking Dawn*. Boston: Little, Brown, 2008.

———. *Twilight*. Boston: Little, Brown, 2005.

Miall, David S. "Affect and Narrative: a Model of Responses to Stories." *Poetics* 17 (1988): 259–72.

———. "Beyond the Schema Given: Affective Comprehension of Literary Narratives." *Cognition and Emotion* 3 (1989): 55–78.

———. "Feeling from the Perspective of the Empirical Study of Literature." *Journal of Literary Theory* (2007): 377–393.

———. "Foregrounding and Feeling in Response to Narrative." *Directions in Empirical Literary Studies: Essays in Honor of Willie van Peer*. Ed. Sonia Zyngier, Marisa Bortolussi, Anna Chesnokova, and Jan Auracher. Amsterdam and Philadelphia: John Benjamins, 2008. 89–102.

———. *Literary Reading: Empirical and Theoretical Studies*. Peter Lang, 2006.

———. "On the necessity of empirical studies of literary reading." *Frame: Utrecht Journal of Literary Theory* 14. 2–3 (2000): 43–59.

Miall, David S. and Don Kuiken. "What is Literariness? Three Components of Literary Reading." *Discourse Processes* 28 (1999): 121–38.

Michie, Elsie B. "The Odd Couple: Anthony Trollope and Henry James." *The Henry James Review* 27. 1 (Winter 2006): 10–23.

Miller, Nancy K. *Getting Personal: Feminist Occasions and Other Autobiographical Acts*. New York: Routledge, 1991.

Minami, Masahiko and Alyssa McCabe. "Rice Balls and Bear Hunts: Japanese and North American Family Narrative Patterns." *Journal of Child Language* 22 (1995): 423–45.

Minsky, Marvin. *The Emotion Machine: Commonsense Thinking, Artificial Intelligence, and the Future of the Human Mind*. New York: Simon and Schuster, 2006.

———. *The Society of Mind*. New York: Simon and Schuster, 1986.

Mistry, Rohinton. *A Fine Balance*. Toronto: McClelland and Stewart, 1995.

Mohr, Lawrence B. *The Causes of Human Behavior: Implications for Theory and Method in the Social Sciences*. Ann Arbor: U Michigan P, 1996.

Moi, Toril. *Sexual/Textual Politics: Feminist Literary Theory*. London and New York: Methuen, 1985.

Moretti, Franco. *Maps, Graphs, Trees: Abstract Models for a Literary History*. London and New York: Verso, 2005.

Morrison, Toni. *Beloved*. New York: Knopf, 1987.

Morse, Deborah Denenholz. "RE: Empathy so intense you stopped reading." Listserv discussion. VICTORIA, 31 January 2016.

———. *Reforming Trollope: Race, Gender, and Englishness in the Novels of Anthony Trollope*. Farnham, Surrey and Burlington, VT: Ashgate, 2013.

Mühlhoff, Rainer. "Affective Resonance and Social Interaction." *Phenomenology and the Cognitive Sciences* 14 (2014): 1001–19.

Muir, John. *Travels in Alaska*. 1915. Rpt. Penguin Nature Library. Ed. Richard Nelson. Harmondsworth: Penguin, 1997.

Mullaney, Julie. *Postcolonial Literatures in Context*. London and New York: Continuum, 2010.

Naipaul, V. S. *A House for Mr. Biswas*. London: Andre Deutsch, 1961.

"narrative, n." 1906. Rev. 2003. *OED Online*. Oxford UP. www.oed.com/view/Entry/125146. 9 April 2022.

Narvaez, Darcia. "Moral Text Comprehension: Implications for Education and Research." *Journal of Moral Education* 30. 1 (2001): 43–54.

Nathanson, Donald L. "Prologue: Affect Imagery Consciousness." Silvan Tomkins' *Affect Imagery Consciousness*, Book One. New York: Springer, 2008. xi–xxvi.

National Endowment for the Arts. *Reading at Risk: A Survey of Literary Reading in America*. Research Division Report #46. Washington, D. C: National Endowment for the Arts, June 2004.

———. *To Read or Not to Read: A Question of National Consequence* Research Report #47. Washington, D. C.: National Endowment for the Arts, Nov. 2007.

———. *Reading on the Rise: A New Chapter in American Literacy*. Washington, D. C.: National Endowment for the Arts, 2009.

Nell, Victor. *Lost in a Book: The Psychology of Reading for Pleasure*. New Haven: Yale UP, 1988.

Neumann, Birgit and Ansgar Nünning. "Metanarration and Metafiction." *the living handbook of narratology*. Ed. Peter Hühn, Peter et al. Hamburg: Hamburg University. www.lhn.uni-hamburg.de/article/metanarration-and-metafiction. 14 Aug. 2021.

Neumann, Birgit, Ansgar Nünning, and Bo Pettersson. Ed. *Narrative and Identity: Theoretical Approaches and Critical Analyses* Trier: Wissenschaftlicher Verlag Trier, 2008.

Ngai, Sianne. *Ugly Feelings*. Cambridge, MA: Harvard UP, 2005.

Nicholson, Christy. "Thinking it Over: fMRI and Psychological Science" *Association for Psychological Science Observer* 19 (9. Sept. 2006). www.psychologicalscience.org/observer/. 10 Mar. 2010.

Noddings, Nel. *Caring: A Feminine Approach to Ethics and Moral Education*. 2nd. ed. Berkeley and London: U of California P, 2003.

Nussbaum, Martha C. *Cultivating Humanity: A Classical Defense of Reform in Liberal Education*. Cambridge: Harvard UP, 1997.

———. *Love's Knowledge: Essays on Philosophy and Literature*. Oxford and New York: Oxford UP, 1990.

———. *Upheavals of Thought: The Intelligence of Emotions* Cambridge: Cambridge UP, 2001.

Oakley, Barbara, Ariel Knafo, Guruprasad Madhavan, and David Sloan Wilson. Ed. *Pathological Altruism*. Oxford and New York: Oxford UP, 2012.

Oatley, Keith. *Such Stuff as Dreams: The Psychology of Fiction*. Malden, MA: Wiley-Blackwell, 2001.

———. "A Taxonomy of the Emotions of Literary Response and a Theory of Identification in Fictional Narrative." *Poetics* 23 (1994): 53–74.

Oatley, Keith, et al. *Understanding Emotions*, 2nd ed. Oxford: Blackwell, 2006.

Odag, Ozen. "Emotional Engagement during Literary Reception: Do Men and Women Differ?" *Cognition & Emotion* (2013): 1–19.

———. "Of Men Who Read Romance and Women Who Read Adventure Stories: An Empirical Reception Study on the Emotional Engagement of Men and Women while Reading Narrative Texts." *New Beginnings in Literary Studies* (2008): 308–29.

Ortner, Sherry B. "Is Female to Male as Nature is to Culture?" *Women, Culture, and Society*. Ed. Michele Zimbalist Rosaldo and Louise Lamphere, Stanford: Stanford UP, 1974. 68–87.

Oxenhandler, Neal. "The Changing Concept of Literary Emotion: A Selective History." *New Literary History* 20. 1 (1988): 105–21.

Page, Ruth E. "Feminist Narratology? Literary and Linguistic Perspectives on Gender and Narrativity." *Language and Literature* 12. 1 (2003): 43–56.

Palmer, Alan. *Fictional Minds*. Lincoln, NE: U Nebraska P, 2004.

———. *Social Minds in the Novel*. Columbus: Ohio State UP, 2010.

Panksepp, Jaak. "Emotions as Natural Kinds in the Brain." *Handbook of Emotions*, 2nd ed. Ed. Michael Lewis and Jeannette M. Haviland-Jones. New York: Guilford P, 2000. 137–56.

Pascal, Roy. *The Dual Voice: Free Indirect Speech and Its Functioning in the Nineteenth-Century European Novel*. Manchester: Manchester UP, 1977.

Pavel, Thomas. *The Poetics of Plot: The Case of English Renaissance Drama*. Manchester: U of Manchester P, 1985.

Pedwell, Carolyn. *Affective Relations: The Transnational Politics of Empathy*. Basingstoke and New York: Palgrave, 2014.

Pennebaker, James W. *Opening Up: The Healing Power of Expressing Emotion*. New York: Guilford, 1997.

———. "Writing about Emotional Experiences as a Therapeutic process." *Psychological Science* 8 (1997): 62–166.

Phelan, James. *Experiencing Fiction: Judgments, Progressions, and the Rhetorical Theory of Narrative*. Columbus: Ohio State UP, 2007.

———. *Living to Tell about It: A Rhetoric and Ethics of Character Narration* Ithaca, NY: Cornell UP, 2005.

———. *Narrative as Rhetoric: Technique, Audiences, Ethics, Ideology*. Columbus: Ohio State UP, 1996

———. *Reading People, Reading Plots: Character, Progression, and the Interpretation of Narrative*. Chicago: U Chicago P, 1989.

Phillips, Natalie M. "Literary Neuroscience and History of Mind: An fMRI Study of Attention and Jane Austen." *The Oxford Handbook for Cognitive Approaches to Literature*. Ed. Lisa Zunshine. Oxford and New York: Oxford UP, 2015. 55–81.

Pinch, Adela. *Thinking About Other People in Nineteenth-Century British Writing*. Cambridge and New York: Cambridge UP, 2010.

Pinker, Steven. *The Better Angels of Our Nature: Why Violence Has Declined*. New York: Viking, 2011.

———. "Taming the Devil Within Us." *Nature* 478 (20 Oct. 2011): 309–11.

Pinker, Steven and Rebecca Goldsmith. "The Seed Salon: Steven Pinker and Rebecca Goldsmith." *Seed* 10 (2004): 44–49, 97–99.

Plamper, Jan. *The History of Emotions: An Introduction*. Oxford: Oxford UP, 2017.

Plutchik, Robert. *Emotion: Theory, Research, and Experience: v. 1. Theories of Emotion*. New York: Academic, 1980.

Popescu, Irina. "The Educational Power of Discomfort." *The Chronicle of Higher Education* (17 Apr. 2016). http://chronicle. com/article/The-Educational-Power-of/236136. 17 Apr. 2016.

Posner, Richard. "Against Ethical Criticism." *Philosophy and Literature* 21 (1997): 1–27.

Preston, Stephanie D. and Frans B. M. de Waal. "Empathy: Its Ultimate and Proximate Bases." *Behavioral and Brain Sciences* 25 (Feb. 2002): 1–20, 49–71.

Price, Leah. *The Anthology and the Rise of the Novel: from Richardson to George Eliot*. Cambridge and New York: Cambridge UP, 2000.

Prinz, Jesse. "Against Empathy." *The Southern Journal of Philosophy* 49. 1 (2011): 214–33.

———. *Gut Reactions: A Perceptual Theory of Emotion*. New York: Oxford UP, 2004.

Pustilnik, Amanda C. "Violence on the Brain: A Critique of Neuroscience in Criminal Law." *Wake Forest Law Review* 44. 1 (2009): 183–237.

Rabinowitz, Peter J. *Before Reading: Narrative Conventions and the Politics of Interpretation*. Ithaca, NY: Cornell, 1987.

Radford, Colin. "How Can We Be Moved by the Fate of Anna Karenina?" *Proceedings of the Aristotelian Society*, Supplemental v. 49 (1975): 67–80.

———. "Tears and Fiction." *Philosophy* 52 (1977): 208–13.

Radway, Janice. *A Feeling for Books: the Book-of-the-Month Club, Literary Taste, and Middle-class Desire*. Chapel Hill: U North Carolina P, 1997.

———. *Reading the Romance: Women, Patriarchy, and Popular Literature*. Chapel Hill: U of North Carolina P, 1984.

Reed, Stephen K. *Cognition: Theory and Applications*, 6th ed. Belmont, CA: Wadsworth, 2004.

Richards, I. A. *Nations and Peace*. New York: Simon and Schuster, 1947.

———. *Principles of Literary Criticism*, 2nd ed. London: Routledge & Kegan Paul, 1926.

———. *Science and Poetry*. London: K. Paul, Trench and Trubner, 1926.

Richardson, Alan. *The Neural Sublime: Cognitive Theories and Romantic Texts*. Baltimore: Johns Hopkins UP, 2010.

Richardson, Brian. "The Other Reader's Response: On Multiple, Divided, and Oppositional Audiences." *Criticism* 38 (1997): 31–53.

———. "Singular Text, Multiple Implied Readers." *Style* 41. 3 (2007): 257–72.

Richter, David. *The Progress of Romance: Literary Historiography and the Gothic Novel*. Columbus: Ohio State UP, 1996.

Robinson, Jenefer. *Deeper than Reason: Emotion and Its Role in Literature, Music, and Art*. Oxford and New York: Oxford UP, 2005.

———. "Emotion and the Understanding of Narrative." *A Companion to the Philosophy of Literature*. Ed. Gary L. Hagberg and Walter Jost, Malden, MA, Oxford and Chichester: Wiley Blackwell, 2010. 71–92.

Rolls, Edmund T. "A Theory of Emotion, Its Functions, and Its Adaptive Value." *Emotions in Humans and Artifacts*. Ed. Robert Trappl, Paolo Petta, and Sabine Payr. Cambridge, MA: MIT P, 2002. 11–34.

Rosen, Howard J., et al. "Emotion Comprehension in the Temporal Variant of Frontotemporal Dementia." *Brain* 125 (Oct. 2002): 2286–95.

Rosenblatt, Louise. *Literature as Exploration*. New York: Appleton, 1938.

———. *Literature as Exploration*. 5th ed. New York. Modern Language Association of America, 1995.

———. *The Reader, the Text, the Poem*. Carbondale and London: Southern Illinois UP, 1978.

Rosenwein, Barbara H. *Emotional Communities in the Early Middle Ages*. Ithaca: Cornell UP, 2006.

———. "Worrying about Emotions in History." *The American Historical Review* 107. 3 (2002): 821–45.

Rothbart, Mary K. and John E. Bates. "Temperament." *Handbook of Child Psychology: Social, Emotional, and Personality Development.* Ed. William Damon and Richard M. Lerner. Hoboken: Wiley, 2006. 99–166.

Rothfuss, Patrick. *The Name of the Wind.* New York: DAW Books, 2007.

———. *The Slow Regard of Silent Things.* New York: DAW Books, 2014.

———. *The Wise Man's Fear.* New York: Rpt. DAW Books, 2014.

Rottenberg, Jonathan, et al. *Handbook of Emotion Elicitation and Assessment.* Ed. James A. Coan and John J. B. Allen. Oxford and New York: Oxford UP, 2007. 9–28.

Rueckert, Linda, Brandon Branch, Tiffany Doan. "Are Gender Differences in Empathy Due to Differences in Emotional Reactivity?" *Psychology* 2 (2011): 574–578.

Rumbaut, Rubén. "Ages, Life Stages, and Generational Cohorts: Decomposing the Immigrant First and Second Generations in the United States." *International Migration Review* (Fall 2004): 1160–1205.

Ryan, Marie Laure. *Narrative as Virtual Reality: Immersion and Interactivity in Literature and Electronic Media.* Baltimore: Johns Hopkins UP, 2001.

Rylance, Rick. *Victorian Psychology and British Culture 1850–1888.* Oxford and New York: Oxford UP, 2000.

Ryman, Geoff. *253: A Novel for the Internet about London Underground in Seven Cars and a Crash.* 1996. www.ryman-novel.com/. 30 Jan. 2012.

Said, Edward. *Culture and Imperialism.* Knopf, New York, 1993.

Sapolsky, Barry and Dolf Zillmann. "Experience and Empathy: Affective Reactions to Witnessing Childbirth." *Journal of Social Psychology* 105 (1978): 133–44.

Sarnecki, John. "The Emergence of Empathy in the Context of Cross-Species Mind Reading." *Origins of Mind.* Ed. Liz Swan. Dordrecht, The Netherlands: Springer, 2013. 129–42.

Savarese, Ralph. "From Neurodiversity to Neurocosmopolitanism: Beyond Mere Acceptance and Inclusion." *Ethics and Neurodiversity.* Ed. C. D. Herrera and Alexandra Perry. Newcastle Upon Tyne: Cambridge Scholars Publishing, 2013. 191–205.

Scarry, Elaine. *Rule of Law, Misrule of Men.* Cambridge, MA: MIT P, 2010.

Schaffer, Kay and Sidonie Smith. *Human Rights and Narrated Lives: The Ethics of Recognition.* New York: Palgrave Macmillan, 2004.

Scheflen, Albert E. "Psychological Terms and Some Problems of Semiotics." *Essays in Semiotics.* Ed. Julia Kristeva, Josette Rey-Debove, and Donna J. Umiker. The Hague: Mouton, 1971. 267–76.

Schneider, Ralf. "Toward a Cognitive Theory of Literary Character: the Dynamics of Mental-Model Construction." *Style* 35 (2001): 607–42.

Schulkin, Jay. *Bodily Sensibility: Intelligent Action.* Oxford and New York: Oxford UP, 2004.

Sedgwick, Eve Kosofsky. *Epistemology of the Closet.* Berkeley: U of California P, 1990.

Sewall, Anna. *Black Beauty: The Autobiography of a Horse.* 1877. Rpt. Oxford and New York: Oxford UP, 2008.

Sheldon, Charles. *In His Steps.* 1896. Rpt. Grand Rapids: Revell, 2012.

Sherman, Nancy. "Empathy and Imagination." *Philosophy of Emotions. Midwest Studies in Philosophy, XXII.* Ed. Peter French and Howard K. Wettstein. Notre Dame, IN: U Notre Dame P, 1998. 82–119.

Shields, Stephanie A. *Speaking from the Heart: Gender and the Social Meaning of Emotion.* Cambridge and New York: Cambridge UP, 2002.

Shouse Eric. "Feeling, Emotion, Affect." *M/C Journal* 8. 6 (2005): http://journal. media-culture. org. au/0512/03-shouse. php. 28 Jan. 2018.

Shriver, Lionel. *We Need To Talk About Kevin*. USA: Counterpoint P, 2003.

Shusterman, Richard. *Body Consciousness: A Philosophy of Mindfulness and Somaesthetics*. New York: Cambridge UP, 2008.

———. *Pragmatist Aesthetics: Living Beauty, Rethinking Art*, 2nd edition. New York: Rowman and Littlefield, 2000.

———. "Somaesthetics and Education: Exploring the Terrain." *Knowing Bodies, Moving Minds: Towards Embodied Teaching and Learning*. Ed. Liora Bressler. Dordrecht: Kluwer, 2004.

Singer, Tania. et al. "Empathy for Pain Involves the Affective but not Sensory Components of Pain." *Science* 303 (20 Feb. 2004): 1157–62.

Slaughter, Joseph R. *Human Rights, Inc: The World Novel, Narrative Form, and International Law*. New York: Fordham UP, 2009.

Slote, Michael. *The Ethics of Care and Empathy*. London and New York. Routledge, 2007.

———. *Morals from Motives*. New York: Oxford UP, 2001.

Smith, Adam. *The Theory of Moral Sentiments*. Ed. D. D. Raphael and A. L. Macfie. *Glasgow Edition of the Works and Correspondence of Adam Smith*, v. 1. Oxford: Clarendon P, 1976.

Smith, Dorothy E. *The Conceptual Practices of Power: A Feminist Sociology of Knowledge*. Toronto: U Toronto P, 1990.

Smith, Murray. "Film Spectatorship and the Institution of Fiction." *Journal of Aesthetics and Art Criticism* 53 (1995): 113–27.

Snow, C. P. "The Two Cultures" *The New Statesman* (6 Oct. 1956). Rpt. www.newstatesman.com/cultural-capital/2013/01/c-p-snow-two-cultures. 14 Aug. 2021.

———. *The Two Cultures and the Scientific Revolution*. Cambridge: Cambridge UP, 1959.

"Special Section: Empathy." *Emotion Review* 4. 1 (2012): 3–97.

Spielberg, Steven. Dir. *Saving Private Ryan*. 1998.

Spivak, Gayatri Chakravorty. "Subaltern Studies: Deconstructing Historiography." 1985. Rpt. *The Spivak Reader: Selected Works of Gayatri Chakravorty Spivak*. Ed. Donna Landry and Gerald MacLean. New York: Routledge, 1996. 203–235.

Spreng, R. C., M. C. McKinnon, R. A. Mar, and B. Levine B. "The Toronto Empathy Questionnaire: A factor-analytic solution to multiple empathy measures." *Journal of Personality Assessment* 91 (2009): 62–71.

Stallybrass, Peter and Allon White. *The Politics and Poetics of Transgression*, Ithaca: Cornell UP, 1986.

Stanzel, F. K. *Narrative Situation in the Novel*. Trans James P. Pusack. Bloomington: Indiana, 1971.

Stearns, Peter N. with Carol Z. Stearns. "Emotionology: Clarifying the History of Emotions and Emotional Standards." *The American Historical Review* 90 (October 1985): 813–36.

Stein, Edith. *On the Problem of Empathy. The Collected Works of Edith Stein*, v. 3 Trans. Watraut Stein. Washington, D. C: ICS Publications, 1989.

Steiner, George. *Real Presences*, Chicago: U Chicago P, 1989.

Stern, Barbara. "Classical and Vignette Television Advertising Dramas: Structural Models, Formal Analysis, and Consumer Effects." *The Journal of Consumer Research* 20 (1994): 601–15.

Sternberg, Meir. "Epilogue: How (not) to Advance toward the Narrative Mind." *Cognitive Poetics: Goals, Gains, and Gaps*. Ed. Geert Brône and Jeroen Vandaele. Berlin and New York: Mouton de Gruyter, 2009. 455–532.

———. *Expositional Modes and Temporal Ordering in Fiction*. Baltimore: Johns Hopkins UP, 1978.

———. "How Narrativity Makes a Difference." *Narrative* 9. 2 (2001): 115–122.

———. "The 'Laokoon' Today: Interart Relations, Modern Projects, and Projections." *Poetics Today* 20. 2 (1999): 291–379.

———. "Narrativity: From Objectivist to Functional Paradigm." *Poetics Today* 31 (2010): 507–659.

———. *The Poetics of Biblical Narrative: Ideological Literature and the Drama of Reading*. Bloomington: Indiana UP, 1985.

———. "Proteus in Quotation-Land: Mimesis and the Forms of Reported Discourse." *Poetics Today* 3. 2 (1982): 107–56.

———. "Telling in Time. II): Chronology, Teleology, Narrativity." *Poetics Today* 13. 3 (1992): 463–541.

———. "Universals of Narrative and Their Cognitivist Fortunes. I," *Poetics Today* 24. 2 (2003): 297–391.

———. "Universals of Narrative and Their Cognitivist Fortunes. II," *Poetics Today* (2003): 517–638.

Sternberg, Robert J. and Michael L. Barnes. Ed. *The Psychology of Love*. New Haven: Yale UP, 1988.

Stockwell, Peter. *Cognitive Poetics: an Introduction*. London: Routledge, 2002.

Storer, Richard. "Richards, Ivor Armstrong. 1893–1979." *Oxford Dictionary of National Biography*. Oxford UP, Oct. 2008. www.oxforddnb.com/view/article/31603. 8 Mar. 2010.

Stotland, Ezra. et al. *Empathy, Fantasy and Helping*. Beverly Hills: Sage, 1978.

Stross, Charles. *Halting State*. NY: Ace Books, 2007.

Sundby, Scott. *A Life and Death Decision: A Jury Weighs the Death Penalty*. Basingstoke: Palgrave Macmillan, 2007.

Sutton-Ramspeck, Beth. Personal correspondence. 5 Feb. 2016.

Sweeney, Sarah. "On the Side of the Angels: Pinker Says the World is Becoming More Peaceful." *Harvard Gazette* (Thursday, 10 Nov. 2011): https://news.harvard.edu/gazette/story/2011/11/on-the-side-of-the-angels/. 14 Aug. 2021.

Tajerian, Maral. "Fight or Flight: The Neuroscience of Survival Horror." *Gamasutra: The Art and Business of Making Games*. www.gamasutra.com/view/feature/172168/fight_or_flight_the_neuroscience_. php. 13 July 2012.

Tamir, Diana I., et al. "Reading Fiction and Reading Minds: The Role of Simulation in the Default Network." *Social, Cognitive, and Affective Neuroscience* 11. 2 (2016): 215–24.

Tan, Ed. *Emotion and the Structure of Narrative Film: Film as an Emotion Machine*. Mahwah, NJ: Lawrence Erlbaum, 1996.

Tan, Ed S. "Film-induced Affect as a Witness Emotion." *Poetics* 23 (1995): 7–32.

Tavris, Carol. *Anger, the Misunderstood Emotion*. MY: Simon and Schuster, 1982.

Taylor, Marjorie, et al. "The Illusion of Independent Agency: Do Adult Fiction Writers Experience Their Characters as having Minds of their Own?" *Imagination, Cognition and Personality* 22 (2002/2003): 361–80.

Tettamanti, Marco, et al. "Listening to Action-related Sentences Activates Fronto–parietal Motor Circuits." *Journal of Cognitive Neuroscience* 17 (Feb. 2005): 273–81.

Thelen, Esther, and Linda B. Smith. *A Dynamic Systems Approach to the Development of Cognition and Action*. Cambridge, MA: MIT P, 1994.

Thiong'o, Ngũgĩ wa. "The Language of African Literature" 1985. Rpt. *Decolonising the Mind*. London: James Currey, 1986. 4–33.

———. *Wizard of the Crow*. New York: Knopf, 2006.

Thomas, Jacky. "Association of Personal Distress with Burnout, Compassion Fatigue and Compassion Satisfaction among Clinical Social Workers." *Journal of Social Service Research*, 39. 3 (2013): 365–79.

Tieje, Arthur Jerrold. *The Theory of Characterization in Prose Fiction Prior to 1740. The University of Minnesota Studies in Language and Literature* 5 (Dec. 1916).

Titchener, Edward Bradford. *A Beginner's Psychology*. New York: Macmillan, 1915.

———. *Lectures on Experimental Psychology of the Thought Processes*. London: Macmillan, 1909.

Todorov, Tzvetan. *The Poetics of Prose*. Trans. Richard Howard. Ithaca: Cornell UP, 1977.

Tolstoy, Leo. *Tolstoi on Art and Its Critics*. Trans. Aylmer Maude. London: H. Milford, 1925.

Tomkins, Silvan S. *Affect, Imagery, and Consciousness*, v. 1. New York: Springer, 1962.

Tompkins, Jane P. *Sensational Designs: The Cultural Work of American Fictions, 1790–1860*. New York and Oxford: Oxford UP, 1985.

Tompkins, Jane. P. Ed. *Reader-Response Criticism: From Formalism to Post-Structuralism*. Baltimore: Johns Hopkins UP, 1980.

Towles, Amor. *A Gentleman in Moscow*. New York: Viking, 2016.

Trollope, Anthony. *An Autobiography*. 1883. Rpt. Oxford World's Classics. Ed. Michael Sadleir and Frederick Page. Oxford and New York: Oxford UP, 2008.

———. *The American Senator*. 1877. Rpt. Oxford World's Classics. Ed. John Halperin. Oxford and New York: Oxford UP, 2008.

———. *Can You Forgive Her?* 1864–65. Rpt. Oxford World's Classics. Ed. Dinah Birch. Oxford and New York: Oxford UP, 2012.

———. *Doctor Thorne*. 1858. Rpt. Oxford World's Classics. Ed. Simon Dentith. Oxford and New York: Oxford UP, 2014.

———. *An Eye for an Eye*. 1879. Rpt. World's Classics. Ed. John Sutherland. Oxford and New York. Oxford UP, 1992.

———. *He Knew He Was Right*. 1868–69. Rpt. Oxford World's Classics. Ed. John Sutherland. Oxford and New York: Oxford UP, 2008.

———. *Orley Farm*. 1860–61. Rpt. Oxford World's Classics. Ed. David Skilton. Oxford and New York: Oxford UP, 2008.

———. *Rachel Ray*. 1863. Rpt. Oxford World's Classics. Ed. P. D. Edwards. Oxford and New York: Oxford UP, 2008.

———. *The Warden*. 1855. Rpt. Oxford World's Classics. Ed. Nicholas Shrimpton. Oxford and New York: Oxford UP, 2014.

———. *The Way We Live Now*. 1875. Rpt. Oxford World's Classics. Ed. John Sutherland. Oxford and New York: Oxford UP, 2008.

Tromp, Marlene. *The Private Rod: Marital Violence, Sensation, and the Law in Victorian Britain*. Charlottesville: UP of Virginia, 2000.

Trounstine, Jean and Robert P. Waxler. *Finding a Voice: The Practice of Changing Lives through Literature*. Ann Arbor: U Michigan P, 2005.

Tsai, J. L. "Culture." *Encyclopedia of Human Emotions*. Ed. David Levinson, James J. Ponzetti, and Peter F. Jorgensen. New York: Macmillan Reference, 1999. 159–66.

Turner, Jonathan H. *On the Origins of Human Emotions: a Sociological Inquiry into the Evolution of Human Affect*. Stanford: Stanford UP, 2000.

The Universal Declaration of Human Rights. The United Nations. 10 Dec. 1948. www.un.org/en/about-us/universal-declaration-of-human-rights. 14 Aug. 2021.

Vaillancort, Dan, et al. "Beauty and Healing." *The International Journal of the Humanities*. 5.4 (2007): 217–32.

van Peer, Willie. "Justice in Perspective." *New Perspectives on Narrative Perspective*. Ed. Willie van Peer and Seymour Chatman. Albany, NY: SUNY P, 2001. 325–38.

———. "Towards a Poetics of Emotion." *Emotion and the Arts*. Ed. Mette Hjort and Sue Laver. Oxford and New York: Oxford UP, 1997. 215–24.

van Peer, Willie and H. Pander Maat. "Perspectivation and Sympathy: Effects of Narrative Point of View." *Empirical Approaches to Literature and Aesthetics*. Ed. Roger J. Kreuz and Mary Sue MacNealy. Norwood, NJ: Ablex, 1996. 143–54.

Vermeule, Blakey. *Why Do We Care about Literary Characters?* Baltimore: Johns Hopkins UP, 2010.

VIDA, *Women in Literary Arts*. "The 2011 Count." www.vidaweb.org/the-2011-count/. 2 July 2012.

Vivas, Eliseo. "A Definition of the Esthetic Experience." *Journal of Philosophy* 34 (1937): 628–34.

———. "A Note on the Emotion in Mr. Dewey's Theory of Art." *The Philosophical Review* 47 (1938): 527–31.

Vordere, Peter, Hans J. Wulff and Mike Friedrichsen. Ed. *Suspense: Conceptualizations, Theoretical Analyses, and Empirical Explorations*. Mahwah, NJ: Lawrence Erlbaum, 1996.

Vygotsky, Lev. *The Psychology of Art*. Cambridge, MA: MIT P, 1971.

Walker, Alice. *Possessing the Secret of Joy*, Orlando: Harcourt, 1992.

Walsh, Richard. *The Rhetoric of Fictionality: Narrative Theory and the Idea of Fiction*, Columbus, OH: Ohio State, 2007.

———. "Why We Wept for Little Nell: Character and Emotional Involvement." *Narrative* 5 (Oct. 1997): 306–21.

Walton, Kendall. "Fearing Fictions." *Journal of Philosophy* 75. 1 (1978): 5–27.

———. *Mimesis as Make-Believe: On the Foundations of the Representational Arts*, Cambridge, MA and London: Harvard UP, 1990.

Ware, Chris. *Building Stories*. New York: Pantheon, 2012.

Warhol, Robyn. "A Feminist Approach to Narrative." *Narrative Theory: Core Concepts and Critical Debates*. Ed. David Herman, James Phelan, Peter J. Rabinowitz, Brian Richardson, and Robyn Warhol. Columbus: The Ohio State UP, 2012. 9–13.

———. *Having a Good Cry: Effeminate Feelings and Pop-Culture Forms*. Columbus: Ohio State UP, 2003.

Waters, Sarah. *The Night Watch*. New York: Riverhead Books, 2006.

Watt, Ian. *The Rise of the Novel: Studies in Defoe, Richardson and Fielding*. Berkeley: U of California P, 1957.

Weisberg, Deena, et al. "The Seductive Allure of Neuroscience Explanations." *Journal of Cognitive Neuroscience* 20. (2008): 470–77.

Williams, Hayden M. Rev. of *So Many Freedoms: A Study of the Major Fiction of Mulk Raj Anand*, by Saros Cowasje. *The Journal of Asian Studies* 39. 2 (Feb. 1980): 411–12.

Williams, Raymond. *The Country and the City*. Oxford and New York: Oxford UP, 1973.

———. *Culture and Society, 1780–1950*. Rpt. New York: Columbia UP, 1983.

———. *Keywords: A Vocabulary of Culture and Society*. 1976. Rev. Ed. Oxford and New York: Oxford UP, 1983.

———. *Marxism and Literature*. Oxford and New York: Oxford UP, 1977.

Wilson, Angus. "Raspberry Jam." *The Wrong Set*, Secker, 1949.

Wimsatt, W. K. and Monroe Beardsley. "The Affective Fallacy." *Sewanee Rev* 54. 3 (1949): 468–88. Rpt. *The Verbal Icon: Studies in the Meaning of Poetry*. Lexington, KY: U of Kentucky P, 1954. 21–39.

Winerman, Lea. "The Mind's Mirror: A New Type of Neuron—Called a Mirror Neuron—Could Help Explain How We Learn Through Mimicry and Why We Empathize with Others." *APA Monitor on Psychology* 36 (2005): 48.

Winter, Sarah. "The Novel and Prejudice." *Comparative Literature Studies* 46. 1 (2009): 76–102.

Wispé, Lauren. "History of the Concept of Empathy." *Empathy and its Development* Ed. Nancy Eisenberg and Janet Strayer. Cambridge and New York: Cambridge UP, 1987. 17–37.

Wood, Marcus. *Slavery, Empathy and Pornography*. Oxford and New York: Oxford, 2002.

Woolf, Virginia. *Mrs Dalloway*. London: Hogarth P, 1925.

Wright, Daniel. "Because I Do: Trollope, Tautology, and Desire." *ELH* 80. 4 (Winter 2013): 1121–1143.

Xu, Xiaojing, et al. "Do You Feel my Pain? Racial Group Membership Modulates Empathic Neural Responses." *Journal of Neuroscience* 29 (2009): 8525–9.

Yanal, Robert J. *The Paradoxes of Emotion and Fiction*. University Park: Pennsylvania State UP, 1999.

Young, Allan. "Empathy, Evolution, and Human Nature." *Empathy: From Bench to Bedside*. Cambridge, MA and London: MIT P, 2012. 21–37.

Young, Kay. *Imagining Minds: Austen, Eliot, Hardy, and the Aesthetic of Consciousness*. Columbus: Ohio State UP, 2009.

———. *Ordinary Pleasures: Couples, Conversation and Comedy*. Columbus: Ohio State UP, 2001.

Zahn-Waxler, Carolyn, et al. "Empathy and Prosocial Patterns in Young MZ and DZ Twins: Development and Genetic and Environmental Influences." *Infancy to Early Childhood: Genetic and Environmental Influences on Developmental Change*. Ed. Robert M. Emde and John K. Hewitt. Oxford and New York: Oxford UP, 2001. 141–62.

Zillmann, Dolf. "Empathy: Affect from Bearing Witness to the Emotions of Others." *Responding to the Screen: Reception and Reaction Processes*. Ed. Dolf Zillmann and Jennings Bryant. Mahwah, NJ: Erlbaum, 1991. 135–67.

———. "Empathy: Affective Reactivity to Others' Emotional Experiences." *Psychology of Entertainment*. Ed. Jennings Bryant and Peter Vorderer. London and NY: Routledge, 2006. 151–82.

———. "Mechanisms of Emotional Reactivity to Media Entertainments." *The Routledge Handbook of Emotions and Mass Media*. Ed. Katrin Döveling, Christian von Scheve, and Elly A. Konijn. London and New York: Routledge, 2010. 101–15.

———. "Mechanisms of Emotional Involvement with Drama." *Poetics* 23 (1994): 33–51.

Zunshine, Lisa. "Richardson's *Clarissa* and a Theory of Mind." *The Work of Fiction: Cognition, Culture, and Complexity* Ed. Alan Richardson and Ellen Spolsky. Aldershot, Hampshire and Burllington, VT: Ashgate, 2004. 127–46.

———. "Theory of Mind and Experimental Representations of Fictional Consciousness." *Narrative* 11 (Oct. 2003): 270–91.

———. *Why We Read Fiction: Theory of Mind and the Novel*. Columbus: Ohio State UP, 2006.

Zwaan, Rolf A. "Effect of Genre Expectations on Text Comprehension." *Journal of Experimental Psychology: Learning, Memory and Cognition* 20 (1994): 920–33.

———. "Embodiment and Language Comprehension: Reframing the Discussion." *Trends in Cognitive Science* 18. 5 (2014): 229–34.

Zwaan, Rolf A., and Lawrence J. Taylor. "Seeing, Acting, Understanding: Motor Resonance in Language Comprehension." *Journal of Experimental Psychology* 135.1 (2006): 1–11.

Zyngier, Sonia, Marisa Bortolussi, Anna Chesnokova, and Jan Auracher. Ed. *Directions in Empirical Literary Studies*. Amsterdam and Philadelphia: John Benjamins, 2008.

INDEX

Made in the USA
Monee, IL
13 September 2026

62980173R10157